Gastric Cancer

Editor

CHIN HUR

GASTROINTESTINAL ENDOSCOPY CLINICS OF NORTH AMERICA

www.giendo.theclinics.com

Consulting Editor
CHARLES J. LIGHTDALE

July 2021 • Volume 31 • Number 3

ELSEVIER

1600 John F. Kennedy Boulevard • Suite 1800 • Philadelphia, Pennsylvania, 19103-2899

http://www.theclinics.com

GASTROINTESTINAL ENDOSCOPY CLINICS OF NORTH AMERICA Volume 31, Number 3
July 2021 ISSN 1052-5157, ISBN-13: 978-0-323-77544-1

Editor: Kerry Holland

Developmental Editor: Jessica Cañaberal

Gastrointestinal Endoscopy Clinics of North America (ISSN 1052-5157) is published quarterly by Elsevier Inc., 360 Park Avenue South, New York, NY 10010-1710. Months of issue are January, April, July, and October. Business and Editorial Offices: 1600 John F. Kennedy Blvd., Suite 1800, Philadelphia, PA, 19103-2899. Periodicals postage paid at New York, NY and additional mailing offices. Subscription prices are $363.00 per year for US individuals, $813.00 per year for US institutions, $100.00 per year for US and Canadian students/residents, $399.00 per year for Canadian individuals, $841.00 per year for Canadian institutions, $476.00 per year for international individuals, $841.00 per year for international institutions, and $245.00 per year for international students/residents. To receive student/resident rate, orders must be accompanied by name of affiliated institution, date of term, and the *signature* of program/residency coordinator on institution letterhead. Orders will be billed at individual rate until proof of status is received. Foreign air speed delivery is included in all *Clinics* subscription prices. All prices are subject to change without notice. **POSTMASTER:** Send address change to *Gastrointestinal Endoscopy Clinics of North America*, Elsevier Health Sciences Division, Subscription Customer Service, 3251 Riverport Lane, Maryland Heights, MO 63043. **Customer Service: 1-800-654-2452 (US). From outside the United States, call 1-314-447-8871. Fax: 1-314-447-8029. E-mail: JournalsCustomerService-usa@elsevier.com (for print support) or JournalsOnlineSupport-usa@elsevier.com (for online support).**

Reprints. For copies of 100 or more, of articles in this publication, please contact the Commercial Reprints Department, Elsevier Inc., 360 Park Avenue South, New York, NY 10010-1710. Tel. 212-633-3874; Fax: 212-633-3820; E-mail: reprints@elsevier.com.

Gastrointestinal Endoscopy Clinics of North America is covered in *Excerpta Medica, MEDLINE/PubMed (Index Medicus), and MEDLINE/MEDLARS.*

Contributors

CONSULTING EDITOR

CHARLES J. LIGHTDALE, MD
Professor of Medicine, Division of Digestive and Liver Diseases, Columbia University Medical Center, New York, New York, USA

EDITOR

CHIN HUR, MD, MPH
Director, Healthcare Innovations Research and Evaluation (HIRE), Professor, Columbia University, Department of Medicine, Columbia University Irving Medical Center, New York, New York, USA

AUTHORS

ANDREW CANAKIS, DO
Department of Medicine, Boston University School of Medicine, Boston Medical Center, Boston, Massachusetts, USA

CHARLOTTE K. CHING, MD
Internal Medicine Resident, Vagelos College of Physicians and Surgeons, Department of Medicine, Columbia University Irving Medical Center, New York, New York, USA

SOO-JEONG CHO, MD, PhD
Associate Professor, Department of Internal Medicine and Liver Research Institute, Seoul National University Hospital, Seoul National University College of Medicine, Seoul, Korea

ANDREW HSU, MD
Chief Fellow, Division of Hematology/Oncology, The Warren Alpert Medical School of Brown University, Lifespan Cancer Institute, Rhode Island Hospital/The Miriam Hospital, Providence, Rhode Island, USA

ROBERT J. HUANG, MD, MS
Division of Gastroenterology and Hepatology, Stanford University, Stanford, California, USA

JOO HA HWANG, MD, PhD
Division of Gastroenterology and Hepatology, Stanford University, Stanford, California, USA

HAEJIN IN, MD, MPH, MBA
Associate Professor of Surgery, Associate Professor of Epidemiology and Population Health, Department of Surgery, Montefiore Medical Center, Departments of Surgery, and Epidemiology and Population Health, Albert Einstein College of Medicine, New York, New York, USA

MANAMI INOUE, MD, PhD
Chief, Division of Prevention, Center for Public Health Sciences, National Cancer Center, Tokyo, Japan

HWOON-YONG JUNG, MD, PhD, AGAF
Department of Gastroenterology, University of Ulsan College of Medicine, Asan Medical Center, Asan Digestive Disease Research Institute, Seoul, Korea

FAY KASTRINOS, MD, MPH
Associate Professor of Medicine, Herbert Irving Comprehensive Cancer Center, Columbia University Medical Center, Division of Digestive and Liver Diseases, Columbia University Irving Medical Cancer, Vagelos College of Physicians and Surgeons, New York, New York, USA

BOKYUNG KIM, MD
Clinical Fellow, Department of Internal Medicine and Liver Research Institute, Seoul National University Hospital, Seoul National University College of Medicine, Seoul, Korea

GA HEE KIM, MD, PhD
Department of Gastroenterology, University of Ulsan College of Medicine, Asan Medical Center, Asan Digestive Disease Research Institute, Seoul, Korea

JUDITH KIM, MD
Post-doctoral Fellow, Department of Medicine, Division of Digestive and Liver Diseases, Columbia University Irving Medical Center, New York, New York, USA

RAYMOND KIM, MD
Division of Gastroenterology and Hepatology, University of Maryland Medical Center, University of Maryland School of Medicine, Baltimore, Maryland, USA

THERESA H. NGUYEN, MD
Clinical Post-doctoral Fellow, Section of Gastroenterology and Hepatology, Department of Medicine, Baylor College of Medicine, Houston, Texas, USA

RICHARD M. PEEK, Jr, MD
Division of Gastroenterology, Hepatology, and Nutrition, Vanderbilt University Medical Center, Nashville, Tennessee, USA

ALEXANDER G. RAUFI, MD
Assistant Professor of Medicine, Division of Hematology/Oncology, The Warren Alpert Medical School of Brown University, Lifespan Cancer Institute, Rhode Island Hospital/The Miriam Hospital, Providence, Rhode Island, USA

SHEILA D. RUSTGI, MD
Assistant Professor of Medicine, Herbert Irving Comprehensive Cancer Center, Columbia University Medical Center, Division of Digestive and Liver Diseases, Columbia University Irving Medical Cancer, Vagelos College of Physicians and Surgeons, New York, New York, USA

SHAILJA C. SHAH, MD, MPH
Division of Gastroenterology, Hepatology, and Nutrition, Vanderbilt University Medical Center, Nashville, Tennessee, USA; Veterans Affairs San Diego Healthcare System, University of California, San Diego, La Jolla, California, USA

IAN SOLSKY, MD, MPH
Department of Surgery, Montefiore Medical Center, New York, New York, USA

AARON P. THRIFT, PhD
Assistant Professor, Section of Epidemiology and Population Sciences, Department of Medicine, Dan L Duncan Comprehensive Cancer Center, Baylor College of Medicine, Houston, Texas, USA

TIMOTHY CRAGIN WANG, MD
Division Chief, Department of Medicine, Division of Digestive and Liver Diseases, Columbia University Irving Medical Center, New York, New York, USA

Contents

Foreword: Turning a Spotlight on Gastric Cancer xiii

Charles J. Lightdale

Preface: Gastric Cancer: An Update on the Rapidly Changing Characteristics and Evolving Opportunities for Interventions xv

Chin Hur

Gastric Cancer Epidemiology 425

Aaron P. Thrift and Theresa H. Nguyen

In the United States, the incidence of gastric cancer has decreased over the past five decades. However, despite overall decreasing trends in incidence rates of gastric cancer, rates of noncardia gastric cancer among adults aged less than 50 years in the United States are increasing, and most cases of gastric cancer still present with advanced disease and poor resultant survival. Epidemiologic studies have identified the main risk factors for gastric cancer, including increasing age, male sex, non-White race, Helicobacter pylori infection, and smoking. This article summarizes the current epidemiologic evidence with implications for primary and secondary prevention of gastric cancer.

Public Health Interventions for Gastric Cancer Control 441

Manami Inoue

Despite its generally decreasing trend in incidence, gastric cancer remains the fifth-most common cancer worldwide. Gastric cancer has substantially declined over the past century, thanks to decreases in risk factors such as Helicobacter pylori infection, tobacco smoking, and salt-preserved food intake. These decreases have resulted from natural interventions and population-based intervention strategies. H pylori eradication for infected patients has potential as a prevention strategy for those at high risk, but warrants a longer follow-up period. The ongoing increase in obesity prevalence may cause an increase in cardia gastric cancer, especially in Western populations, and should be carefully monitored.

***Helicobacter* pylori and Gastric Cancer** 451

Judith Kim and Timothy Cragin Wang

Helicobacter pylori is present in approximately one-half of the world's population. There are significant differences in prevalence based on region, age, race/ethnicity, and socioeconomic status. H pylori is the most common cause of infection-related cancers. Studies have demonstrated the relationship between H pylori infection and gastric adenocarcinoma and mucosa-associated lymphoid tissue lymphoma. H pylori has features and enzymatic properties allowing it to survive in the acidic stomach environment, and has specific virulence factors that promote an increased risk

of gastric pathology. Eradication of H pylori is first-line therapy for mucosa-associated lymphoid tissue lymphoma and decreases the risk of gastric adenocarcinoma.

Inherited Predisposition to Gastric Cancer **467**

Sheila D. Rustgi, Charlotte K. Ching, and Fay Kastrinos

Approximately 10% of patients with gastric cancer show familial aggregation and up to 3% are related to various inherited cancer syndromes. There are multiple germline pathogenic variants and cancer syndromes associated with an increased risk of gastric cancer. Appropriate assessment of familial and genetic risk may allow a personalized approach to gastric cancer prevention through screening and risk-reducing surgeries. The ability to better identify carriers with pathogenic genetic variants associated with gastric cancer before a diagnosis of cancer requires effective genetic risk assessment and testing, followed by optimal screening and surveillance recommendations or prophylactic surgery to further reduce the associated morbidity and mortality.

Endoscopic Screening and Surveillance for Gastric Cancer **489**

Bokyung Kim and Soo-Jeong Cho

Gastric cancer is one of the most common cancers worldwide. Gastric cancer is a multifactorial disease, and the incidence varies widely by geographic region, with half of new cases occurring in East Asia. Population-based nationwide screening for gastric cancer has been implemented in some Eastern Asian countries such as South Korea and Japan. In these countries, endoscopic screening decreased gastric cancer mortality. Endoscopic screening seems to be a cost-effective modality in countries with high incidence of gastric cancer. However, the usefulness of population-based screening has not yet been proved in countries with low incidence of gastric cancer.

Improving the Early Diagnosis of Gastric Cancer **503**

Robert J. Huang and Joo Ha Hwang

Video content accompanies this article at http://www.giendo.theclinics.com.

Gastric cancer (GC) remains a leading cause of cancer morbidity and mortality worldwide. Outcomes from GC remain poor, especially in Western nations where cancer diagnosis is usually at advanced stages where curative resection is not possible. By contrast, nations of East Asia have adopted methods of population-level screening with improvements in stage of diagnosis and survival. In this review, the authors discuss the epidemiology of GC in Western populations, highlight at-risk populations who may benefit from screening, overview screening modalities, and discuss promising approaches to early GC detection.

Chemoprevention Against Gastric Cancer **519**

Shailja C. Shah and Richard M. Peek Jr.

Gastric cancer is the fifth most common cause of cancer and the third leading cause of cancer-related deaths globally. The number of gastric

cancer-related deaths is projected to increase, attributable primarily to the expanding aging population. Prevention is a mainstay of gastric cancer control programs, particularly in the absence of accurate, noninvasive modalities for screening and early detection, and the absence of an infrastructure for this purpose in the majority of countries worldwide. Herein, we discuss the evidence for several chemopreventive agents, along with putative mechanisms. There remains a clear, unmet need for primary chemoprevention trials for gastric cancer.

Endoscopic Advances for Gastric Neoplasia Detection **543**

Andrew Canakis and Raymond Kim

This article explores advances in endoscopic neoplasia detection with supporting clinical evidence and future aims. The ability to detect early gastric neoplastic lesions amenable to curative endoscopic submucosal dissection provides the opportunity to decrease gastric cancer mortality rates. Newer imaging techniques offer enhanced views of mucosal and microvascular structures and show promise in differentiating benign from malignant lesions and improving targeted biopsies. Conventional chromoendoscopy is well studied and validated. Narrow band imaging demonstrates superiority over magnified white light. Autofluorescence imaging, i-scan, flexible spectral imaging color enhancement, and bright image enhanced endoscopy show promise but insufficient evidence to change current clinical practice.

Endoscopic Resection of Gastric Cancer **563**

Ga Hee Kim and Hwoon-Yong Jung

Video content accompanies this article at http://www.giendo.theclinics.com.

With improvements in the early detection of early gastric cancer (EGC) and advances in therapeutic techniques, endoscopic resection (ER) for EGC has become widely adopted in East Asian and Western countries. Endoscopic submucosal dissection has higher rates of en bloc, complete, and curative resections with lower rates of local recurrence than that of endoscopic mucosal resection. ER is a minimally invasive method with low morbidity that provides excellent outcomes. ER for EGC is a safe, effective method, preserving organ function and thus maintaining the patient's quality of life, and is recognized as the first-line treatment of EGC in selected patients.

Surgical Treatment for Gastric Cancer **581**

Ian Solsky and Haejin In

Video content accompanies this article at http://www.giendo.theclinics.com.

Surgery is an essential component of curative-intent treatment strategies for gastric cancer. However, the care of each patient with gastric cancer must be individualized based on patients and tumor characteristics. It is important that all physicians who will be caring for patient with gastric cancer understand the current best practices of surgical management to

provide patients with the highest quality of care. This article aims to provide this information while acknowledging areas of surgical management that are still controversial.

Advances in Systemic Therapy for Gastric Cancer **607**

Andrew Hsu and Alexander G. Raufi

Gastric cancer represents a major global health problem. Approximately half of patients are diagnosed with early stage disease and surgical resection is potentially curative. The addition of combination chemotherapy, with or without radiotherapy, to surgery has been shown to improve outcomes. In metastatic disease, combination chemotherapy in the form of 2- or 3-drug regimens has been used. The aim of this chapter is to summarize currently approved systemic treatment options for gastric cancer and to highlight several promising treatments currently under investigation.

GASTROINTESTINAL ENDOSCOPY CLINICS OF NORTH AMERICA

FORTHCOMING ISSUES

October 2021
Optimizing Endoscopic Operations
John Vargo and Sunguk N. Jang, *Editors*

January 2022
Gastrointestinal Cancers and Genetic Testing
Fay Kastrinos, *Editor*

RECENT ISSUES

April 2021
Video Capsule Endoscopy
David R. Cave, *Editor*

January 2021
Advances in Barrett's Esophagus
Sachin Wani, *Editor*

RELATED CLINICS SERIES

Gastroenterology Clinics
(www.gastro.theclinics.com)
Clinics in Liver Disease
(www.liver.theclinics.com)

Foreword

Turning a Spotlight on Gastric Cancer

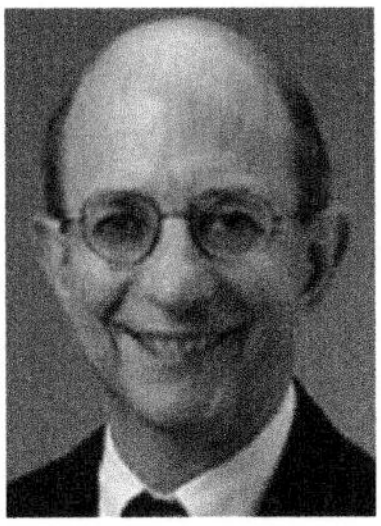

Charles J. Lightdale, MD
Consulting Editor

Gastric adenocarcinoma is a common and highly lethal cancer worldwide. The disease is of lower incidence in the United States and other western countries. The lower incidence is probably related in part to the decreasing incidence of gastric *Helicobacter pylori* infections in the west. A reverse effect of the decline in *H pylori* in the west has been the dramatic rise in Barrett's esophagus and esophageal adenocarcinoma primarily affecting white men. Adenocarcinoma of the stomach, on the other hand, excluding esophagogastric junction cancer, more commonly occurs in blacks, Hispanics, and Asians, creating health disparities in western countries. As immigration has led to more diversity in western populations, there is an increasing need to pay attention to the relatively "neglected" adenocarcinomas of the stomach.

A fascinating finding is that the precursor to gastric adenocarcinoma on pathology is intestinal metaplasia, the same type of tissue that characterizes Barrett's esophagus. On pathology examination, the incomplete type of intestinal metaplasia has the highest potential for malignant transformation in the stomach. The distribution of intestinal metaplasia in the stomach, usually distal in patients with *H pylori* infection, can be patchy and irregular and difficult to identify on endoscopy. Another challenge is that the surface area of the stomach is much larger than the tubular esophagus and takes longer to thoroughly examine. The earliest changes of dysplasia and intramucosal cancer, often subtle, pale, flat, or slightly raised or depressed lesions, can also be very difficult to find. Random biopsies by the dozens can still miss these lesions. Endoscopists in high-incidence regions have in recent decades trained their eyes to detect these lesions with experience and training not yet widely available in the west. The newest endoscopes with high-resolution white light and electronic chromoendoscopy with magnification have been clearly an advance in examination of the stomach for detection of intestinal metaplasia and early neoplasia.

Gastrointest Endoscopy Clin N Am 31 (2021) xiii–xiv
https://doi.org/10.1016/j.giec.2021.04.003
1052-5157/21/© 2021 Published by Elsevier Inc.

Dr Chin Hur, the Editor for this issue of the *Gastrointestinal Endoscopy Clinics of North America*, is an internationally recognized expert in cancer screening and prevention for gastrointestinal cancers. He has assembled an outstanding group of experts to create an issue that shines a bright spotlight on gastric cancer, providing a comprehensive state-of-the-art review. I urge all general gastroenterologists and gastrointestinal endoscopists to read this issue. It is time for us to up our game for the prevention, early detection, and treatment of adenocarcinoma of the stomach.

Charles J. Lightdale, MD
Division of Digestive and Liver Diseases
Columbia University Irving Medical Center
161 Fort Washington Avenue
New York, NY 10032, USA

E-mail address:
cjl18@cumc.columbia.edu

Preface

Gastric Cancer: An Update on the Rapidly Changing Characteristics and Evolving Opportunities for Interventions

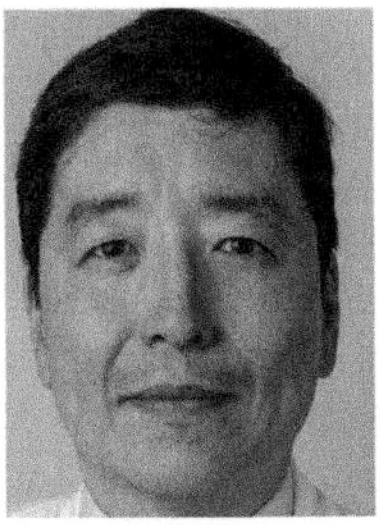

Chin Hur, MD, MPH
Editor

Gastric cancer (GC), specifically gastric adenocarcinoma, is the fifth most common cancer and the third leading cause of cancer death globally and has been categorized as a *neglected cancer* by the World Health Organization.[1,2] Usually diagnosed at advanced stages, GC has a 5-year survival rate of ∼30%.[3] In the United States, there are stark disparities, with blacks, Hispanics, and Asians having a nearly 2-fold greater risk of developing or dying from GC compared with whites,[4] reflecting differences in risk factors, such as *Helicobacter pylori* infection and smoking, as well as access to primary prevention[5] and care.[6] Several factors are changing the landscape of GC prevention, including a better understanding of the disease's natural history,[7–9] new evidence on prevention from prospective studies,[10–14] and anticipated results from ongoing randomized controlled trials.[15] As early GC detection can improve survival by allowing for curative surgical or noninvasive endoscopic resection,[16] new targeted approaches to GC prevention have the potential to markedly improve population health and reduce GC disparities within the United States.

Although *H pylori* has been the primary focus of global GC prevention efforts to date,[1,2] substantial variation by subpopulation in *H pylori* prevalence in the United States and the world has accentuated the need to optimize *H pylori* screen-and-treat interventions for vulnerable groups.[17–20] Early detection of GC or precancerous lesions can further reduce GC burden. For example, surveillance of individuals with gastric

Gastrointest Endoscopy Clin N Am 31 (2021) xv–xviii
https://doi.org/10.1016/j.giec.2021.04.002
1052-5157/21/© 2021 Published by Elsevier Inc.
giendo.theclinics.com

intestinal metaplasia (IM), a precursor lesion with a high progression risk to gastric neoplasia, is currently recommended in many countries.[21,22] However, as gastric IM is often asymptomatic, most of the 5% to 10% of US adults with this condition remain undiagnosed.[9,23] In addition, an increase in GC incidence among younger individuals has been observed, particularly in young women.[24–27] A critical need exists to identify effective and cost-effective strategies to address these clinical challenges in the United States, as well as globally.

I would like to express my gratitude to Dr Charlie Lightdale for providing me the opportunity to serve as a guest editor for this issue of *Gastrointestinal Endoscopy Clinics of North America*. I am deeply indebted to all the authors who have written superb articles that distill the current state of the spectrum of GC knowledge ranging from biology to epidemiology and therapy. To our readers, we hope and trust that our efforts have produced a useful resource for clinical care, research, and cancer control interventions.

Chin Hur, MD, MPH
Director, Healthcare Innovations Research
and Evaluation (HIRE)
Professor, Columbia University
Department of Medicine
Columbia University Irving Medical Center
622 W 168th Street, PH9-105C
New York, NY 10032, USA

E-mail address:
Chin.hur@columbia.edu

REFERENCES

1. Herrero R, Parsonnet J, Greenberg ER. Prevention of gastric cancer. JAMA 2014; 312(12):1197–8. https://doi.org/10.1001/jama.2014.10498.
2. IARC Helicobacter pylori Working Group. Helicobacter pylori eradication as a strategy for preventing gastric cancer. Lyon (France): International Agency for Research on Cancer (IARC Working Group Reports, No. 8); 2014. Available at: http://www.iarc.fr/en/publications/pdfs-online/wrk/wrk8/index.php.
3. Siegel R, Naishadham D, Jemal A. Cancer statistics, 2012. CA Cancer J Clin 2012;62(1):10–29. https://doi.org/10.3322/caac.20138.
4. CancerDisparitiesProgressReport.org [Internet]. American Association for Cancer Research. ©2020. Available at: http://www.CancerDisparitiesProgressReport.org/. Accessed January 11, 2021.
5. Florea A, Brown HE, Harris RB, et al. Ethnic disparities in gastric cancer presentation and screening practice in the United States: analysis of 1997-2010 surveillance, epidemiology, and end results—Medicare data. Cancer Epidemiol Biomarkers Prev 2019;28(4):659–65. https://doi.org/10.1158/1055-9965.EPI-18-0471.
6. Ikoma N, Cormier JN, Feig B, et al. Racial disparities in preoperative chemotherapy use in gastric cancer patients in the United States: analysis of the National Cancer Data Base, 2006-2014. Cancer 2018;124(5):998–1007. https://doi.org/10.1002/cncr.31155.
7. Kumar S, Metz DC, Ellenberg S, et al. Risk factors and incidence of gastric cancer after detection of Helicobacter pylori infection: a large cohort study. Gastroenterology 2020;158(3):527–36.e7. https://doi.org/10.1053/j.gastro.2019.10.019.

8. Li D, Bautista MC, Jiang SF, et al. Risks and predictors of gastric adenocarcinoma in patients with gastric intestinal metaplasia and dysplasia: a population-based study. Am J Gastroenterol 2016;111(8):1104–13. https://doi.org/10.1038/ajg.2016.188.
9. Sonnenberg A, Genta RM. Changes in the gastric mucosa with aging. Clin Gastroenterol Hepatol 2015;13(13):2276–81. https://doi.org/10.1016/j.cgh.2015.02.020.
10. Piazuelo MB, Bravo LE, Mera RM, et al. The Colombian Chemoprevention Trial: 20-Year Follow-Up of a Cohort of Patients With Gastric Precancerous Lesions. Gastroenterology 2020;160(4):1106–17 e3.
11. Choi IJ, Kook MC, Kim YI, et al. Helicobacter pylori therapy for the prevention of metachronous gastric cancer. N Engl J Med 2018;378(12):1085–95. https://doi.org/10.1056/NEJMoa1708423.
12. Choi IJ, Kim CG, Lee JY, et al. Family history of gastric cancer and Helicobacter pylori treatment. N Engl J Med 2020;382(5):427–36. https://doi.org/10.1056/NEJMoa1909666.
13. Li WQ, Ma JL, Zhang L, et al. Effects of Helicobacter pylori treatment on gastric cancer incidence and mortality in subgroups. J Natl Cancer Inst 2014;106(7):dju116. https://doi.org/10.1093/jnci/dju116.
14. Ma JL, Zhang L, Brown LM, et al. Fifteen-year effects of Helicobacter pylori, garlic, and vitamin treatments on gastric cancer incidence and mortality. J Natl Cancer Inst 2012;104(6):488–92. https://doi.org/10.1093/jnci/djs003.
15. Pan KF, Zhang L, Gerhard M, et al. A large randomised controlled intervention trial to prevent gastric cancer by eradication of Helicobacter pylori in Linqu County, China: baseline results and factors affecting the eradication. Gut 2016;65(1):9–18. https://doi.org/10.1136/gutjnl-2015-309197.
16. Choi KS, Jun JK, Suh M, et al. Effect of endoscopy screening on stage at gastric cancer diagnosis: results of the National Cancer Screening Programme in Korea. Br J Cancer 2015;112(3):608–12. https://doi.org/10.1038/bjc.2014.608.
17. Committee ASoP, Evans JA, Early DS, et al, Standards of Practice Committee of the American Society for Gastrointestinal E. The role of endoscopy in Barrett's esophagus and other premalignant conditions of the esophagus. Gastrointest Endosc 2012;76(6):1087–94. https://doi.org/10.1016/j.gie.2012.08.004.
18. Yeh JM, Hur C, Schrag D, et al. Contribution of H pylori and smoking trends to US incidence of intestinal-type noncardia gastric adenocarcinoma: a microsimulation model. PLoS Med 2013;10(5):e1001451. https://doi.org/10.1371/journal.pmed.1001451.
19. Group HaCC. Gastric cancer and Helicobacter pylori: a combined analysis of 12 case control studies nested within prospective cohorts. Gut 2001;49(3):347–53. https://doi.org/10.1136/gut.49.3.347.
20. Bray F, Ferlay J, Soerjomataram I, et al. Global cancer statistics 2018: GLOBOCAN estimates of incidence and mortality worldwide for 36 cancers in 185 countries. CA Cancer J Clin 2018;68(6):394–424. https://doi.org/10.3322/caac.21492.
21. Pimentel-Nunes P, Libanio D, Marcos-Pinto R, et al. Management of epithelial precancerous conditions and lesions in the stomach (MAPS II): European Society of Gastrointestinal Endoscopy (ESGE), European Helicobacter and Microbiota Study Group (EHMSG), European Society of Pathology (ESP), and Sociedade Portuguesa de Endoscopia Digestiva (SPED) guideline update 2019. Endoscopy 2019;51(4):365–88. https://doi.org/10.1055/a-0859-1883.
22. Banks M, Graham D, Jansen M, et al. British Society of Gastroenterology guidelines on the diagnosis and management of patients at risk of gastric adenocarcinoma. Gut 2019;68(9):1545–75. https://doi.org/10.1136/gutjnl-2018-318126.

23. Sonnenberg A, Lash RH, Genta RM. A national study of Helicobactor pylori infection in gastric biopsy specimens. Gastroenterology 2010;139(6):1894–901.e2. https://doi.org/10.1053/j.gastro.2010.08.018 [quiz: e12].
24. Merchant SJ, Kim J, Choi AH, et al. A rising trend in the incidence of advanced gastric cancer in young Hispanic men. Gastric Cancer 2017;20(2):226–34. https://doi.org/10.1007/s10120-016-0603-7.
25. He XK, Sun LM. The increasing trend in the incidence of gastric cancer in the young population, not only in young Hispanic men. Gastric Cancer 2017;20(6): 1010. https://doi.org/10.1007/s10120-017-0752-3.
26. De B, Rhome R, Jairam V, et al. Gastric adenocarcinoma in young adult patients: patterns of care and survival in the United States. Gastric Cancer 2018;21(6): 889–99. https://doi.org/10.1007/s10120-018-0826-x.
27. Anderson WF, Rabkin CS, Turner N, et al. The changing face of noncardia gastric cancer incidence among US non-Hispanic whites. J Natl Cancer Inst 2018; 110(6):608–15. https://doi.org/10.1093/jnci/djx262.

Gastric Cancer Epidemiology

Aaron P. Thrift, PhD[a,*], Theresa H. Nguyen, MD[b]

KEYWORDS

• Incidence • Survival • Risk factors • Genetics • Environment

KEY POINTS

- Globally, gastric cancer remains the fifth most common cancer and the third leading cause of cancer-related mortality.
- In the United States, despite overall decreasing rates over the past five decades, incidence of noncardia gastric cancer is increasing among adults less than 50 years.
- *Helicobacter pylori* is the main cause of gastric cancer, accounting for approximately 89% of distal gastric cancer cases worldwide.
- Population-based programs of screening and surveillance and *H pylori* screening and eradication hold greatest promise for reducing the burden of gastric cancer.

INTRODUCTION

Gastric cancer is the fifth most common cancer worldwide and the third leading cause of cancer-related mortality.[1] There are two main topographic types of gastric cancer: cardia gastric cancer (arising in the area of the stomach adjoining the esophagogastric junction) and noncardia gastric cancer (arising from more distal regions of the stomach). The epidemiology of the two topographic types is distinct. Furthermore, according to the Lauren classification, there are two histologic types of gastric cancer: intestinal and diffuse. Both histologic subtypes are associated with *Helicobacter pylori* infection. The diffuse type contains diffuse carcinoma cells that lack cohesion and invade tissues independently or in small clusters. The intestinal type of adenocarcinoma forms glands or tubules lined by epithelium with cohesion among tumor cells that resemble the intestinal mucosa. The intestinal type is the most frequent type found in high gastric cancer incidence populations. A prolonged precancerous process occurs before the development of the intestinal type of adenocarcinoma, known as the Correa cascade, with well-defined, consecutive stages.[2] The process is initiated with *H pylori* infection causing chronic active gastritis. With sustained infection for decades, gastric mucosal inflammation may lead to glandular loss, known as chronic atrophic gastritis. Atrophy typically first occurs in the incisura angularis and

[a] Section of Epidemiology and Population Sciences, Department of Medicine, Dan L Duncan Comprehensive Cancer Center, Baylor College of Medicine, Houston, TX 77030, USA; [b] Baylor Clinic, 6620 Main Street, MS: BCM620, Room 110D, Houston, TX, 77030, USA
* Corresponding author. Baylor College of Medicine, One Baylor Plaza, MS: 307, Room 621D, Houston, TX 77030.
E-mail address: aaron.thrift@bcm.edu

Gastrointest Endoscopy Clin N Am 31 (2021) 425–439
https://doi.org/10.1016/j.giec.2021.03.001
1052-5157/21/

then extends over time to the anterior and posterior gastric walls. Atrophy is then replaced with intestinal metaplastic cells, initially with small intestinal complete phenotype, then eventually to large intestinal (incomplete or colonic) phenotype. Following incomplete intestinal metaplasia, dysplasia then develops (first low grade, then high grade), after which invasive carcinoma is the final stage. This article describes the descriptive epidemiology of gastric cancer, its main risk factors, and opportunities and challenges for primary and secondary prevention.

INCIDENCE AND MORTALITY

Worldwide Trends

According to GLOBOCAN estimates, there were 1,033,701 new cases of gastric cancer worldwide and 782,685 deaths related to gastric cancer in 2018.[3] Gastric cancer was the fifth-most commonly diagnosed cancer type in 2018 (representing 5.7% of all cancer cases diagnosed) and was responsible for 8.2% of all deaths from cancer in 2018, making it the third-most common cause of cancer-related death after lung (18.4% of deaths) and colorectal (9.2% of deaths) cancers.[3] In 2018, the global age-standardized incidence and mortality rates for gastric cancer were 11.1 and 8.2 per 100,000, respectively. Gastric cancer incidence rates increase with increasing age and are two-fold to three-fold higher for men than women. Gastric cancer was the fourth most commonly diagnosed cancer type in men (incidence rate, 15.7 per 100,000) and the seventh most commonly diagnosed cancer type in women (incidence rate, 7.0 per 100,000) in 2018.[3] Recent studies examining global trends in incidence and mortality rates for gastric cancer have confirmed a continued decline worldwide[4–6]; however, these studies also highlight the global variability in incidence and mortality rates and differences in secular trends. Approximately 86% (885,119 of 1,033,701) of new gastric cancer cases in 2018 occurred in regions with high and very high Human Development Index. Environmental factors likely explain this, particularly *H pylori* infection because highly virulent strains of *H pylori* are found in Eastern and South Eastern Asia, regions with high Human Development Index level and where 64% (657,254 cases) of new gastric cancer cases were diagnosed in 2018 (**Fig. 1**).[1,7] The highest incidence rates for gastric cancer are observed in Eastern Asia (32.1 per 100,000 men; 13.2 per

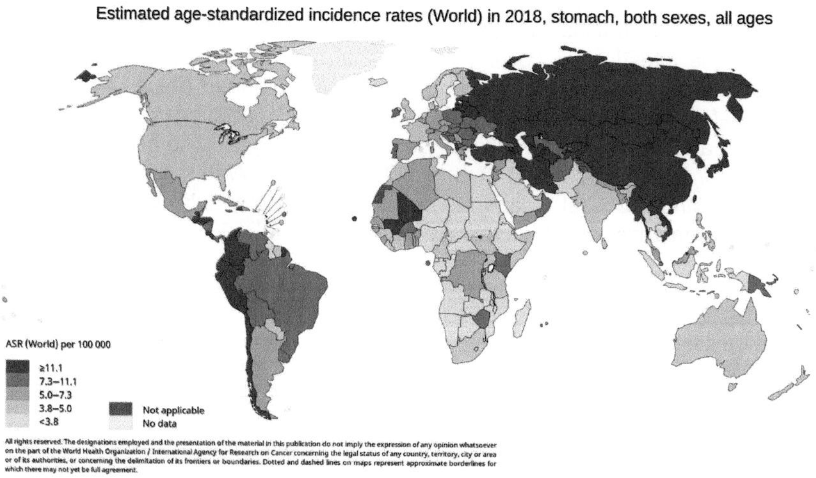

Fig. 1. Worldwide age-standardized incidence rate per 100,000 for gastric cancer in 2018. (*From* GLOBOCAN 2020; Graph production: IARC (http://gco.iarc.fr/today) World Health Organization.)

100,000 women), Central and Eastern Europe (17.1 per 100,000 men; 7.5 per 100,000 women), and South America (12.7 per 100,000; 6.9 per 100,000 women), whereas the lowest incidence rates are observed in North America (5.6 per 100,000 men; 2.8 per 100,000 women) and Africa (~5 per 100,000 men and 3–4 per 100,000 women).[1] There has been a steady decline in incidence and mortality rates for gastric cancer in Western populations since the middle of the twentieth century. In Japan and Korea, countries with historically high gastric cancer incidence rates, delayed but similar decreasing trends have been observed in recent years.[8] The highest mortality rates for gastric cancer are observed in Eastern Asia (15.9 per 100,000).[1] High mortality rates are also observed in Central and Eastern Europe and South America, whereas lowest mortality rates for gastric cancer are seen in Northern America (1.8 per 100,000).[1]

United States Trends

The epidemiology of gastric cancer in the United States has changed dramatically over time,[9] with a linear decline in incidence rates in recent decades.[10,11] For the purpose of this review, the most recent data were analyzed from the US National Cancer Institute's Surveillance, Epidemiology, and End Results (SEER) nine registries[12] (covering approximately 10% of the US population) in which 89,066 cases of invasive gastric cancer (defined using International Classification of Diseases for Oncology, Third Edition, site codes C160–C169 and histology type, excluding 9050–9055, 9140, and 9590–9992) were diagnosed between 1975 and 2017. Gastric cancer incidence rates decreased from 11.7 per 100,000 in 1975 to 6.6 per 100,000 in 2017 (**Fig. 2**). During that period, incidence of gastric cancer decreased at a rate of 1.49% per year (average annual percent change [AAPC], −1.49%; 95% confidence interval [CI], −1.43% to −1.55%). Among all gastric cancer cases in the SEER database diagnosed between 1975 and 2017, 61.4% were in men. Between 1975 and

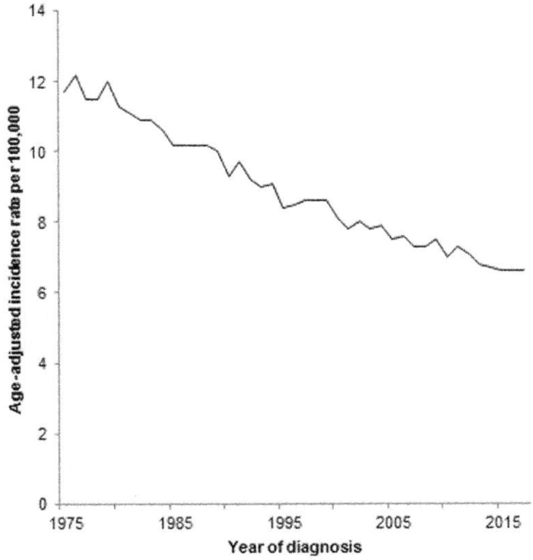

Fig. 2. Age-adjusted incidence rates of gastric cancer in the United States, 1975 to 2017. (*From* Surveillance, Epidemiology, and End Results (SEER) Program (www.seer.cancer.gov) SEER*Stat Database: Incidence - SEER Research Data, 9 Registries, Nov 2019 Sub (1975-2017) - Linked To County Attributes - Time Dependent (1990-2017) Income/Rurality, 1969-2017 Counties, National Cancer Institute, DCCPS, Surveillance Research Program, released April 2020, based on the November 2019 submission.)

2017, gastric cancer incidence rates in the United States decreased in men (AAPC, −1.70%; 95% CI, −1.64% to −1.77%) and women (AAPC, −1.34%; 95% CI, −1.21% to −1.47%). The lifetime risk of gastric cancer in the United States is approximately 1 in 95 men and 1 in 154 women.[10]

Incidence rates for gastric cancer in the United States increase with increasing age, with, historically, low rates of gastric cancer among adults aged less than 50 years.[10] However, although rates of noncardia gastric cancer in the United States continue to decrease among adults aged greater than or equal to 50 years, the incidence of noncardia gastric cancer among persons aged less than 50 years is increasing.[13–15] In addition to established sex disparities, incidence rates for gastric cancer vary among different ethnic groups within the United States.[10] Compared with non-Hispanic Whites, incidence rates for gastric cancer are two-fold higher among Hispanics, non-Hispanic Blacks, and Asian and Pacific Islanders in the United States.[10] Divergent secular trends in gastric cancer rates by cancer stage at diagnosis between non-Hispanic Whites and Hispanics aged less than 50 years have also been reported in the United States.[10,11] Among non-Hispanic Whites, rates of localized-stage noncardia gastric cancer increased by 5.28% (95% CI, 3.94%–6.64%) per year between 2001 and 2014. Conversely, during the same period, the rates of regional- and distant-staged noncardia gastric cancer among non-Hispanic Whites aged less than 50 years decreased and remained unchanged, respectively. By contrast, there was a significant increase in distant-staged noncardia gastric cancers among Hispanics aged less than 50 years (AAPC, 1.78%; 95% CI, 0.66%–2.91%).[14]

Geographic differences in overall gastric cancer incidence rates and trends over time have been observed in the United States.[15] Data from the US Cancer Statistics registry (covering 100% of the US population in 2015)[16] show that the highest incidence rates for gastric cancer in 2001 to 2002, 2006 to 2007, and 2011 to 2012 were found in Hawaii (14.4, 10.6, and 9.1 per 100,000, respectively), whereas by 2016 to 2017 the highest rates were found in New York (8.7 per 100,000). In 2001 to 2002, 12 of the 50 states had incidence rates less than or equal to 5.7 per 100,000; this number increased to 22 states by 2016 to 2017. By contrast, the number of states with incidence rates greater than 8.4 per 100,000 decreased from seven states (Hawaii, Alaska, New York, Rhode Island, New Jersey, Connecticut, Louisiana) in 2001 to 2002 to one (New York) by 2016 to 2017 (**Fig. 3**).

For gastric cancer cases in the SEER 18 registries,[17] median relative survival has increased from 10.3 months in 2000 to 17.6 months for persons diagnosed in 2016. Overall 5-year observed survival rates increased from 18.8% for patients diagnosed with gastric cancer in 2000 to 28.4% for patients diagnosed in 2012. The greatest absolute improvement in survival trends occurred in patients with gastric cancer diagnosed with localized disease. Approximately 46% of patients diagnosed with localized gastric cancer in 2000 survived 5 years after their diagnosis, whereas the 5-year observed survival rate for patients diagnosed with localized gastric cancer in 2012 was 61% (**Fig. 4**). However, one-third of patients with gastric cancer are still diagnosed with distant-stage disease and there has been little improvement in 5-year survival rates for these patients (2.3% for patients diagnosed in 2000 vs 5.4% for those diagnosed in 2012).

RISK FACTORS

Helicobacter pylori Infection

Chronic infection with *H pylori* is the main cause of gastric cancer, accounting for approximately 89% of distal gastric cancer cases worldwide.[18] In 1994, the International Agency for Research on Cancer classified *H pylori* as a class I carcinogen for

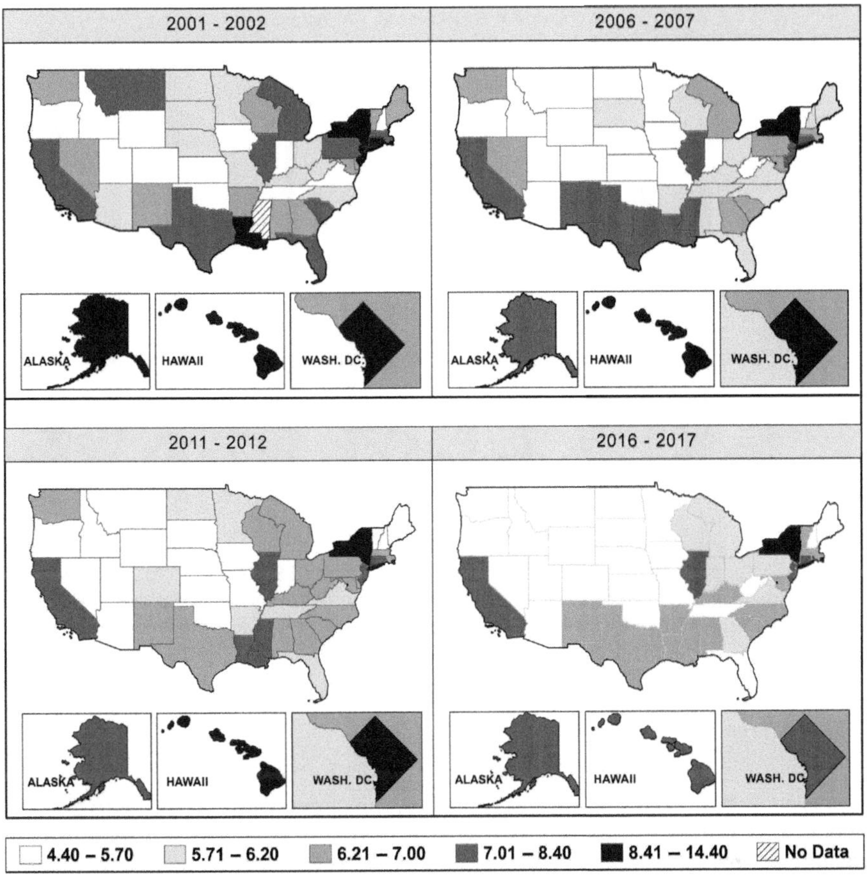

Fig. 3. State-level heat maps showing age-adjusted incidence rates of gastric cancer in the United States, 2001 to 2017. (*From* National Program of Cancer Registries and Surveillance, Epidemiology, and End Results SEER*Stat Database: NPCR and SEER Incidence - U.S. Cancer Statistics 2001-2017 Public Use Research Database, 2019 Submission (2001-2017), United States Department of Health and Human Services, Centers for Disease Control and Prevention and National Cancer Institute. Released June 2020. Accessed at www.cdc.gov/cancer/uscs/public-use.)

noncardia gastric cancer and reconfirmed this classification in 2009.[19] Most *H pylori* infections are acquired during childhood and, once established, usually persist for life unless treated. There is substantial regional variation in prevalence,[20] with highest prevalence in Central and South America and in parts of Asia and Eastern Europe, regions with highest rates of gastric cancer.[20] A stronger effect of *H pylori* on the risk of noncardia gastric cancer is observed among individuals with the CagA-positive *H pylori* strain compared with the CagA-negative strain.[21] Likely because of a reduced bacterial load in severe corpus atrophy, positive low CagA antibody titers may confer higher risk for noncardia gastric cancer (relative risk [RR], 3.9; 95% CI, 2.1–7.0) than high antibody titers (RR, 2.0; 95% CI, 1.3–3.2).[22] Geographic variation in noncardia gastric cancer incidence may be explained by global variability in the prevalence of CagA-positive *H pylori* strains, and by functional differences in CagA tyrosine phosphorylation sites between Eastern and Western CagA-positive *H pylori* strains.[23]

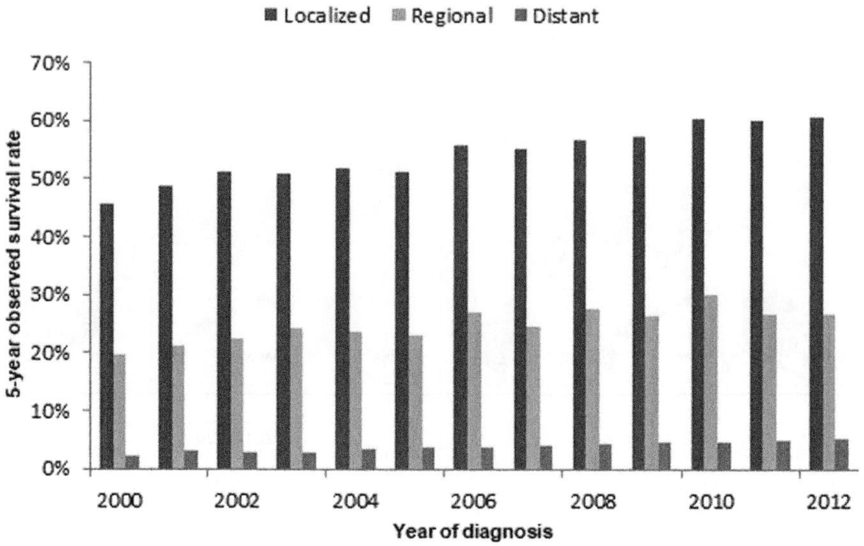

Fig. 4. Five-year survival rates for gastric cancer in the United States, 2000 to 2012, by stage at diagnosis (localized, regional, and distant stage). (*From* Surveillance, Epidemiology, and End Results (SEER) Program (www.seer.cancer.gov) SEER*Stat Database: Incidence - SEER Research Data, 18 Registries, Nov 2019 Sub (2000-2017) - Linked To County Attributes - Time Dependent (1990-2017) Income/Rurality, 1969-2018 Counties, National Cancer Institute, DCCPS, Surveillance Research Program, released April 2020, based on the November 2019 submission.)

Studies show that the CagA EPIYA-D in East Asian strains of *H pylori* bind to the pro-oncogenic SHP2 phosphatase two-fold more strongly than the CagA EPIYA-C in Western strains.[24] However, a case-control study found that the odds of noncardia gastric cancer in CagA seropositives was higher in non-Japanese Brazilians (odds ratio [OR], 4.5; 95% CI, 2.6–7.9) than in Japanese Brazilians (OR, 2.1; 95% CI, 1.2–3.6), which may reflect geographic variations in the frequency rather than oncogenic potential of CagA-positive *H pylori* strains.[25]

Cigarette Smoking

In 2002, International Agency for Research on Cancer concluded that there was sufficient evidence for a causal relationship between smoking and gastric cancer.[26] In a meta-analysis, compared with never smoking, current smoking was associated with increased risk of cardia gastric cancer (RR, 1.87; 95% CI, 1.31–2.67; nine studies) and noncardia gastric cancer (RR, 1.60; 95% CI, 1.41–1.80; nine studies).[27] A recent pooled analysis of data from 10,290 gastric cancer cases and 26,145 control subjects in the Stomach Cancer Pooling Project (StoP) found that current smokers had 25% higher risk of gastric cancer compared with never smokers (OR, 1.25; 95% CI, 1.11–1.40).[28] Smoking conferred increased risk regardless of tumor location; however, the magnitude of association seemed stronger for cardia gastric cancer than noncardia gastric cancer. Risk increased linearly with increasing number of cigarettes per day (P for trend <0.01) and duration of smoking (P for trend <0.01). Importantly, this study found evidence that, among ever smokers, gastric cancer risk declined with increased years of smoking cessation (P for trend <0.01). Gastric cancer risk in former smokers became similar to that of never smokers after 10 years of smoking cessation.[28] Other forms of tobacco use have been associated with an increased risk of gastric cancer, although this has not been consistent across studies.[29]

Excess Body Weight

Studies examining the association between excess body weight and gastric cancer risk have reported conflicting results. A meta-analysis of 13 cohort and three case-control studies found that obesity (body mass index [BMI] $\geq$30 kg/m^2; OR, 1.13; 95% CI, 1.03–1.24) was associated with a modest increased risk for gastric cancer.[30] When examined separately by tumor location, obesity was associated with increased risk for cardia gastric cancer (OR, 1.61; 95% CI, 1.15–2.24) but not noncardia gastric cancer (OR, 0.83; 95% CI, 0.68–1.01).[30] Notably, a meta-analysis of 10 cohort studies found that excess body weight (using the World Health Organization classification of overweight and obese) was associated with an increased risk of gastric cancer in non-Asians (BMI $\geq$25; OR, 1.24; 95% CI, 1.14–1.36), but not in Asians (OR, 1.17; 95% CI, 0.88–1.56).[31] Using the Asia-Pacific classification system of obesity (BMI $\geq$25 kg/m^2), a meta-analysis of seven Asian cohort studies found that obesity was associated with only 3% increased risk of gastric cancer (RR, 1.03; 95% CI, 1.01–1.06).[32]

Dietary Factors

There is strong evidence that diet influences risk of cancer; however, reported associations of dietary factors with gastric cancer are conflicting. These variations might reflect true differences in exposure–disease outcome associations but might also be a result of inherent challenges in the design and conduct of nutritional epidemiology studies. For example, when stratified by study design, a meta-analysis found that red meat was associated with increased risk for gastric cancer in 24 case-control studies (RR, 1.67; 95% CI, 1.36–2.05) but there was no association in four cohort studies (RR, 1.14; 95% CI, 0.97–1.34).[33] Similarly, increased white meat consumption was associated with lower risk of gastric cancer when assessed in population-based case-control studies (RR, 0.75; 95% CI, 0.61–0.93; nine studies) but not in cohort studies (RR, 0.85; 95% CI, 0.63–1.16; five studies).[34] There is, however, stronger evidence for processed meat. In a meta-analysis, high consumption of processed meat was associated with increased risk for gastric cancer whether assessed in cohort (RR, 1.21; 95% CI, 1.04–1.41; seven studies) or case-control (RR, 2.17; 95% CI, 1.51–3.11; 12 studies) studies.[34] When stratified by anatomic subtype, high processed meat consumption conferred increased risk for noncardia gastric cancer but not cardia gastric cancer. Given the association between a diet high in processed meats and increased risk of noncardia gastric cancer, attention has been placed on nitrates and nitrites, and, in particular, *N*-nitrosodimethylamine (NDMA), a type of nitrosamine produced by chemical reactions of nitrates and nitrites. NDMA occurs in dietary foods as a food additive often used in processed meats and is a potential carcinogen.[35] A meta-analysis of seven cohort and four case-control studies found that those with the highest NDMA consumption had 34% increased risk of gastric cancer compared with lowest intake (RR, 1.34; 95% CI, 1.02–1.76).[36] A nonlinear trend toward gastric cancer risk was seen with increasing NDMA intake greater than 0.12 μg/day (*P* for nonlinearity $<$0.001).

High salt intake has been hypothesized to promote gastric mucosal damage, hypergastrinemia, and cell proliferation, and several prospective studies have been performed to evaluate the relationship between salt intake and risk of gastric cancer.[37] A meta-analysis of seven cohort studies found that high salt intake was associated with 68% higher risk of gastric cancer compared with low intake (RR, 1.68; 95% CI, 1.17–2.41).[38] Stratified analysis was not performed for anatomic subtype of gastric cancer in the meta-analysis; however, a large case-control study from Portugal found that high salt intake (>3960.1 mg/day) was associated with increased risk of noncardia gastric cancer (OR, 2.26; 95% CI, 1.27–4.04) compared with low intake (<3067.5 mg/day), whereas no association was found for cardia gastric cancer.[39] Although these data suggest that salt intake is a risk factor for gastric cancer, only one study in the meta-analysis adjusted for *H pylori* infection, and the positive association may be caused by confounding because those ethnicities with high prevalence of *H pylori* infection may also have diets high in salt.[38,40]

Decreasing trends in the incidence of gastric cancer has been hypothesized to be partly caused by the increased availability of fresh fruit and vegetables. A meta-analysis of six cohort studies found an inverse relationship with high white vegetable consumption versus low (RR, 0.67; 95% CI, 0.47–0.95), but no association was seen with total vegetables and gastric cancer risk (22 studies; RR, 0.98; 95% CI, 0.91–1.05) and stratified by cardia and noncardia cancer.[41] Total fruit consumption was found to be inversely associated with risk of gastric cancer in pooled analysis of 30 cohort studies (RR, 0.93; 95% CI, 0.89–0.98); however, this was not seen in pooled analyses stratified by cardia (RR, 1.08; 95% CI, 0.93–1.26; seven studies) and noncardia (RR, 0.98; 95% CI, 0.82–1.16; seven studies).[41]

Alcohol Consumption

Alcohol may affect gastric cancer cell proliferation[42] and has been examined as a risk factor for gastric cancer with inconsistent results. A meta-analysis of 23 cohort studies published through 2016 found some evidence for a modest increased risk of gastric cancer associated with ever alcohol consumption (RR, 1.17; 95% CI, 1.00–1.34; I^2 = 79.6%).[43] Among alcohol drinkers, risk increased by 7% with every 10 g/day increment in alcohol consumption (RR, 1.07; 95% CI, 1.02–1.12).[43] Likewise, a meta-analysis of 56 case-control and 17 cohort studies also reported increased risk of gastric cancer with high alcohol consumption (vs low; RR, 1.25; 95% CI, 1.15–1.37) with a curvilinear dose-response.[44] Notably, subgroup analysis for type of alcohol demonstrated increased risk of gastric cancer with high consumption of beer (RR, 1.13; 95% CI, 0.98–1.39) and liquor (RR, 1.22; 95% CI, 1.06–1.40), but not wine. When stratified by anatomic subtype, there was a significant association between high alcohol consumption and risk of noncardia gastric cancer (18 studies; RR, 1.19; 95% CI, 1.01–1.40) but not cardia gastric cancer (15 studies; RR, 1.16; 95% CI, 0.98–1.39).[44] In pooled analyses of data from StoP, heavy alcohol drinking (>6 drinks/day) conferred increased risk for cardia (OR, 1.61; 95% CI, 1.11–2.34) and noncardia (OR, 1.28; 95% CI, 1.13–1.45) gastric cancer.[45]

Medications

Nonsteroidal anti-inflammatory drugs (NSAIDs), including nonselective NSAIDs (aspirin), have been proposed as potential chemopreventive therapy for gastric cancer given increased cyclooxygenase-2 expression found in gastric cancer tissue.[46] A meta-analysis of 24 studies demonstrated that any NSAID use was associated with 22% lower risk of gastric cancer compared with never use (RR, 0.78; 95% CI, 0.72–0.85).[47] For every 2 years of incremental NSAID use, gastric cancer risk decreased by 11% (RR, 0.89; 95% CI, 0.83–0.96). Aspirin alone was also inversely related to gastric cancer risk (RR, 0.70; 95% CI, 0.62–0.89). In subgroup analysis for anatomic subtype, any NSAID use was associated with lower risk of noncardia gastric cancer (RR, 0.70; 95% CI, 0.59–0.84), with evidence for a dose–response relationship (per 2-year increments; RR, 0.83; 95% CI, 0.72–0.96; *P* for linear trend <0.01), but not associated with cardia gastric cancer.[47] However, a meta-analysis of nine randomized controlled trials found no statistically significant association between NSAID use and gastric cancer risk (RR, 0.84; 95% CI, 0.65–1.10).[48]

Statins (HMG CoA reductase inhibitors), one of the most widely used medications for hyperlipidemia, have also been proposed as chemopreventive therapy, because studies have shown that statins have antiproliferative, proapoptotic, antiangiogenic, and immunomodulatory effects in human gastric cancer–derived cell lines.[49] A meta-analysis of six case-control studies demonstrated an inverse relationship between statin use and risk of gastric cancer (OR, 0.83; 95% CI, 0.76–0.90; $I^2 = 0\%$).[50] Pooled analysis of three case-control studies found a dose-duration response with long statin duration use (≥2 years of daily use) having more chemopreventive effect (OR, 0.35; 95% CI, 0.16–0.76) than short statin duration use (<2 years of daily use; OR, 0.73; 95% CI, 0.51–1.05).[50] Another meta-analysis of 26 randomized controlled trials found that statin use was associated with 27% lower risk of gastric cancer (RR, 0.73; 95% CI, 0.58–0.92), which was attenuated but remained significant after excluding subjects with diabetes (RR, 0.85; 95% CI, 0.80–0.91).[51]

Genetics

Although most gastric cancers are sporadic, risk of gastric cancer is up to 10-fold higher in persons with a family history of gastric cancer.[52] Gastric cancer may also develop as part of a familial cancer syndrome, such as hereditary diffuse gastric cancer syndrome, Lynch syndrome (in particular patients with an MLH1 or MSH2 mutation),[53] familial adenomatous polyposis, Peutz-Jeghers syndrome, and Li-Fraumeni syndrome.[54]

Other

Up to 10% of gastric cancers are attributed to less common causes, including infection with Epstein-Barr virus (EBV), autoimmune gastritis, and Ménétrier disease. A recent international pooled analysis of 15 studies reported that approximately 8% of gastric cancers harbor EBV,[55] but there is insufficient epidemiologic evidence of a clear etiologic role for EBV in gastric carcinogenesis.[19]

PREVENTION

Gastric cancer maintains a high case fatality rate of 75% throughout most of the world[56] and is a main contributor to global disability-adjusted life-year burden.[57] Mass screening for gastric cancer is generally not included in national strategies for cancer prevention because of high cost; decreasing incidence; and a lack of data on whom, when, and how to screen. To date, the clinical practice of gastric cancer prevention has focused on screening and surveillance and *H pylori* screening and eradication. However, incorporating multiple risk factors into a clinical prediction rule could lead to more efficient selection for screening of patients at risk for gastric cancer. Several models have been developed[58]; however, none of these models is perfect and they require further examination in larger, external populations before clinical implementation is recommended.[59]

Primary Prevention with Helicobacter pylori Screening and Eradication

A systematic review and meta-analysis of six international randomized controlled trials found that adults who have tested positive for *H pylori* and received eradication therapy had 34% lower risk of developing incident gastric cancer compared with *H pylori*–positive control subjects who received placebo or no therapy (RR, 0.66; 95% CI, 0.46–0.95)[60]; corresponding to a number needed to treat to prevent one gastric cancer of 124 (95% CI, 78–843).[60] A phase 3 randomized controlled trial in school-aged *H pylori*–naive children reported successful prevention of *H pylori* infection with a prophylactic oral *H pylori* vaccine (vaccine efficacy, 71.8%).[61] A large community-based intervention trial in China demonstrated that *H pylori* eradication is feasible and acceptable; however, eradication was not uniformly achieved in the population.[62]

These studies show that under conditions of low bacterial burden and acute infection, persistent *H pylori* infection can be prevented, and eradication of *H pylori* may lead to reduced incidence of gastric cancer. Additionally, under various assumptions about effectiveness and costs, population-based screening and eradication of *H pylori* has been shown to be cost-effective.[63,64] In particular, for geographic regions with high gastric cancer burden, population-based *H pylori* serology screening is cost-effective when performed in persons aged greater than 50 years. There is some evidence that population-based *H pylori* serology screening is cost-effective for populations with gastric cancer rates as low as 4.2 per 100,000.[64] Further studies are needed to establish whether screening in high-risk subpopulations residing in countries with low gastric cancer incidence, such as the United States, is cost-effective.[65]

Secondary Prevention with Screening and Surveillance

Upper gastrointestinal endoscopy studies have shown the highest detection rates among the screening modalities and are considered the gold standard for the diagnosis of gastric cancer.[66] Although the available evidence shows that endoscopic population screening is cost-effective in areas with high gastric cancer burden,[64] further studies are needed to evaluate the impact of this technique before recommending its broad use as a primary screening test.[67] Upper gastrointestinal series has continuously been analyzed as a rivaling modality for cancer detection but has not shown clear benefits over endoscopy.[68]

Several countries have implemented national screening programs. For example, in South Korea, the Korean Gastric Cancer Association and National Cancer Center established national guidelines for gastric cancer screening in 2001. These guidelines recommend biennial gastric cancer screening via upper endoscopy or upper gastrointestinal series for men and women aged greater than or equal to 40 years, which started in 2002.[69] In 2013, the Japanese government approved insurance coverage for a gastric cancer prevention program that includes *H pylori* screening and treatment (primary prevention) and post–*H pylori* treatment surveillance (secondary prevention for people with atrophic gastritis).[70] In the United States, there are no population-based mass screening programs aimed at reducing the incidence of gastric cancer.

FUTURE DIRECTIONS

Biomarkers for screening and risk triaging and clinical prediction rules that combine these biomarkers with established clinical and lifestyle factors for risk stratification need to be derived, optimized, and then validated in external populations. Future biomarker studies should aim to state the *a priori* plan for building statistical models; consider interactions, transformations, and splines; refrain from categorizing predictors; use and report model coefficients; aim for external validation; use informed and *a priori* stated criteria for desired sensitivity and specificity; and assess model performance by incorporating population disease risk. Finally, at the public health level and clinically, risk communication should be a central feature of research and implementation.

SUMMARY

Further improvements in screening, treatment, and early diagnosis are needed for gastric cancer, which remains the third most common cause of cancer-related mortality worldwide. Although mass screening strategies could be beneficial, current modalities are not yet readily implementable in organized screening settings. Conversely, because the population risk (based on histology) can change rapidly, and *H pylori* eradication is effective, population-based programs of screening and treatment of *H pylori* may hold greatest promise for reducing the burden of gastric cancer.[61]

CLINICS CARE POINTS

- Although rates of noncardia gastric cancer in the United States continue to decrease among adults aged $\geq$50 years, the incidence of noncardia gastric cancer among persons aged less than 50 years is increasing, particularly among Hispanics, non-Hispanic Blacks, and Asian and Pacific Islanders.
- Chronic infection with *H pylori* is the main cause of gastric cancer, accounting for approximately 89% of distal gastric cancer cases worldwide, and data demonstrate that eradicating *H pylori* reduces the incidence of gastric cancer.
- Although studies show that endoscopic population screening is cost-effective in areas with high gastric cancer burden, further studies are needed before recommending the broad use of upper endoscopy as a primary screening test in the United States and other low-incidence countries.

DISCLOSURE

The authors have nothing to disclose.

REFERENCES

1. Ferlay J, Ervik M, Lam F. Global cancer observatory: cancer today, vol. 2020. Lyon (France): International Agency for Research on Cancer; 2018.
2. Correa P. Gastric cancer: overview. Gastroenterol Clin North Am 2013;42:211–7.
3. Bray F, Ferlay J, Soerjomataram I, et al. Global cancer statistics 2018: GLOBOCAN estimates of incidence and mortality worldwide for 36 cancers in 185 countries. CA Cancer J Clin 2018;68:394–424.
4. Luo G, Zhang Y, Guo P, et al. Global patterns and trends in stomach cancer incidence: age, period and birth cohort analysis. Int J Cancer 2017;141:1333–44.
5. Arnold M, Karim-Kos HE, Coebergh JW, et al. Recent trends in incidence of five common cancers in 26 European countries since 1988: analysis of the European Cancer Observatory. Eur J Cancer 2015;51:1164–87.
6. Ferro A, Peleteiro B, Malvezzi M, et al. Worldwide trends in gastric cancer mortality (1980-2011), with predictions to 2015, and incidence by subtype. Eur J Cancer 2014;50:1330–44.
7. Fidler MM, Soerjomataram I, Bray F. A global view on cancer incidence and national levels of the human development index. Int J Cancer 2016;139:2436–46.
8. Ferlay J, Colombet M, Bray F. Cancer incidence in five continents, CI5plus: International Agency for Research on Cancer CancerBase No. 9. Lyon (France): 2018.
9. Anderson WF, Camargo MC, Fraumeni JF Jr, et al. Age-specific trends in incidence of noncardia gastric cancer in US adults. JAMA 2010;303:1723–8.

10. Thrift AP, El-Serag HB. Burden of gastric cancer. Clin Gastroenterol Hepatol 2020; 18:534–42.
11. U.S. Cancer Statistics Working Group. U.S. Cancer Statistics Data Visualizations Tool. U.S. Department of Health and Human Services, Centers for Disease Control and Prevention and National Cancer Institute; www.cdc.gov/cancer/dataviz.
12. Surveillance, Epidemiology, and End Results (SEER) Program (www.seer.cancer.gov) SEER*Stat Database: Incidence - SEER Research Data, 9 Registries, Nov 2019 Sub (1975- 2017) - Linked To County Attributes - Time Dependent (1990-2017) Income/Rurality, 1969- 2017 Counties, National Cancer Institute, DCCPS, Surveillance Research Program, released April 2020, based on the November 2019 submission.
13. Anderson WF, Rabkin CS, Turner N, et al. The changing face of noncardia gastric cancer incidence among US non-Hispanic Whites. J Natl Cancer Inst 2018;110: 608–15.
14. Wang Z, El-Serag HB, Thrift AP. Increasing incidence of advanced non-cardia gastric cancers among younger Hispanics in the USA. Dig Dis Sci 2020.
15. Wang Z, Graham DY, Khan A, et al. Incidence of gastric cancer in the USA during 1999 to 2013: a 50-state analysis. Int J Epidemiol 2018;47:966–75.
16. U.S. Cancer Statistics Working Group. U.S. Cancer Statistics Data Visualizations Tool, based on 2019 submission data (1999-2017): U.S. Department of Health and Human Services, Centers for Disease Control and Prevention and National Cancer Institute; www.cdc.gov/cancer/dataviz.
17. Surveillance, Epidemiology, and End Results (SEER) Program (www.seer.cancer.gov) SEER*Stat Database: Incidence - SEER Research Data, 18 Registries, Nov 2019 Sub (2000-2017) - Linked To County Attributes - Time Dependent (1990-2017) Income/Rurality, 1969-2018 Counties, National Cancer Institute, DCCPS, Surveillance Research Program, released April 2020, based on the November 2019 submission.
18. Plummer M, Franceschi S, Vignat J, et al. Global burden of gastric cancer attributable to *Helicobacter pylori*. Int J Cancer 2015;136:487–90.
19. IARC Working Group on the Evaluation of Carcinogenic Risks to Humans. Biological agents. Volume 100 B. A review of human carcinogens. IARC Monogr Eval Carcinog Risks Hum. 2012;100(Pt B):1-441.
20. Peleteiro B, Bastos A, Ferro A, et al. Prevalence of *Helicobacter pylori* infection worldwide: a systematic review of studies with national coverage. Dig Dis Sci 2014;59:1698–709.
21. Akopyants NS, Clifton SW, Kersulyte D, et al. Analyses of the cag pathogenicity island of *Helicobacter pylori*. Mol Microbiol 1998;28:37–54.
22. Suzuki G, Cullings H, Fujiwara S, et al. Low-positive antibody titer against *Helicobacter pylori* cytotoxin-associated gene A (CagA) may predict future gastric cancer better than simple seropositivity against *H. pylori* CagA or against *H. pylori*. Cancer Epidemiol Biomarkers Prev 2007;16:1224–8.
23. Higashi H, Tsutsumi R, Fujita A, et al. Biological activity of the *Helicobacter pylori* virulence factor CagA is determined by variation in the tyrosine phosphorylation sites. Proc Natl Acad Sci U S A 2002;99:4428–33.
24. Hayashi T, Senda M, Suzuki N, et al. Differential mechanisms for SHP2 binding and activation are exploited by geographically distinct *Helicobacter pylori* CagA oncoproteins. Cell Rep 2017;20:2876–90.
25. Tatemichi M, Hamada GS, Nishimoto IN, et al. Ethnic difference in serology of *Helicobacter pylori* CagA between Japanese and non-Japanese Brazilians for non-cardia gastric cancer. Cancer Sci 2003;94:64–9.

26. IARC Working Group on the Evaluation of Carcinogenic Risks to Humans. Tobacco smoke and involuntary smoking. IARC Monogr Eval Carcinog Risks Hum 2004;83:1–1438.
27. Ladeiras-Lopes R, Pereira AK, Nogueira A, et al. Smoking and gastric cancer: systematic review and meta-analysis of cohort studies. Cancer Causes Control 2008;19:689–701.
28. Praud D, Rota M, Peluchi C, et al. Cigarette smoking and gastric cancer in the Stomach Cancer Pooling (StoP) Project. Eur J Cancer Prev 2018;27:124–33.
29. Sadjadi A, Derakhshan MH, Yazdanbod A, et al. Neglected role of hookah and opium in gastric carcinogenesis: a cohort study on risk factors and attributable fractions. Int J Cancer 2014;134:181–8.
30. Lin X-J, Wang C-P, Liu X-D, et al. Body mass index and risk of gastric cancer: a meta-analysis. Jpn J Clin Oncol 2014;44:783–91.
31. Yang P, Zhou Y, Chen B, et al. Overweight, obesity and gastric cancer risk: results from a meta-analysis of cohort studies. Eur J Cancer 2009;45:2867–73.
32. Bae J-M. Body mass index and risk of gastric cancer in Asian adults: a meta-epidemiological meta-analysis of population-based cohort studies. Cancer Res Treat 2020;52:369–73.
33. Zhao Z, Yin Z, Zhao Q. Red and processed meat consumption and gastric cancer risk: a systematic review and meta-analysis. Oncotarget 2017;8:30563–75.
34. Kim SR, Kim K, Lee SA, et al. Effect of red, processed, and white meat consumption on the risk of gastric cancer: an overall and dose-response meta-analysis. Nutrients 2019;11:826.
35. Tricker AR, Preussmann R. Carcinogenic N-nitrosamines in the diet: occurrence, formation, mechanisms and carcinogenic potential. Mutat Res 1991;259:277–89.
36. Song P, Wu L, Guan W. Dietary nitrates, nitrites, and nitrosamines intake and the risk of gastric cancer: a meta-analysis. Nutrients 2015;7:9872–95.
37. Furihata C, Ohta H, Katsuyama T. Cause and effect between concentration-dependent tissue damage and temporary cell proliferation in rat stomach mucosa by NaCl, a stomach tumor promoter. Carcinogenesis 1996;17:401–6.
38. D'Elia L, Rossi G, Ippolito R, et al. Habitual salt intake and risk of gastric cancer: a meta-analysis of prospective studies. Clin Nutr 2012;31:489–98.
39. Peleteiro B, Lopes C, Figueiredo C, et al. Salt intake and gastric cancer risk according to *Helicobacter pylori* infection, smoking, tumour site and histological type. Br J Cancer 2011;104:198–207.
40. Firestone MJ, Beasley J, Kwon SC, et al. Asian American dietary sources of sodium and salt behaviors compared with other racial/ethnic groups, NHANES, 2011-2012. Ethn Dis 2017;27:241–8.
41. Fang X, Wei J, He X, et al. Landscape of dietary factors associated with risk of gastric cancer: a systematic review and dose-response meta-analysis of prospective cohort studies. Eur J Cancer 2015;51:2820–32.
42. Jelski W, Chrostek L, Zalewski B, et al. Alcohol dehydrogenase (ADH) isoenzymes and aldehyde dehydrogenase (ALDH) activity in the sera of patients with gastric cancer. Dig Dis Sci 2008;53:2101–5.
43. Han X, Xiao L, Yu Y, et al. Alcohol consumption and gastric cancer risk: a meta-analysis of prospective cohort studies. Oncotarget 2017;8:83237–45.
44. Wang P-L, Xiao F-T, Gong B-C, et al. Alcohol drinking and gastric cancer risk: a meta-analysis of observational studies. Oncotarget 2017;8:99013–23.
45. Rota M, Pelucchi C, Bertuccio P, et al. Alcohol consumption and gastric cancer risk: a pooled analysis within the StoP project consortium. Int J Cancer 2017;141:1950–62.

46. Lim HY, Joo HJ, Choi JH, et al. Increased expression of cyclooxygenase-2 protein in human gastric carcinoma. Clin Cancer Res 2000;6:519–25.
47. Huang X-Z, Chen Y, Wu J, et al. Aspirin and non-steroidal anti-inflammatory drug use reduce gastric cancer risk: a dose-reponse meta-analysis. Oncotarget 2017; 8:4781–95.
48. Niikura R, Hirata Y, Hayakawa Y, et al. Effect of aspirin use on gastric cancer incidence and survival: a systematic review and meta-analysis. JGH Open 2019;4: 117–25.
49. Follet J, Corco L, Baffet G, et al. The association of statins and taxanes: an efficient combination trigger of cancer cell apoptosis. Br J Cancer 2012;106:685–92.
50. Singh PP, Singh S. Statins are associated with reduced risk of gastric cancer: a systematic review and meta-analysis. Ann Oncol 2013;24:1721–30.
51. Wu X-D, Zeng K, Xue F-Q, et al. Statins are associated with reduced risk of gastric cancer: a meta-analysis. Eur J Clin Pharmacol 2013;69:1855–60.
52. Gonzalez CA, Agudo A. Carcinogenesis, prevention and early detection of gastric cancer: where we are and where we should go. Int J Cancer 2012;130: 745–53.
53. Capelle LG, Van Grieken NCT, Lingsma HF, et al. Risk and epidemiological time trends of gastric cancer in Lynch syndrome carriers in the Netherlands. Gastroenterology 2010;138:487–92.
54. Oliveira C, Seruca R, Carneiro F. Genetics, pathology, and clinics of familial gastric cancer. Int J Surg Pathol 2006;14:21–33.
55. Camargo MC, Murphy G, Koriyama C, et al. Determinants of Epstein-Barr virus-positive gastric cancer: an international pooled analysis. Br J Cancer 2011;105: 38–43.
56. Fock KM. Review article: the epidemiology and prevention of gastric cancer. Aliment Pharmacol Ther 2014;40:250–60.
57. Soerjomataram I, Lortet-Tieulent J, Maxwell Parkin D, et al. Global burden of cancer in 2008: a systematic analysis of disability-adjusted life-years in 12 world regions. Lancet 2012;380:1840–50.
58. Cai Q, Zhu C, Yuan Y, et al. Development and validation of a prediction rule for estimating gastric cancer risk in the Chinese high-risk population: a nationwide multicentre study. Gut 2019;68:1576–87.
59. Thrift AP, Kanwal F, El-Serag HB. Prediction models for gastrointestinal and liver diseases: too many developed, too few validated. Clin Gastroenterol Hepatol 2016;14:1678–80.
60. Ford AC, Forman D, Hunt RH, et al. *Helicobacter pylori* eradication therapy to prevent gastric cancer in healthy asymptomatic infected individuals: systematic review and meta-analysis of randomised controlled trials. BMJ 2014;348:g3174.
61. Zeng M, Mao X-H, Li J-X, et al. Efficacy, safety, and immunogenicity of an oral recombinant *Helicobacter pylori* vaccine in children in China: a randomised, double-blind, placebo-controlled, phase 3 trial. Lancet 2015;386:1457–64.
62. Pan K-f, Zhang L, Gerhard M, et al. A large randomised controlled intervention trial to prevent gastric cancer by eradication of *Helicobacter pylori* in Linqu County, China: baseline results and factors affecting the eradication. Gut 2016; 65:9–18.
63. IARC Helicobacter pylori Working Group (2014). Helicobacter pylori Eradication as a Strategy for Preventing Gastric Cancer. Lyon, France: International Agency for Research on Cancer (IARC Working Group Reports, No. 8). Available from: http://www.iarc.fr/en/publications/pdfsonline/wrk/wrk8/index.php

64. Areia M, Carvalho R, Cadime AT, et al. Screening for gastric cancer and surveillance of premalignant lesions: a systematic review of cost-effectiveness studies. Helicobacter 2013;18:325–37.
65. El-Serag HB, Kao JY, Kanwal F, et al. Houston consensus conference on testing for *Helicobacter pylori* infection in the United States. Clin Gastroenterol Hepatol 2018;16:992–1002.
66. Karimi P, Islami F, Anandasabapathy S, et al. Gastric cancer: descriptive epidemiology, risk factors, screening, and prevention. Cancer Epidemiol Biomarkers Prev 2014;23:700–13.
67. Choi KS, Jun JK, Park E-C, et al. Performance of different gastric cancer screening methods in Korea: a population-based study. PLoS One 2012;7:e50041.
68. Tashiro A, Sano M, Kinameri K, et al. Comparing mass screening techniques for gastric cancer in Japan. World J Gastroenterol 2006;12:4873–4.
69. Choi KS, Suh M. Screening for gastric cancer: the usefulness of endoscopy. Clin Endosc 2014;47:490–6.
70. Asaka M. A new approach for elimination of gastric cancer deaths in Japan. Int J Cancer 2013;132:1272–6.

Public Health Interventions for Gastric Cancer Control

Manami Inoue, MD, PhD

KEYWORDS

• Gastric cancer • Risk factor • Prevention • Intervention

KEY POINTS

- Gastric cancer incidence has decreased substantially over the past century, by decreases in Helicobacter pylori infection, tobacco smoking and salt-preserved food intake.
- *Helicobacter pylori* eradication for infected patients has potential as a prevention strategy for those at high risk but warrants a longer follow-up period.
- The increase in obesity prevalence may cause an increase in cardia gastric cancer, especially in Western populations, and should be carefully monitored.

INTRODUCTION AND BACKGROUND

Despite the generally decreasing trend in incidence, gastric cancer still contributes to the global burden of cancer, remaining the fifth-most common cancer worldwide with more than 1 million incident cases in 2018.[1] Gastric cancer incidence is characterized by large geographic variation, with high rates in East Asia, Eastern Europe, and some South American countries, which in turn provides insights into how to approach risk factors and primary prevention of gastric cancer. Gastric cancer can be divided by anatomic origin into 2 subtypes, cardia and noncardia, which share some risk factors, but have others that are specific to each. Noncardia gastric cancer is more common than cardia gastric cancer in East Asian populations, where gastric cancer rates are generally high, whereas cardia gastric cancer is more common in Western populations. These differences again provide important clues to the differences in etiology of these 2 cancer subtypes.

The most important risk factor for gastric cancer is *Helicobacter pylori* (*H pylori*) infection, particularly for noncardia gastric cancer. The prevalence of *H pylori* varies widely by geographic area, socioeconomic status, and birth cohort.[2] Generally, countries and regions with high gastric cancer rates tend to have a high seroprevalence of *H pylori* infection. The recent global reduction in gastric cancer is attributed in large part to a decrease in *H pylori* infection. This decline in *H pylori* has coincided with a decrease in the incidence of noncardia gastric cancer and an increase in the incidence of cardia gastric cancer.[3] Stated differently, *H pylori* is a significant risk factor for

Conflict of Interest: None declared.

Division of Prevention, Center for Public Health Sciences, National Cancer Center, 5-1-1 Tsukiji, Chuo-ku, Tokyo 104-0045, Japan
E-mail address: mnminoue@ncc.go.jp

Gastrointest Endoscopy Clin N Am 31 (2021) 441–449
https://doi.org/10.1016/j.giec.2021.03.002

noncardia gastric cancer, but is inversely associated with the risk of cardia gastric cancer.[4]

However, a decrease in gastric cancer was evident in many countries even before this bacterium was discovered. This finding suggests that gastric cancers result from a variety of environmental causes, both related and unrelated to *H pylori* infection, and that both directed and nonspecific interventions impacting these causes might have led to this decline. Here, the risk factors of gastric cancer and its population-level prevention are discussed.

RISK FACTORS OF GASTRIC CANCER

With the increasing importance of evidence-based cancer prevention approaches, various international bodies have continued a series of risk factor assessments over recent decades that use both systematic review and meta-analysis. From the current evidence base, *H pylori* infection and tobacco smoking are known causes of gastric cancer, with sufficient evidence for categorization as group 1 carcinogens by the International Agency for Research on Cancer (IARC).[5] Apart from these 2 factors, the Continuous Update Project of the World Cancer Research Fund (WCRF) summarizes the most recently updated evaluation of risk factors for gastric cancer.[3] In its project report focusing on gastric cancer, the panel judged that high consumption of alcoholic drinks (>45 g ethanol/d) and foods preserved by salting is a probable cause of gastric cancer and that a greater amount of body fat or a higher body mass index (BMI) is a probable cause of cardia gastric cancer. Nonstarchy vegetables, allium vegetables, and fruit, judged in its previous 2007 report as probably decreasing this risk,[6] have been downgraded owing to limited evidence. The updated report states that there is only limited evidence to suggest that consumption of grilled (broiled) or barbecued (charbroiled) meat and fish increases the risk of gastric cancer or consumption of processed meat increases the risk of noncardia gastric cancer, or that low consumption of fruit increases the risk of gastric cancer or low consumption of citrus fruit increases the risk of cardia gastric cancer. **Table 1** summarizes the risk factors for gastric cancer.

H PYLORI INFECTION

H pylori is, above all others, the most important cause of gastric cancer, especially noncardia gastric cancer. The acquisition of *H pylori* infection generally occurs during childhood, usually before 5 years of age. Infection status is, therefore, strongly suggested to depend on environmental hygiene during childhood and eating behavior, such as mouth-to-mouth feeding. Such lifestyle factors during infancy greatly reflect the infection rate in adulthood.[2] It is notable that, in Japan, where gastric cancer has been the most common cancer for the last century, the prevalence of *H pylori* infection has decreased with a birth cohort effect,[2,7] peaking at approximately 70% to 80% for those born around 1930 to 1940 and decreasing with age to reach approximately 5% for those born around 2000, with no substantial change of infection rate during the lifetime for each birth cohort (**Fig. 1**). This finding implies that gastric cancer prevention strategies confer generational effects. Countries with a similar experience should consider risk-stratified approaches to gastric cancer prevention over the next few decades. A decreasing trend has also been observed in Korea, suggesting the importance of *H pylori* infection management at a younger age.[8] Although screen-and-treat strategies are recommended in communities at high risk of gastric cancer, their use in children and adolescents is controversial, and further evidence is awaited.[9] Going forward, improvements in hygiene and socioeconomic conditions will foster a

Table 1
Summary of risk factors for gastric cancer

Evidence Level		Risk Factor (Positive Association)
Strong evidence	Convincing/ established cause	*H pylori* infection (noncardia) Tobacco smoking
	Probable	Body fatness (cardia) Alcoholic beverages (intake above 45 g of ethanol per day) Food preserved by salting
Limited evidence	Limited—suggestive	Processed meat (noncardia) Grilled (broiled) or barbecued (charbroiled) meat and fish Low fruit intake Low citrus fruit intake (cardia)

Data from Refs.[3,17,18]

substantial decrease in the overall prevalence of *H pylori* infection in all age groups and even in countries with a high prevalence of infection, eventually reaching the level of a rare event and leading to an overall decrease in gastric cancers.

H pylori eradication for infected individuals has been considered a possible preventive measure for gastric cancer, despite incurring side effects such as gastroesophageal reflux disease and antibiotic resistance.[10] The effectiveness of eradication is considered dependent on whether it can reverse precancerous lesions, such as atrophic gastritis or intestinal metaplasia, before the point of no return, namely the irreversible point of progression to gastric cancer.[11] One meta-analysis indicated that eradication of *H pylori* is not effective in patients with intestinal metaplasia and dysplasia.[12] Accordingly, eradication of *H pylori* at an early stage is considered effective in preventing gastric cancer onset by inhibiting the progression of these precancerous lesions. A recent Cochrane systematic review assessed the effectiveness of *H*

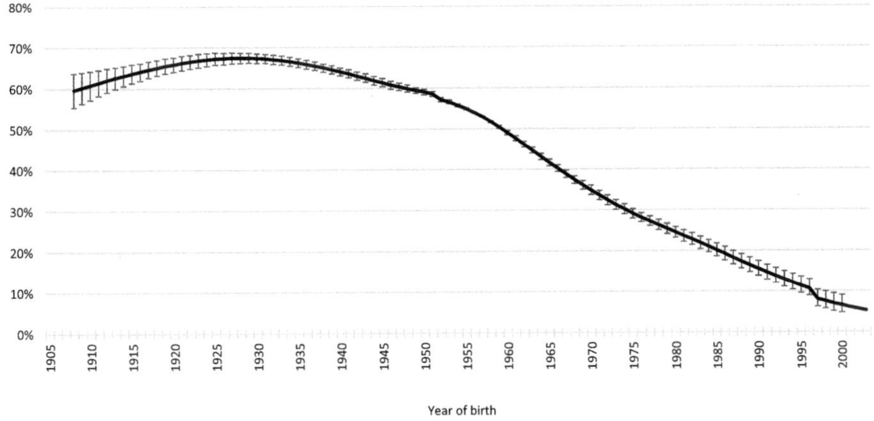

Fig. 1. Declining trends in the prevalence of *H pylori* infection by birth year in a Japanese population (meta-regression analysis of 170,752 Japanese participants). (*Adapted from* Wang C, Nishiyama T, Kikuchi S et al. Changing trends in the prevalence of H. pylori infection Japan (1908-2003): a systematic review and meta-regression analysis of 170,752 individuals. Sci Rep. 2017;7(1):15491; with permission.)

pylori eradication among healthy, asymptomatic individuals in the general population in decreasing the incidence of gastric cancer. The results provided moderately certain evidence that eradication decreases the incidence of gastric cancer and mortality in healthy, asymptomatic infected Asian individuals; however, the authors noted that these results cannot necessarily be extrapolated to other populations.[13] An earlier systematic review mentioned that large-scale eradication has been performed mostly for benign conditions in Japan, where the effects of eradication in preventing gastric cancer are conceivably greater than would be seen in multinational, mixed populations with differing screening quality and disease progression.[14] To date, most studies investigating the incidence of gastric cancer after *H pylori* eradication had relatively short periods of about 10 years, and whether the effect extends beyond 10 years remains unclear.[15] A study in Japan with follow-up beyond 10 years reported that patients with mild to moderate gastric atrophy at baseline had a greater risk of developing diffuse-type gastric cancer with longer follow-up and that endoscopic surveillance should be continued accordingly beyond 10 years after cure of *H pylori,* irrespective of the severity of gastric atrophy.[16] Additional studies with long follow-up periods are required.

TOBACCO SMOKING

From the current evidence base, tobacco smoking is a known cause of gastric cancer,[17] with sufficient evidence for categorization as a group 1 carcinogen by the IARC.[18] A systematic review and meta-analysis of prospective studies showed a significantly increased risk for both men and women and both cardia and noncardia gastric cancer in Asians, Europeans, and Americans. Compared with those who never smoked, current smokers had a 1.2- to 1.9-fold increased risk of gastric cancer, in a dose-responsive manner.[19] There was insufficient evidence for different risks between cardia and noncardia subsites, or by histologic type. It was also estimated that 16.5% of gastric cancers among male patients and 1.9% among female patients were attributable to tobacco smoking globally in 2020, having decreased from respective 2012 estimates of 19.5% and 3.0%, respectively.[20]

Several mechanisms are suggested to explain the specific effect of tobacco smoking on gastric cancer. Nicotine, nitrosamines, and other nitroso compounds in cigarette smoke affect gastric physiology.[21] Also, tobacco smoking is related to an increased risk of transition to dysplasia and intestinal metaplasia and to a delay in both stomach emptying and alcohol absorption.[22] Tobacco smoking increases the risk of gastroesophageal reflux disease, which is associated with cardia gastric cancer.[23]

Because active and secondhand smoking are known to increase the risk of major diseases, including many sites of cancer, prevention of active and secondhand smoking has long been targeted as both global and national health policies, and many countries have already regulated tobacco smoke.[24] Obviously, tobacco smoking is a major risk factor for cancer. Measures to prevent smoking will prevent not only the target gastric cancer but also other smoking-related cancers.

ALCOHOL CONSUMPTION

The WCRF has summarized the most updated evaluation of risk factors for gastric cancer in its Continuous Update Project.[3] In the project report, the panel judged that greater consumption of alcoholic beverages is a probable cause of gastric cancer, based on evidence for intake of greater than 45 g ethanol/d (approximately 3 drinks per day).

A nonlinear dose–response meta-analysis showed that daily consumption of 45 g of ethanol and above particularly and significantly increased the risk of gastric cancer. No difference was observed between cardia and noncardia gastric cancers.

Alcoholic beverages and the acetaldehyde associated with their consumption are classified in the IARC monograph evaluation as group 1 carcinogens to humans.[5] Ethanol is fat soluble and acts as a solvent, enhancing the penetration of carcinogens into cells, causing damage to the gastric mucosa.[25] Its metabolite acetaldehyde can have a local toxic effect, which may be related to the occurrence of gastric cancer. The pathogenic effect of ethanol in causing gastric mucosal damage is associated with disruption of the balance of gastric mucosal defense and external invasion. Genetic polymorphisms, such as alcohol dehydrogenase-2 polymorphism, are more common in Japanese and East Asian populations[26] and influence susceptibility to alcohol.[3]

To prevent gastric cancer, a decrease in alcohol consumption to less than 45 g/d may be effective,[3] albeit that no consumption at all is recommended considering total cancer prevention.[27]

SALT-PRESERVED FOODS

Salt intake in general terms is known to be associated not only with gastric cancer, but also with hypertension and stroke.[28] These diseases were historically the 2 most common conditions in Japan. Interestingly, although the amount of salt intake tends to be associated with an increased risk of stroke, the intake of highly salt-concentrated preserved foods instead increases the risk of gastric cancer.[29] The WCRF concluded that greater consumption of salt-preserved foods is a probable cause of gastric cancer.[3] Highly salt-concentrated preserved foods are irritating to the delicate lining of the stomach, which makes *H pylori* infection more likely or more severe and leads to gastric cancer.[30]

Salt reduction indicates both a decrease in the amount of salt intake and in the intake of highly salt-concentrated preserved foods. Salt-preserved foods in general were more commonly consumed before the availability of refrigeration.[31,32] The dissemination of refrigeration about a century ago had a major impact on the decrease in gastric cancer mortality in some developed countries. In addition, the expansion of industrial refrigeration in both storage and transportation resulted in an increased intake of fresh food.[31,32] It also decreased the need for salting and pickling, which are positively associated with gastric cancer. Home refrigeration increased the shift from salt preservation to frozen storage.[32] In Japan, the number of households with electric refrigerators increased rapidly after 1960, a trend that was strongly inversely correlated with gastric cancer decline.[31]

Bolstering this natural unplanned triumph through the widespread adoption of refrigeration,[31] many countries such as in Finland and the UK have adopted population-based salt reduction strategies.[33] These interventions have proved effective in terms of both health and financial cost.[30] These countries based their strategies on a gradual and sustained decrease in the amount of salt added to food by food manufacturers, plus a sustained mass media campaign aimed at encouraging dietary change within households and communities. In contrast, countries in which consumption derives mostly from salt added during cooking or from sauces require public health campaigns to encourage consumers to use less salt.

Japan has achieved a decrease in salt consumption at the community level. In the late 1950s, deaths from stroke in Japan were the highest in the world. It became apparent that salt consumption was particularly high in the northern regions and that the number of strokes in different parts of the country was directly related to the amount of salt consumption. The Japanese government initiated a campaign to reduce salt intake, which proved effective over the following decade. A consequent decrease in blood pressure was seen in both adults and children, along with a substantial decreased in stroke mortality[30] and eventually in gastric cancer incidence and mortality. Beginning in the 1970s, Finland aimed to decrease salt intake in the whole population in collaboration with the food industry. In the following 30 years, salt intake has been decreased by one-third, and cardiovascular disease and gastric cancer mortality has substantially declined.[30] More recently, in the UK, the Consensus Action on Salt and Health, a nongovernmental organization, and the Food Standards Agency, a quasigovernmental organization, developed a program for voluntary salt reduction in 2003 in collaboration with the food industry that has resulted in a reduction of salt intake in the UK population.[34] Cost estimates reveal that a decrease in salt intake is equally or more cost effective to tobacco control in terms of decreasing cardiovascular disease, the leading cause of death and disability worldwide.[33] Overall, it is evident that a modest reduction in population-level salt intake worldwide would result in a major improvement in public health, owing not only to the prevention of cancer, but also to that of other major diseases.

BODY FATNESS

Greater body fatness, as marked by BMI, was not recognized as a risk factor for gastric cancer until recent risk assessments. A meta-analysis by the WCRF of the relative risk of gastric cancer by anatomic subsite showed a 23% increase in risk of cardia gastric cancer per 5 kg/m^2 increase in BMI (relative risk, 1.23; 95% confidence interval, 1.07–1.40), although no significant association was observed with noncardia gastric cancer (relative risk, 0.93; 95% confidence interval, 0.85–1.02 per 5 kg/m^2 increase in BMI). This effect of greater body fatness was especially apparent in men and non-Asians.

Obesity may introduce inflammation of the stomach lining via tumor necrosis factor-α, IL-6, and monocyte chemoattractant protein-1. According to the increasing cardia gastric cancer rate in Western populations, accumulating evidence suggests that greater body fatness or higher BMI are probable causes of cardia gastric cancer.[35]

This status of greater body fatness or obesity as probable risk factors for cardia gastric cancer but not noncardia gastric cancer is notable. In some reports, the overall decrease in gastric cancer in these decades is mainly attributable to a decline in noncardia gastric cancer.[36,37] There are exceptions, however, in which cardia gastric cancer has been absolutely or relatively increasing in countries with previously low rates, such as the United States.[38,39] The burden of gastric cancer attributed to higher BMI was not high in regions with a high overall gastric cancer rate. The current global pattern shows that cardia gastric cancer rates are similar to or higher than noncardia rates in populations with a low noncardia gastric cancer incidence.[40]

Obesity is increasing globally[41,42] and will positively affect cardia gastric cancer incidence. This is particularly evident in Western populations, in which gastric cancer rates are conventionally low. As with tobacco smoking and alcoholic beverage consumption, prevention strategies targeting obesity impact not only gastric cancer, but also many other major diseases. Decreasing the obesity burden requires a combined approach of individual interventions and changes in the environment and society.[43] At the same time, the trend in cardia gastric cancer should also be monitored, namely not only regarding the relative proportion but also the absolute rate in both high and low gastric cancer incidence countries.

SUMMARY AND PERSPECTIVES

Gastric cancer has substantially declined over the past century, thanks to decreases in risk factors such as *H pylori* infection, tobacco smoking, and salt-preserved food intake resulting from both general improvements in hygiene and food storage after the dissemination of refrigeration and population-based intervention strategies, including prevention of tobacco smoking, decreases in salt intake, and obesity control. *H pylori* eradication for infected subjects has potential as a prevention strategy for those at high risk, but warrants a longer follow-up period. The ongoing increase in obesity may cause increases in cardia gastric cancer, especially in Western populations, and this possibility should be carefully monitored in both Western and Asian populations.

ACKNOWLEDGMENT

The author have received grant from National Cancer Center Research and Development Fund (grant number 2021-A-16) and from Practical Research for Innovative Cancer Control, Japan Cancer Research Project, Japan Agency for Medical Research and Development (grant number 20CK0106561h0001).

REFERENCES

1. Ferlay J, Ervik M, Lam F, et al. Global cancer observatory: cancer today. Lyon (France): International Agency for Research on Cancer; 2018.
2. Inoue M. Changing epidemiology of Helicobacter pylori in Japan. Gastric Cancer 2017;20:3–7.
3. Continuous Update Expert Report 2018. Diet, nutrition, physical activity and stomach cancer. [homepage on the Internet]; c2018. Available at: dietandcancerreport.org. Accessed November 1, 2020.
4. Kamangar F, Dawsey SM, Blaser MJ, et al. Opposing risks of gastric cardia and noncardia gastric adenocarcinomas associated with Helicobacter pylori seropositivity. J Natl Cancer Inst 2006;98:1445–52.
5. Agents Classified by the IARC Monographs, Volumes 1–127 [homepage on the Internet]. Lyon, France. Available at: https://monographs.iarc.fr/agents-classified-by-the-iarc/. Accessed November 1, 2020.
6. World Cancer Research Fund/American Institute for Cancer Research. Food, nutrition, physical activity and the prevention of cancer: a global perspective 2007. Second Expert Report.
7. Wang C, Nishiyama T, Kikuchi S, et al. Changing trends in the prevalence of H. pylori infection in Japan (1908-2003): a systematic review and meta-regression analysis of 170,752 individuals. Sci Rep 2017;7:15491.
8. Lim SH, Kwon JW, Kim N, et al. Prevalence and risk factors of Helicobacter pylori infection in Korea: nationwide multicenter study over 13 years. BMC Gastroenterol 2013;13:104.
9. Okuda M, Lin Y, Kikuchi S. Helicobacter pylori infection in children and adolescents. Adv Exp Med Biol 2019;1149:107–20.
10. Fischbach W, Malfertheiner P. Helicobacter Pylori infection. Dtsch Arztebl Int 2018;115:429–36.
11. Watari J, Chen N, Amenta PS, et al. Helicobacter pylori associated chronic gastritis, clinical syndromes, precancerous lesions, and pathogenesis of gastric cancer development. World J Gastroenterol 2014;20:5461–73.

12. Chen HN, Wang Z, Li X, et al. Helicobacter pylori eradication cannot reduce the risk of gastric cancer in patients with intestinal metaplasia and dysplasia: evidence from a meta-analysis. Gastric Cancer 2016;19:166–75.
13. Ford AC, Yuan Y, Forman D, et al. Helicobacter pylori eradication for the prevention of gastric neoplasia. Cochrane Database Syst Rev 2020;(7):CD005583.
14. Sugano K. Effect of Helicobacter pylori eradication on the incidence of gastric cancer: a systematic review and meta-analysis. Gastric Cancer 2019;22:435–45.
15. Sugimoto M, Murata M, Kawai T. How long should patients be surveyed for gastric cancer risk after Helicobacter pylori eradication therapy? 10 years is no longer enough. J Gastroenterol 2020;55:577–8.
16. Take S, Mizuno M, Ishiki K, et al. Risk of gastric cancer in the second decade of follow-up after Helicobacter pylori eradication. J Gastroenterol 2020;55:281–8.
17. Surgeon General. The health consequences of smoking: a report of the surgeon general. Atlanta (GA): U.S. Department of Health and Human Services, Centers for Disease Control and Prevention, National Center for Chronic Disease Prevention and Health Promotion, Office on Smoking and Health; 2004.
18. IARC Working Group on the Evaluation of Carcinogenic Risks to Humans. Personal habits and indoor combustions. Volume 100 E. A review of human carcinogens. IARC Monogr Eval Carcinog Risks Hum 2012;100:1–538.
19. Ladeiras-Lopes R, Pereira AK, Nogueira A, et al. Smoking and gastric cancer: systematic review and meta-analysis of cohort studies. Cancer Causes Control 2008;19:689–701.
20. Peleteiro B, Castro C, Morais S, et al. Worldwide burden of gastric cancer attributable to tobacco smoking in 2012 and predictions for 2020. Dig Dis Sci 2015;60: 2470–6.
21. Sasazuki S, Sasaki S, Tsugane S, et al, Japan Public Health Center Study Group. Cigarette smoking, alcohol consumption and subsequent gastric cancer risk by subsite and histologic type. Int J Cancer 2002;101:560–6.
22. Johnson RD, Horowitz M, Maddox AF, et al. Cigarette smoking and rate of gastric emptying: effect on alcohol absorption. BMJ 1991;302:20–3.
23. Ness-Jensen E, Lagergren J. Tobacco smoking, alcohol consumption and gastro-oesophageal reflux disease. Best Pract Res Clin Gastroenterol 2017;31: 501–8.
24. World Health Organization. WHO report on the global tobacco epidemic 2019: offer help to quit tobacco use. Geneva (Switzerland): 2019.
25. Ma K, Baloch Z, He TT, et al. Alcohol consumption and gastric cancer risk: a meta-analysis. Med Sci Monit 2017;23:238–46.
26. Tramacere I, Negri E, Pelucchi C, et al. A meta-analysis on alcohol drinking and gastric cancer risk. Ann Oncol 2012;23:28–36.
27. World Cancer Research Fund/American Institute for Cancer Research. Diet, nutrition, physical activity and cancer: a global perspective. The Third Expert Report; 2018.
28. Aburto NJ, Ziolkovska A, Hooper L, et al. Effect of lower sodium intake on health: systematic review and meta-analyses. BMJ 2013;346:f1326.
29. Takachi R, Inoue M, Shimazu T, et al. Consumption of sodium and salted foods in relation to cancer and cardiovascular disease: the Japan Public Health Center-based Prospective Study. Am J Clin Nutr 2010;91:456–64.
30. He FJ, MacGregor GA. A comprehensive review on salt and health and current experience of worldwide salt reduction programmes. J Hum Hypertens 2009; 23:363–84.

31. Howson CP, Hiyama T, Wynder EL. The decline in gastric cancer: epidemiology of an unplanned triumph. Epidemiol Rev 1986;8:1–27.
32. Tominaga S, Kuroishi T. An ecological study on diet/nutrition and cancer in Japan. Int J Cancer 1997;(Suppl 10):2–6.
33. He FJ, MacGregor GA. Reducing population salt intake worldwide: from evidence to implementation. Prog Cardiovasc Dis 2010;52:363–82.
34. He FJ, Brinsden HC, MacGregor GA. Salt reduction in the United Kingdom: a successful experiment in public health. J Hum Hypertens 2014;28:345–52.
35. Petryszyn P, Chapelle N, Matysiak-Budnik T. Gastric cancer: where are we heading? Dig Dis 2020;38:280–5.
36. Nicolas C, Sylvain M, Come L, et al. Trends in gastric cancer incidence: a period and birth cohort analysis in a well-defined French population. Gastric Cancer 2016;19:508–14.
37. Holster IL, Aarts MJ, Tjwa ET, et al. Trend breaks in incidence of non-cardia gastric cancer in the Netherlands. Cancer Epidemiol 2014;38:9–15.
38. Devesa SS, Blot WJ, Fraumeni JF Jr. Changing patterns in the incidence of esophageal and gastric carcinoma in the United States. Cancer 1998;83: 2049–53.
39. Abrams JA, Gonsalves L, Neugut AI. Diverging trends in the incidence of reflux-related and Helicobacter pylori-related gastric cardia cancer. J Clin Gastroenterol 2013;47:322–7.
40. Colquhoun A, Arnold M, Ferlay J, et al. Global patterns of cardia and non-cardia gastric cancer incidence in 2012. Gut 2015;64:1881–8.
41. Chooi YC, Ding C, Magkos F. The epidemiology of obesity. Metabolism 2019; 92:6–10.
42. Seidell JC, Halberstadt J. The global burden of obesity and the challenges of prevention. Ann Nutr Metab 2015;66(Suppl 2):7–12.
43. Bluher M. Obesity: global epidemiology and pathogenesis. Nat Rev Endocrinol 2019;15:288–98.

Helicobacter pylori and Gastric Cancer

Judith Kim, MD*, Timothy Cragin Wang, MD

KEYWORDS

- *Helicobacter pylori* • Gastric cancer • Gastric adenocarcinoma • MALT lymphoma

KEY POINTS

- *Helicobacter pylori* prevalence varies based on geography, age, race/ethnicity, and socioeconomic status.
- Multiple case-control and prospective studies in humans and animal models have investigated the relationship between *H pylori* and gastric cancer.
- The mechanism for *H pylori*–associated gastric carcinogenesis is complex, and likely involves the interaction of bacterial factors, host factors, and environmental factors.
- Eradication of *H pylori* decreases the risk of gastric cancer, although population-based screening and treating is not recommended universally.

INTRODUCTION

Helicobacter pylori is a spiral shaped, gram-negative bacterium and the most common chronic bacterial infection in humans. This bacterium is present in approximately one-half of the world's population, although there is significant variation based on region, age, race/ethnicity, and socioeconomic status.[1,2] *H pylori* is associated with multiple gastrointestinal diseases, including gastritis, peptic ulcer disease, and gastric cancer. The vast majority of patients are asymptomatic, although about 10% develop peptic ulcer disease, 1% to 3% develop gastric adenocarcinoma, and 0.1% develop mucosa-associated lymphoid tissue (MALT) lymphoma. In 1994, *H pylori* was recognized as a class I carcinogen in 1994 by the World Health Organization and International Agency for Research on Cancer based on the growing evidence establishing the role of *H pylori* in gastric carcinogenesis.[3] Since then, numerous preclinical studies have shown the direct carcinogenicity of *H pylori* in susceptible animal species. The bacterium is considered a necessary but insufficient cause of gastric cancer; only a minority of *H pylori*–infected individuals develop cancer. Disease pathogenesis likely represents a complex interaction

Department of Medicine, Division of Digestive and Liver Diseases, Columbia University Irving Medical Center, New York, NY, USA
* Corresponding author.
E-mail address: jk3848@cumc.columbia.edu

Gastrointest Endoscopy Clin N Am 31 (2021) 451–465
https://doi.org/10.1016/j.giec.2021.03.003 giendo.theclinics.com
1052-5157/21/

between bacterial, host, and environmental factors that has been the subject of intense investigation since the discovery of *H pylori*.

EPIDEMIOLOGY

H pylori is ubiquitous, but its distribution is heterogenous throughout the world. The prevalence of infection is greater in developing countries than developed countries. The wide variation in international and national prevalence is likely related to risk factors such as socioeconomic status, level of hygiene, and household crowding.[4–6] The transmission of *H pylori* is most likely person to person via the fecal–oral or oral–oral route.[7] Children are often infected by strains identical to their parents, suggesting transmission within families in early childhood.[8]

In developing countries, *H pylori* prevalence can reach more than 80% in older adults.[1,9] The incidence of *H pylori* infection has generally decreased over time with improving sanitation and standards of living in many countries. In Japan, the prevalence of *H pylori* infection has drastically decreased with rising economic status. Older generations born in the 1950's have a prevalence greater than 80%, decreasing to 10% for those born in the 1990s and 2% for those born after 2000.[10] In the United States, the prevalence of *H pylori* is estimated to be 30% to 40%, which has been decreasing steadily over time since World War II. However, in the last decade, there has been a significant increase in gastric cancer in patients under the age of 40.[11,12] Furthermore, there is significant variation among different ethnic groups. Blacks and Hispanics have a higher prevalence of infection compared with non-Hispanic Whites.[1,6,13] Asians in the United States also have much higher rates of *H pylori* infection compared with Whites.[14,15]

H PYLORI AND GASTRIC ADENOCARCINOMA

The association between *H pylori* and the development of noncardia gastric cancer has been well-established. The majority of those infected with *H pylori* remain asymptomatic, but an estimated 1% to 3% develop gastric adenocarcinoma and 0.1% develop MALT lymphoma. Approximately 90% of all gastric cancers can be attributable to *H pylori*.[1] It is considered the most common cause of infection-related cancers, representing 5.5% of the cancer burden.[16]

About 90% of gastric tumors are adenocarcinomas. Gastric adenocarcinoma is further classified into 2 main histologic types, intestinal or diffuse type. *H pylori* is associated with both subtypes of gastric cancer, although it is more frequently associated with and better characterized in the development of intestinal adenocarcinoma.[17] Intestinal type-tumors are characterized by corpus-dominant gastritis with gastric atrophy and intestinal metaplasia, whereas diffuse type are characterized by gastritis throughout the stomach without atrophy. Intestinal tumors are more common than diffuse cancers, comprising 82% of gastric adenocarcinomas in the United States.[18] There has been a marked decline in intestinal-type gastric cancers in the past 50 years, correlating to improved sanitation and food preservation, in addition to the decreasing prevalence of *H pylori*.[18,19] In contrast, the incidence of diffuse type cancers in Western countries has been increasing, particularly in young (<40 year old) individuals, largely in women with tumors in the gastric corpus.[20,21]

The stepwise development of intestinal-type adenocarcinoma, also known as the Correa cascade, has been well-described (**Fig. 1**).[22] Chronic inflammation leads to the transition of normal mucosa to chronic gastritis, which can further develop into atrophic gastritis, intestinal metaplasia, dysplasia, and finally cancer. *H pylori* infection is the best studied trigger that can lead to chronic active gastritis in this pathway. This

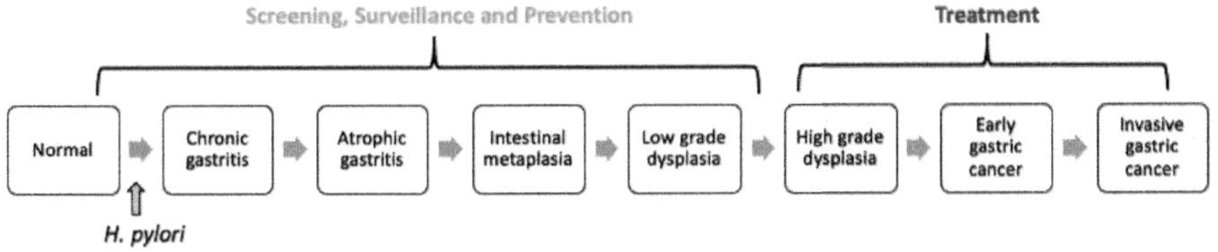

Fig. 1. Correa cascade for gastric intestinal adenocarcinoma.

chronic inflammation leads to the destruction of parietal and chief cells of the stomach, resulting in achlorhydria and atrophic gastritis. The loss of parietal and chief cells, which normally secrete signals that modulate the growth and differentiation of the gastric progenitors, leads to the proliferation and accumulation of undifferentiated gastric progenitor cells as well as intestinal metaplasia. Intestinal metaplasia is a premalignant lesion that harbors the undifferentiated progenitors that can give rise to dysplasia and carcinoma.[23–25] An in vivo study in 1998 using Mongolian gerbils helped to directly demonstrate that *H pylori* induces gastric adenocarcinoma.[26] In this study, long-term inoculation with *H pylori* resulted in intestinal metaplasia and then adenocarcinoma in 37% of the infected animals, whereas no significant changes were found in the uninfected cohort. Similar studies were carried out in mice (INS-GAS), demonstrating directly the carcinogenicity of *H pylori*.[27]

Two landmark studies in 1991 established the relationship between *H pylori* and gastric adenocarcinoma in humans. Parsonnet and colleagues[28] performed a nested case-control study from a cohort of 128,992 patients in California. In this study, 109 patients with histologically confirmed gastric adenocarcinoma were matched with control patients. Serum samples were tested for IgG antibodies to *H pylori*. The authors found that 84% of the patients with gastric cancer had previously been infected with *H pylori* as compared with 61% of the matched control subjects. Prior infection with *H pylori* was associated with 3.6 times the odds of gastric adenocarcinoma than no infection (odds ratio [OR], 3.6; 95% confidence interval [CI], 1.8–7.3).[28] Nomura and colleagues[29] performed a nested case-control study from a cohort of 11,148 Japanese American men in Hawaii. One hundred nine patients with histologically confirmed gastric cancer cases were identified and matched with 109 controls. Of the patients with gastric cancer, 94% had *H pylori* antibodies in the serum compared with the matched control subjects. Prior *H pylori* infection was associated with a 6.0 times odds for gastric cancer compared with no *H pylori* infection (OR, 6.0; 95% CI, 2.1–17.3).[29]

In 2001, one of the largest prospective long-term study evaluating the development of gastric cancer in *H pylori* infected patients was published. This study followed 1526 Japanese patients with duodenal ulcers, gastric ulcers, gastric hyperplasia, or nonulcer dyspepsia, of which 1246 had *H pylori* infection. After a median duration of follow-up of 7.8 years, 36 patients in the infected group and none in the noninfected group developed gastric cancer ($P<.001$).[30] Numerous subsequent studies worldwide have affirmed this relationship, establishing *H pylori* as a primary factor in the pathogenesis of gastric cancer.[6,31–34]

H PYLORI INFECTION AND MUCOSA-ASSOCIATED LYMPHOID TISSUE LYMPHOMA

Another important role of *H pylori* is in the pathogenesis of MALT lymphoma. The first evidence for this association came from histopathological assessment of patients infected with *H pylori*. Lymphoid tissue is absent from the normal gastric mucosa, but is seen in patients with *H pylori*–associated gastritis.[35,36] *H pylori* triggers T-cell–mediated, B-cell expansion through the CD40 pathway. The chronic proliferation of B cells and chronic inflammation induces additional oncogenic events that leads to development of MALT lymphoma.[37]

In a 1991 cohort study, 92% of 110 patients with gastric MALT were found to have *H pylori* infection. Subsequent trials showed that eradication of *H pylori* infection led to a regression of gastric MALT lymphoma.[38,39] One meta-analysis including 34 studies with 1271 patients with MALT lymphoma found that gastric lymphoma remission was achieved in 77.8% of 1250 patients who were successfully cured of *H pylori* infection.[39] Although rare case reports have noted regression of extragastric MALT lymphoma lesions, gastric MALT lymphoma is the only malignancy for which antibiotics are the first choice of therapy with curative intent.

MECHANISM OF *H PYLORI*

The molecular mechanism by which *H pylori* induces gastric cancer is not completely understood, but is likely a combination of virulence factors, host genetic predisposition, and environmental factors.

H pylori was first discovered in patients with gastritis in 1982 by J. Robin Warren and Barry Marshall, who were awarded the Nobel Prize in Physiology or Medicine for their work.[40] *H pylori* are unique bacteria that have adapted to survive in the harsh, acidic environment of the stomach. *H pylori* has multiple characteristics that allow it to survive in the stomach.[41] Its spiral shape and flagella optimize its motility, allowing passage through the mucosa to the gastric epithelium. Bacterial surface adhesins recognize and bind to host receptors on gastric epithelial cells. *H pylori* produces the enzyme urease, which hydrolyzes gastric urea to form ammonia. Ammonia neutralizes gastric acid, allowing the bacterium to penetrate the gastric mucosa, and damages epithelial cells. Urease also stimulates inflammatory cells leading to further cellular injury.[42] *H pylori* produces more catalase enzyme than most other bacteria, which is an antioxidant that neutralizes reactive oxygen metabolites produced by inflammatory cells and may help the organism to survive in the inflamed mucosa. These diverse characteristics allow *H pylori* to reach close proximity to the gastric epithelium and subsequently deliver bacterial factors that modulate its activity to cause cellular damage. *H pylori* isolates demonstrate significant genetic diversity and strain-specific properties are thought to contribute to the ability to cause a variety of diseases.[43]

Two virulence factors, cytotoxin-associated antigen A (CagA) and vacuolating cytotoxin (VacA), are the best defined and associated with an increased risk of gastric pathology. CagA is a bacterial protein that is associated with cell injury and more severe gastrointestinal disease.[44,45] Virulent strains of *H pylori* encode cag pathogenicity island, which expresses a type IV secretion system that allows for the injection of virulence factors like CagA into the host target cells. CagA has multiple effects on gastric epithelial cells, including increasing cell proliferation, decreasing cell apoptosis, and altering cell polarity, which all promote tumor development.

Infection with cagA-positive *H pylori* strains compared with cagA-negative strains are associated with an increased risk for development of gastric adenocarcinoma. One meta-analysis of 16 studies with 2284 gastric cancer cases and 2770 matched controls evaluated the relationship between cagA positivity and gastric cancer.[46] *H pylori* infection was associated with a 2.28-fold increased risk of gastric cancer (OR, 2.28; 95% CI, 1.71–3.05). In *H pylori*–positive populations, cagA seropositivity increased the risk for noncardia gastric cancer (OR, 2.01; 95% CI, 1.21–3.32). These results suggest that patients with cagA-positive strains of *H pylori* are at a greater risk for developing gastric cancer than cagA-negative strains. In 2008, the first study demonstrated a potential causal link between cagA and carcinogenesis in vivo through the generation of transgenic mice expressing CagA throughout the body or predominantly in the stomach. The functional overexpression of phosphorylated CagA-induced gastric epithelial hyperplasia, as well as rare adenocarcinomas of the stomach and small intestine indicating the potential directly oncogenicity of CagA.[47]

VacA is another important virulence factor that promotes the formation of acidic vacuoles in the cytoplasm of gastric epithelial cells. VacA acts as a urea transporter that can increase the permeability of the gastric epithelium to urea and so optimizes urease activity.[48] VacA also induces apoptosis and disrupts the epithelial cell tight junctions to cause cellular collapse. In addition, VacA acts as an immunosuppressant that inhibits T-cell proliferation and alters the host immune response thereby enabling the persistent colonization of the stomach by *H pylori*. All *H pylori* strains contain vacA genes, but certain allelic forms of VacA, such as s1/m1, are associated with an increased risk of developing peptic ulcer disease and gastric cancer.[48,49]

Early on, *H pylori* was thought to colonize primarily the gastric pits. More recently, the potential relationship between *H pylori* and stem cells in disease development has been investigated. Studies by Sigal and colleagues[50] using quantitative confocal microscopy and 3-D reconstruction of gastric glands have shown that *H pylori* colonizes deep in the stomach glands may interact directly with progenitor cells in gastric glands, thereby impacting carcinogenesis. *H pylori* can directly activate and induce proliferation Lgr5+ cells, thus expanding the stem cell compartment, in part through upregulation of R-spondin-3 in stromal cells. However, *H pylori* tends to disappear in late-stage gastric preneoplasia, and there has been no evidence to date that cagA is present dysplastic gastric glands. Patients with gastric cancer and *H pylori* infection overexpress leucine-rich repeat-containing G-coupled receptor 5 cells, which comprise both stem and secretory cells in the gastric antrum, and seem to have antimicrobial activity.[51] *H pylori*–infected patients also have been found to have increased DNA damage in leucine-rich repeat-containing G-coupled receptor cells.[52,53] *H pylori*–related inflammation can also lead to recruitment of bone marrow–derived stem cells to the gastric mucosa.[54,55] Finally, more recently, mouse models of *Helicobacter* infection have revealed the *Helicobacter* sp. can activate CCK2R+ antral stem cells and induce symmetric cell division that predisposes to antral carcinogenesis.[56]

HOST FACTORS AND *H PYLORI*

H pylori elicits a strong inflammatory and immune response from its host. Certain host gene polymorphisms in cytokines have been associated with an increased susceptibility to noncardia gastric adenocarcinoma. IL-1ß, which is a proinflammatory cytokine and inhibitor of gastric acid secretion, is upregulated by the presence of *H pylori*. Proinflammatory genotypes of the IL-1 loci that upregulate IL-1ß concentrations have been associated with an increased likelihood of gastric cancer.[57] Enhanced IL-1ß concentrations lead to an inhibition of acid secretion and increase the spread of *H pylori*–induced inflammation from the antrum to the corpus of the stomach. Proinflammatory genotypes of tumor necrosis factor α and IL-10 were also associated with an increased risk of noncardia gastric adenocarcinoma.[58] The host immune response is likely the major factor that influences the risk of developing gastric cancer, as IL-1ß –driven inflammation alone can induce gastric cancer, even in the absence of

Helicobacter infection,[59] indicating a complex interaction between genetic and bacterial factors in disease carcinogenesis.

ENVIRONMENTAL FACTORS AND *H PYLORI*

Significant geographic variations in the incidence of gastric cancer suggest that environmental factors impact *H pylori* and gastric carcinogenesis. High dietary salt intake has been associated with an increased risk of gastric cancer in prospective cohort studies.[60,61] In 1 study, a higher median urine salt excretion level was correlated with an increased mortality rate of stomach cancer.[62] In vitro and in vivo studies have also described mechanisms by which salt may influence gastric carcinogenesis. The cultivation of *H pylori* in high-salt conditions leads to alterations in the proteome, including increased expression of CagA.[63,64] In 1 study, Mongolian gerbils infected with wild-type cagA+ *H pylori* strains fed a high-salt diet all developed gastric adenocarcinoma compared with one-half of the animals fed a regular diet. Those fed the high-salt diet had more severe gastric inflammation, increased parietal cell loss, increased gastric expression of IL-1ß, and increased cagA transcription compared with those on a regular diet.[65]

Ascorbic acid, an important dietary antioxidant, has also been associated with *H pylori* and gastric cancer. It is thought to decrease the risk of cancer by decreasing the formation of carcinogenic nitrites in the stomach and limit damage from free radicals and reactive oxygen species.[22,66] Lower levels of ascorbic acid are seen in patients with *H pylori*, whereas the eradication of *H pylori* increases these levels.[67] Ascorbic acid ingestion has been associated with a decreased risk of gastric cancer in case-control studies.[68–70] However, studies on the impact of vitamin C supplementation on *H pylori* eradication and gastric cancer have shown conflicting results.[66,71,72] Furthermore, in mouse models of *Helicobacter* infection, vitamin C supplementation does not protect vitamin C–deficient mice from *H pylori*–induced gastritis and gastric cancer.[73] In contrast, supplementation with folic acid does prevent *Helicobacter*-associated gastric cancer in mice, possibly through increasing global DNA methylation and thus decreasing inflammation.[74]

DIAGNOSIS OF *H PYLORI*

There are multiple tests to diagnose active *H pylori* infection, either invasive with upper endoscopy or noninvasive (**Table 1**). There are 4 diagnostic tests that can be performed with upper endoscopy. Gastric biopsies for histology taken at the antrum and body of the stomach can diagnose *H pylori* infection as well as associated gastric pathology. The sensitivity and specificity of histology for diagnosis are approximately 95% and 99%, respectively.[75] Gastric biopsy urease testing can also be performed to test for the production of ammonia. The sensitivity and specificity for biopsy urease testing are about 90% and 95%, respecitvely.[76] Gastric biopsies can also be obtained for bacterial culture and antibiotic sensitivity testing. Bacterial culture has a high specificity, approaching 100%, but a lower sensitivity of 85% to 95% because *H pylori* is difficult to culture.[76] Biopsy for culture and sensitivity should be performed for patients with persistent *H pylori* infection after 2 courses of antibiotic treatment. Quantitative polymerase chain reaction testing on gastric biopsies can detect low amounts of bacteria. Polymerase chain reaction testing has a high specificity and sensitivity (>95%), but its use is limited by higher cost.[76]

Noninvasive tests for active *H pylori* infection are urea breath testing and stool antigen testing. The urea breath test detects for the hydrolysis of urea by *H pylori* to produce carbon dioxide and ammonia. The sensitivity and specificity for this test are both

Table 1
Diagnostic tests for *H* pylori infection

Test	Strengths/Weaknesses	Estimated Sensitivity and Specificity
Biopsy histology	High accuracy, requires invasive endoscopy	95%, 99%[75]
Biopsy urease testing	High accuracy, requires invasive endoscopy	90%, 95%[76]
Biopsy bacterial culture	High specificity, but lower sensitivity as difficult to culture, requires invasive endoscopy	100%, 85%–95%[76]
Biopsy polymerase chain reaction	Expensive, requires invasive endoscopy	95%, 95%[76]
Urea breath test	Noninvasive	95%, 95%[77]
Stool antigen assay	Noninvasive, less expensive	94%, 97%[78]
Serology antibody testing	Indicates either active or prior infection	85%, 79%[79]

approximately 95%.[77] The stool antigen assay is another option that tests for the presence of bacterial antigen, which indicates active infection. The sensitivity and specificity are, respectively, estimated to be 94% and 97%.[78] Serology testing for *H pylori* IgG antibodies can also be performed, although a positive result can be interpreted as either active or prior infection. The sensitivity and specificity for serology testing have been estimated as 85% and 79%, respectively.[79]

H PYLORI ERADICATION

Antibiotic eradication of *H pylori* infection can decrease the risk of gastric cancer. A meta-analysis of 24 studies including 715 incidence gastric cancers among a total of 48,064 patients assessed the effects of antibiotic eradication on gastric cancer risk.[80] Patients with *H pylori* eradication had a lower incidence of gastric cancer than those who did not receive treatment (pooled incidence rate ratio, 0.53; 95% CI, 0.44–0.64). The benefits of antibiotic eradication increased in populations with higher baseline cancer incidence. The relative risk for gastric cancer with *H pylori* treatment in low, intermediate, and high incidence regions were 0.80, 0.49, and 0.45, respectively.

A randomized controlled trial in 2020 from South Korea investigated whether treatment to eradicate *H pylori* decreases the risk of gastric cancer in people with a family history of gastric cancer.[81] One thousand eight hundred thirty-eight patients with first-degree relatives with gastric cancer were randomized to receive either eradication therapy with antibiotics or placebo. During a median follow-up of 9.2 years, the treatment of *H pylori* infection significantly decrease the risk of gastric cancer compared with placebo in patients with a family history of gastric cancer.

It is important to recognize that the antibiotic regimens used in these studies are not specific for *H pylori*, but in fact result in broad decreases and alterations in the gut microbiome. In late stages of gastric disease, *H pylori* colonization decreases and even disappears, and it has been hypothesized the bacterial overgrowth by non–*H pylori* species can contribute to gastric cancer progression. Indeed, the absence of commensal flora in *H pylori*–infected INS-GAS mice prevents progression to high-grade dysplasia/gastric cancer,[82] whereas the additional colonization with a restricted commensal microbiota (eg, Schaedler's flora) is able to restore progression to high-grade dysplasia.[83] These observations on the importance of commensal bacteria was supported by human studies by Li and colleagues,[84] show showed that antibiotic eradication treatment was able to reduce gastric cancer incidence, even in the absence of *H pylori* elimination. Thus, antibiotics prevent gastric cancer through effects on both *H pylori* and commensal bacteria.

OPTIMAL TIMING OF *H PYLORI* ERADICATION

Lee and associates[85] examined the efficacy of *H pylori* eradication in preventing the progression of gastritis to gastric cancer in *H pylori* infected transgenic mice. *H pylori* eradication at 8, 12, and 22 weeks after infection decrease the severity of dysplasia ($P<.01$) compared with untreated mice. The development of neoplasia was prevented by *H pylori* eradication at 8 weeks ($P<.001$) and less effectively at 12 and 22 weeks ($P<.05$). *H pylori* eradication seems to be most effective at preventing cancer when given at an earlier point in the course of the infection.[85]

In 2004, a prospective randomized controlled trial of 1630 healthy carriers of *H pylori* infection from China were randomly assigned to receive *H pylori* eradication or placebo.[86] All patients had an endoscopy at the start of the trial. There were 18 cases of gastric cancer that developed during the 7.5-year follow-up, with no difference between subjects who received eradication or treatment ($P = .33$). However, in the subgroup of patients who did not have any precancerous lesions (gastric atrophy, intestinal metaplasia, and dysplasia) on initial presentation, no patient who received *H pylori* eradication developed cancer compared with those who received placebo (0 vs 6; $P = .02$). Earlier eradication may be more effective in preventing *H pylori*–associated gastric cancer.

There has been controversy regarding whether *H pylori* eradication is effective at stopping carcinogenesis in patients who already have advanced precursor lesions, such as atrophic gastritis or intestinal metaplasia. Atrophic gastritis with or without intestinal metaplasia has often been considered the point of no return, regardless of *H pylori* treatment. However, several studies have shown that *H pylori* eradication can lead to the regression of precancerous lesions, such as atrophic gastritis and intestinal metaplasia.[72,87,88] In addition, *H pylori* eradication can prevent metachronous gastric cancers as well. Patients with early gastric cancers are thought to be at high risk for subsequent gastric cancers owing to advanced glandular atrophy in the stomach. In 1 study published in 2018, 396 patients who underwent endoscopic resection of early gastric cancer or high-grade adenoma received either *H pylori* eradication or placebo.[89] During a median follow-up of 5.9 years, 14 patients developed metachronous cancers compared with 27 in the placebo group (hazard ratio, 0.50; 95% CI, 0.26–0.94). In addition, in a subgroup of 327 patients who underwent endoscopic biopsy at the 3-year follow-up, more patients in the treatment group had an improvement in the atrophy grade than in the placebo group (48.4% vs 15.0%; $P<.001$).

POPULATION-BASED *H PYLORI* SCREENING AND TREATMENT

Although *H pylori* eradication decreases the risk of preneoplastic lesions and gastric cancer, population-based screening and treatment is not universally recommended owing to its cost.[90] However, in high-risk populations, screening and treatment may be cost-effective in high-risk populations[91,92] and is recommended by Asian and European guidelines given the clinical and economic benefits of gastric cancer prevention.[93–95] Other outcomes such as peptic ulcer and lymphoma prevention are additional benefits that would make *H pylori* eradication more cost effective.

Given the evolutionary cohabitation of *H pylori* with humans, it has been postulated that there may be some protective benefits with infection. *H pylori* infection has been associated with a lower incidence of gastroesophageal reflux disease and gastric and esophageal cardia cancers. *H pylori* has also been negatively associated with asthma and other allergic diseases.[96,97] Another potential concern for population-based treatment is the risk of increasing antibiotic resistance.

The International Agency for Research on Cancer has recommended that countries should explore the possibility of introducing population-based *H pylori* screen-and-treat programs based on disease burden and cost effectiveness.[97] Guidelines in the United States recommend that all patients with a positive test for *H pylori* be offered treatment, but state that there is insufficient evidence to support routine testing for and treatment of *H pylori* in asymptomatic individuals.[98]

SUMMARY

H pylori is present in approximately one-half of the world's population and is thought to have coevolved with humans. There are significant differences in prevalence based on region, age, race/ethnicity, and socioeconomic status. The vast majority of infected individuals remain asymptomatic, but *H pylori* can cause multiple gastrointestinal diseases, including gastritis, peptic ulcer disease, and gastric cancer. It is the most common cause of infection-related cancers, representing 5.5% of the world cancer burden. Several case-control and prospective studies have demonstrated the relationship between *H pylori* infection and gastric adenocarcinoma and MALT lymphoma.

The molecular mechanism by which *H pylori* induces gastric cancer is not completely understood but is likely a combination of virulence factors, host genetic predisposition, and environmental factors. *H pylori* isolates demonstrate significant genetic diversity and strain-specific properties are thought to contribute to the ability to cause a wide variety of diseases of differing severity in its hosts. *H pylori* has numerous features and enzymatic properties that allow it to survive in the acidic environment of the stomach, and has specific virulence factors, such as cagA and vacA, that promote an increased risk of gastric pathology. However, host inflammatory responses are likely the major factor driving gastric cancer progression, modified in part by dietary factors that may also contribute to *H pylori*–induced gastric carcinogenesis. Finally, similar to other cancers, the host non–*H pylori* microbiome is likely to be a critical factor but at present requires further study.

The eradication of *H pylori* is the first-line therapy for MALT lymphoma. The eradication of *H pylori* also decreases the risk of developing gastric adenocarcinoma, and the benefits may be increased in populations with a higher baseline cancer incidence. Population-based screening and treatment is not universally recommended owing to its cost, although it may be beneficial in populations at high risk for gastric cancer. Given the heterogeneity of *H pylori* infection and gastric cancer incidence, screening programs should be considered based on disease risk and cost effectiveness.

CLINICS CARE POINTS

- *H pylori* is present in 50% of the world's population though most are asymptomatic without clinical disease.
- The prevalence of *H pylori* is higher in developing countries than developed countries, although there is significant variation depending on socioeconomic factors and race/ethnicity.

- *H pylori* is considered a type I carcinogen by the World Health Organization and is a primary factor in the pathogenesis of gastric adenocarcinoma and MALT lymphoma.
- *H pylori* related carcinogenesis is likely a combination of bacterial properties, host genetic factors, and environmental risk factors.
- *H pylori* are unique bacteria with special characteristics and virulence factors that lead to disease pathogenesis.
- There are various methods for the diagnosis of *H pylori,* including invasive by upper endoscopy and noninvasive tests.
- The eradication of *H pylori* likely decreases the risk of initial and recurrent gastric cancer and is recommended in all patients who test positive for infection.

DISCLOSURE

The authors have nothing to disclose.

REFERENCES

1. Hooi JKY, Lai WY, Ng WK, et al. Global prevalence of Helicobacter pylori infection: systematic review and meta-analysis. Gastroenterology 2017;153:420–9.
2. Venerito M, Vasapolli R, Rokkas T, et al. Gastric cancer: epidemiology, prevention, and therapy. Helicobacter 2018;23(Suppl 1):e12518.
3. Schistosomes, liver flukes and Helicobacter pylori. IARC Working Group on the Evaluation of Carcinogenic Risks to Humans. Lyon, 7-14 June 1994. IARC Monogr Eval Carcinog Risks Hum 1994;61:1–241.
4. Goodman KJ, Correa P. Transmission of Helicobacter pylori among siblings. Lancet 2000;355:358–62.
5. Ford AC, Forman D, Bailey AG, et al. Effect of sibling number in the household and birth order on prevalence of Helicobacter pylori: a cross-sectional study. Int J Epidemiol 2007;36:1327–33.
6. Everhart JE, Kruszon-Moran D, Perez-Perez GI, et al. Seroprevalence and ethnic differences in Helicobacter pylori infection among adults in the United States. J Infect Dis 2000;181:1359–63.
7. Megraud F. Transmission of Helicobacter pylori: faecal-oral versus oral-oral route. Aliment Pharmacol Ther 1995;9(Suppl 2):85–91.
8. Farinha P, Gascoyne RD. Helicobacter pylori and MALT lymphoma. Gastroenterology 2005;128:1579–605.
9. Wang AY, Peura DA. The prevalence and incidence of Helicobacter pylori-associated peptic ulcer disease and upper gastrointestinal bleeding throughout the world. Gastrointest Endosc Clin N Am 2011;21:613–35.
10. Inoue M. Changing epidemiology of Helicobacter pylori in Japan. Gastric Cancer 2017;20:3–7.
11. Anderson WF, Camargo MC, Fraumeni JF Jr, et al. Age-specific trends in incidence of noncardia gastric cancer in US adults. JAMA 2010;303:1723–8.
12. Camargo MC, Anderson WF, King JB, et al. Divergent trends for gastric cancer incidence by anatomical subsite in US adults. Gut 2011;60:1644–9.
13. Grad YH, Lipsitch M, Aiello AE. Secular trends in Helicobacter pylori seroprevalence in adults in the United States: evidence for sustained race/ethnic disparities. Am J Epidemiol 2012;175:54–9.
14. Choi CE, Sonnenberg A, Turner K, et al. High prevalence of gastric preneoplastic lesions in East Asians and Hispanics in the USA. Dig Dis Sci 2015;60:2070–6.

15. Lee E, Liu L, Zhang J, et al. Stomach cancer disparity among Korean Americans by Tumor Characteristics: comparison with Non-Hispanic Whites, Japanese Americans, South Koreans, and Japanese. Cancer Epidemiol Biomarkers Prev 2017;26:587–96.
16. Plummer M, Franceschi S, Vignat J, et al. Global burden of gastric cancer attributable to Helicobacter pylori. Int J Cancer 2015;136:487–90.
17. Hansson LR, Engstrand L, Nyren O, et al. Prevalence of Helicobacter pylori infection in subtypes of gastric cancer. Gastroenterology 1995;109:885–8.
18. Wu H, Rusiecki JA, Zhu K, et al. Stomach carcinoma incidence patterns in the United States by histologic type and anatomic site. Cancer Epidemiol Biomarkers Prev 2009;18:1945–52.
19. Crew KD, Neugut AI. Epidemiology of gastric cancer. World J Gastroenterol 2006;12:354–62.
20. Cho SY, Park JW, Liu Y, et al. Sporadic early-onset diffuse gastric cancers have high frequency of somatic CDH1 alterations, but low frequency of somatic RHOA mutations compared with late-onset cancers. Gastroenterology 2017;153: 536–49.e6.
21. Blaser MJ, Chen Y. A new gastric cancer among us. J Natl Cancer Inst 2018;110: 549–50.
22. Correa P. Human gastric carcinogenesis: a multistep and multifactorial process–First American Cancer Society Award Lecture on Cancer Epidemiology and Prevention. Cancer Res 1992;52:6735–40.
23. Correa P. A human model of gastric carcinogenesis. Cancer Res 1988;48: 3554–60.
24. Blaser MJ. Helicobacter pylori and the pathogenesis of gastroduodenal inflammation. J Infect Dis 1990;161:626–33.
25. Fox JG, Wang TC. Inflammation, atrophy, and gastric cancer. J Clin Invest 2007; 117:60–9.
26. Watanabe T, Tada M, Nagai H, et al. Helicobacter pylori infection induces gastric cancer in Mongolian gerbils. Gastroenterology 1998;115:642–8.
27. Fox JG, Rogers AB, Ihrig M, et al. Helicobacter pylori-associated gastric cancer in INS-GAS mice is gender specific. Cancer Res 2003;63:942–50.
28. Parsonnet J, Friedman GD, Vandersteen DP, et al. Helicobacter pylori infection and the risk of gastric carcinoma. N Engl J Med 1991;325:1127–31.
29. Nomura A, Stemmermann GN, Chyou PH, et al. Helicobacter pylori infection and gastric carcinoma among Japanese Americans in Hawaii. N Engl J Med 1991; 325:1132–6.
30. Uemura N, Okamoto S, Yamamoto S, et al. Helicobacter pylori infection and the development of gastric cancer. N Engl J Med 2001;345:784–9.
31. Helicobacter, Cancer Collaborative Group. Gastric cancer and Helicobacter pylori: a combined analysis of 12 case control studies nested within prospective cohorts. Gut 2001;49:347–53.
32. An international association between Helicobacter pylori infection and gastric cancer. The EUROGAST Study Group. Lancet 1993;341:1359–62.
33. Barreto-Zuniga R, Maruyama M, Kato Y, et al. Significance of Helicobacter pylori infection as a risk factor in gastric cancer: serological and histological studies. J Gastroenterol 1997;32:289–94.
34. Hsu PI, Lai KH, Hsu PN, et al. Helicobacter pylori infection and the risk of gastric malignancy. Am J Gastroenterol 2007;102:725–30.
35. Stolte M, Eidt S. Lymphoid follicles in antral mucosa: immune response to Campylobacter pylori? J Clin Pathol 1989;42:1269–71.

36. Wotherspoon AC, Ortiz-Hidalgo C, Falzon MR, et al. Helicobacter pylori-associated gastritis and primary B-cell gastric lymphoma. Lancet 1991;338: 1175–6.
37. Sagaert X, Van Cutsem E, De Hertogh G, et al. Gastric MALT lymphoma: a model of chronic inflammation-induced tumor development. Nat Rev Gastroenterol Hepatol 2010;7:336–46.
38. Wotherspoon AC, Doglioni C, Diss TC, et al. Regression of primary low-grade B-cell gastric lymphoma of mucosa-associated lymphoid tissue type after eradication of Helicobacter pylori. Lancet 1993;342:575–7.
39. Zullo A, Hassan C, Andriani A, et al. Eradication therapy for Helicobacter pylori in patients with gastric MALT lymphoma: a pooled data analysis. Am J Gastroenterol 2009;104:1932–7 [quiz: 1938].
40. Warren JR, Marshall B. Unidentified curved bacilli on gastric epithelium in active chronic gastritis. Lancet 1983;1:1273–5.
41. Amieva MR, El-Omar EM. Host-bacterial interactions in Helicobacter pylori infection. Gastroenterology 2008;134:306–23.
42. Mobley HL. The role of Helicobacter pylori urease in the pathogenesis of gastritis and peptic ulceration. Aliment Pharmacol Ther 1996;10(Suppl 1):57–64.
43. Alm RA, Ling LS, Moir DT, et al. Genomic-sequence comparison of two unrelated isolates of the human gastric pathogen Helicobacter pylori. Nature 1999;397: 176–80.
44. Censini S, Lange C, Xiang Z, et al. cag, a pathogenicity island of Helicobacter pylori, encodes type I-specific and disease-associated virulence factors. Proc Natl Acad Sci U S A 1996;93:14648–53.
45. Blaser MJ, Perez-Perez GI, Kleanthous H, et al. Infection with Helicobacter pylori strains possessing cagA is associated with an increased risk of developing adenocarcinoma of the stomach. Cancer Res 1995;55:2111–5.
46. Huang JQ, Zheng GF, Sumanac K, et al. Meta-analysis of the relationship between cagA seropositivity and gastric cancer. Gastroenterology 2003;125: 1636–44.
47. Ohnishi N, Yuasa H, Tanaka S, et al. Transgenic expression of Helicobacter pylori CagA induces gastrointestinal and hematopoietic neoplasms in mouse. Proc Natl Acad Sci U S A 2008;105:1003–8.
48. Cover TL, Blanke SR. Helicobacter pylori VacA, a paradigm for toxin multifunctionality. Nat Rev Microbiol 2005;3:320–32.
49. Letley DP, Rhead JL, Twells RJ, et al. Determinants of non-toxicity in the gastric pathogen Helicobacter pylori. J Biol Chem 2003;278:26734–41.
50. Sigal M, Rothenberg ME, Logan CY, et al. Helicobacter pylori activates and expands Lgr5(+) stem cells through direct colonization of the gastric glands. Gastroenterology 2015;148:1392–404.e21.
51. Sigal M, Reines MDM, Mullerke S, et al. R-spondin-3 induces secretory, antimicrobial Lgr5(+) cells in the stomach. Nat Cell Biol 2019;21:812–23.
52. Uehara T, Ma D, Yao Y, et al. H. pylori infection is associated with DNA damage of Lgr5-positive epithelial stem cells in the stomach of patients with gastric cancer. Dig Dis Sci 2013;58:140–9.
53. Yamanoi K, Fukuma M, Uchida H, et al. Overexpression of leucine-rich repeat-containing G protein-coupled receptor 5 in gastric cancer. Pathol Int 2013; 63:13–9.
54. Houghton J, Stoicov C, Nomura S, et al. Gastric cancer originating from bone marrow-derived cells. Science 2004;306:1568–71.

55. Varon C, Dubus P, Mazurier F, et al. Helicobacter pylori infection recruits bone marrow-derived cells that participate in gastric preneoplasia in mice. Gastroenterology 2012;142:281–91.
56. Chang W, Wang H, Kim W, et al. Hormonal suppression of stem cells inhibits symmetric cell division and gastric tumorigenesis. Cell Stem Cell 2020;26:739–54.e8.
57. El-Omar EM, Carrington M, Chow WH, et al. Interleukin-1 polymorphisms associated with increased risk of gastric cancer. Nature 2000;404:398–402.
58. El-Omar EM, Rabkin CS, Gammon MD, et al. Increased risk of noncardia gastric cancer associated with proinflammatory cytokine gene polymorphisms. Gastroenterology 2003;124:1193–201.
59. Tu S, Bhagat G, Cui G, et al. Overexpression of interleukin-1beta induces gastric inflammation and cancer and mobilizes myeloid-derived suppressor cells in mice. Cancer Cell 2008;14:408–19.
60. D'Elia L, Rossi G, Ippolito R, et al. Habitual salt intake and risk of gastric cancer: a meta-analysis of prospective studies. Clin Nutr 2012;31:489–98.
61. Shikata K, Kiyohara Y, Kubo M, et al. A prospective study of dietary salt intake and gastric cancer incidence in a defined Japanese population: the Hisayama study. Int J Cancer 2006;119:196–201.
62. Tsugane S, Tsuda M, Gey F, et al. Cross-sectional study with multiple measurements of biological markers for assessing stomach cancer risks at the population level. Environ Health Perspect 1992;98:207–10.
63. Loh JT, Friedman DB, Piazuelo MB, et al. Analysis of Helicobacter pylori cagA promoter elements required for salt-induced upregulation of CagA expression. Infect Immun 2012;80:3094–106.
64. Voss BJ, Loh JT, Hill S, et al. Alteration of the Helicobacter pylori membrane proteome in response to changes in environmental salt concentration. Proteomics Clin Appl 2015;9:1021–34.
65. Gaddy JA, Radin JN, Loh JT, et al. High dietary salt intake exacerbates Helicobacter pylori-induced gastric carcinogenesis. Infect Immun 2013;81:2258–67.
66. Mei H, Tu H. Vitamin C and Helicobacter pylori infection: current knowledge and future prospects. Front Physiol 2018;9:1103.
67. Ruiz B, Rood JC, Fontham ET, et al. Vitamin C concentration in gastric juice before and after anti-Helicobacter pylori treatment. Am J Gastroenterol 1994; 89:533–9.
68. You WC, Zhang L, Gail MH, et al. Gastric dysplasia and gastric cancer: Helicobacter pylori, serum vitamin C, and other risk factors. J Natl Cancer Inst 2000; 92:1607–12.
69. Lam TK, Freedman ND, Fan JH, et al. Prediagnostic plasma vitamin C and risk of gastric adenocarcinoma and esophageal squamous cell carcinoma in a Chinese population. Am J Clin Nutr 2013;98:1289–97.
70. Block G. Vitamin C and cancer prevention: the epidemiologic evidence. Am J Clin Nutr 1991;53:270S–82S.
71. Chuang CH, Sheu BS, Huang AH, et al. Vitamin C and E supplements to lansoprazole-amoxicillin-metronidazole triple therapy may reduce the eradication rate of metronidazole-susceptible Helicobacter pylori infection. Helicobacter 2002;7:310–6.
72. You WC, Brown LM, Zhang L, et al. Randomized double-blind factorial trial of three treatments to reduce the prevalence of precancerous gastric lesions. J Natl Cancer Inst 2006;98:974–83.

73. Lee CW, Wang XD, Chien KL, et al. Vitamin C supplementation does not protect L-gulono-gamma-lactone oxidase-deficient mice from Helicobacter pylori-induced gastritis and gastric premalignancy. Int J Cancer 2008;122:1068–76.
74. Gonda TA, Kim YI, Salas MC, et al. Folic acid increases global DNA methylation and reduces inflammation to prevent Helicobacter-associated gastric cancer in mice. Gastroenterology 2012;142:824–33.e7.
75. Lee JY, Kim N. Diagnosis of Helicobacter pylori by invasive test: histology. Ann Transl Med 2015;3:10.
76. Wang YK, Kuo FC, Liu CJ, et al. Diagnosis of Helicobacter pylori infection: current options and developments. World J Gastroenterol 2015;21:11221–35.
77. Ferwana M, Abdulmajeed I, Alhajiahmed A, et al. Accuracy of urea breath test in Helicobacter pylori infection: meta-analysis. World J Gastroenterol 2015;21:1305–14.
78. Gisbert JP, de la Morena F, Abraira V. Accuracy of monoclonal stool antigen test for the diagnosis of H. pylori infection: a systematic review and meta-analysis. Am J Gastroenterol 2006;101:1921–30.
79. Loy CT, Irwig LM, Katelaris PH, et al. Do commercial serological kits for Helicobacter pylori infection differ in accuracy? A meta-analysis. Am J Gastroenterol 1996;91:1138–44.
80. Lee YC, Chiang TH, Chou CK, et al. Association between Helicobacter pylori eradication and gastric cancer incidence: a systematic review and meta-analysis. Gastroenterology 2016;150:1113–24.e5.
81. Choi IJ, Kim CG, Lee JY, et al. Family history of gastric cancer and Helicobacter pylori treatment. N Engl J Med 2020;382:427–36.
82. Lofgren JL, Whary MT, Ge Z, et al. Lack of commensal flora in Helicobacter pylori-infected INS-GAS mice reduces gastritis and delays intraepithelial neoplasia. Gastroenterology 2011;140:210–20.
83. Lertpiriyapong K, Whary MT, Muthupalani S, et al. Gastric colonisation with a restricted commensal microbiota replicates the promotion of neoplastic lesions by diverse intestinal microbiota in the Helicobacter pylori INS-GAS mouse model of gastric carcinogenesis. Gut 2014;63:54–63.
84. Li WQ, Ma JL, Zhang L, et al. Effects of Helicobacter pylori treatment on gastric cancer incidence and mortality in subgroups. J Natl Cancer Inst 2014;106.
85. Lee CW, Rickman B, Rogers AB, et al. Helicobacter pylori eradication prevents progression of gastric cancer in hypergastrinemic INS-GAS mice. Cancer Res 2008;68:3540–8.
86. Wong BC, Lam SK, Wong WM, et al. Helicobacter pylori eradication to prevent gastric cancer in a high-risk region of China: a randomized controlled trial. JAMA 2004;291:187–94.
87. Ohkusa T, Fujiki K, Takashimizu I, et al. Improvement in atrophic gastritis and intestinal metaplasia in patients in whom Helicobacter pylori was eradicated. Ann Intern Med 2001;134:380–6.
88. Mera R, Fontham ET, Bravo LE, et al. Long term follow up of patients treated for Helicobacter pylori infection. Gut 2005;54:1536–40.
89. Choi IJ, Kook MC, Kim YI, et al. Helicobacter pylori therapy for the prevention of metachronous gastric cancer. N Engl J Med 2018;378:1085–95.
90. Hogh MB, Kronborg C, Hansen JM, et al. The cost effectiveness of Helicobacter pylori population screening-economic evaluation alongside a randomised controlled trial with 13-year follow-up. Aliment Pharmacol Ther 2019;49:1013–25.

91. Parsonnet J, Harris RA, Hack HM, et al. Modelling cost-effectiveness of Helicobacter pylori screening to prevent gastric cancer: a mandate for clinical trials. Lancet 1996;348:150–4.
92. Han Y, Yan T, Ma H, et al. Cost-effectiveness analysis of Helicobacter pylori eradication therapy for prevention of gastric cancer: a Markov model. Dig Dis Sci 2020;65:1679–88.
93. Talley NJ, Fock KM, Moayyedi P. Gastric cancer consensus conference recommends Helicobacter pylori screening and treatment in asymptomatic persons from high-risk populations to prevent gastric cancer. Am J Gastroenterol 2008; 103:510–4.
94. Malfertheiner P, Megraud F, O'Morain CA, et al. Management of Helicobacter pylori infection-the Maastricht V/Florence Consensus Report. Gut 2017;66:6–30.
95. Du Y, Zhu H, Liu J, et al. Consensus on eradication of Helicobacter pylori and prevention and control of gastric cancer in China (2019, Shanghai). J Gastroenterol Hepatol 2020;35:624–9.
96. Fox JG, Wang TC. Helicobacter pylori–not a good bug after all. N Engl J Med 2001;345:829–32.
97. Herrero R, Parsonnet J, Greenberg ER. Prevention of gastric cancer. JAMA 2014; 312:1197–8.
98. Chey WD, Leontiadis GI, Howden CW, et al. ACG clinical guideline: treatment of Helicobacter pylori infection. Am J Gastroenterol 2017;112:212–39.

Inherited Predisposition to Gastric Cancer

Sheila D. Rustgi, MD[a,b,c], Charlotte K. Ching, MD, MA[c,d], Fay Kastrinos, MD, MPH[a,b,c,*]

KEYWORDS

- Gastric cancer • Genetic testing • Hereditary diffuse gastric cancer
- Lynch syndrome

KEY POINTS

- Approximately 10% of gastric cancer cases involve familial aggregation and up to 3% are related to an inherited cancer syndrome.
- Several pathogenic variants and cancer syndromes, including hereditary diffuse gastric cancer, Lynch syndrome, and gastric adenocarcinoma and proximal polyposis syndrome, are associated with increased risk of gastric cancer.
- Appropriately identifying patients for genetic counseling and testing for pathogenic germline variants informs the patient's and the family members' risks of gastric and other cancers and guides appropriate surveillance and treatment.

INTRODUCTION

Gastric cancer, notably gastric adenocarcinoma, is the fifth most common cancer diagnosed worldwide.[1] In the United States, it is highly lethal, with a median 5-year survival rate of only 32%.[1,2] Although most cases are sporadic, up to 10% of gastric cancers show familial aggregation and arise in individuals with a strong family history of the malignancy, and up to 3% are related to an inherited cancer syndrome.[3–5] There are multiple germline pathogenic variants and cancer syndromes that are associated with an increased risk of gastric cancer.[6–8]

Although family history of gastric cancer is a risk factor for gastric cancer, it is not always clear whether this is caused by shared environmental factors, a genetic predisposition, or a multifactorial cause that may include these factors and others. For example, a recent prospective study found that eradication of the carcinogen *Helicobacter pylori* decreases the risk of gastric cancer among patients with a first-degree relative with gastric cancer.[9]

In the United States, screening for gastric cancer is not recommended because of its low prevalence in the general population. However, a recent systematic review

[a] Herbert Irving Comprehensive Cancer Center, Columbia University Medical Center, New York, NY, USA; [b] Division of Digestive and Liver Diseases, Columbia University Irving Medical Cancer, New York, NY, USA; [c] Vagelos College of Physicians and Surgeons, New York, NY, USA; [d] Department of Medicine, Columbia University Irving Medical Center, New York, NY, USA
* Corresponding author. 161 Fort Washington Avenue, Suite 862, New York, NY 10032.
E-mail address: Fk18@columbia.edu

Gastrointest Endoscopy Clin N Am 31 (2021) 467–487
https://doi.org/10.1016/j.giec.2021.03.010
giendo.theclinics.com

suggests that screening patients at high risk for gastric cancer, whether because of precancerous conditions such as intestinal metaplasia, family history, or known genetic mutations, may be cost-effective.[10]

HISTOLOGY

The most common and worldwide histologic classifications for gastric cancer are the Lauren and World Health Organization (WHO) classifications. Classically, there are 2 histologic subtypes of gastric cancer, first described by Lauren[11] in 1965, the diffuse and intestinal types. The diffuse type is characterized by poorly cohesive cells, highly invasive disease, and occasionally signet cells, so named for their similarities to signet rings on histology because the mucus pushes the nucleus to the edge of the cell.[12] These abnormal cells infiltrate the stroma either alone or in small groups, leading to a population of scattered tumor cells. This cancer type more often affects young women. Furthermore, peritoneal spread before the identification of a precursor lesion is common and therefore has a worse prognosis. In contrast, the intestinal type includes cohesive gland formations and is often associated with intestinal metaplasia. Unlike diffuse gastric cancer, intestinal tumors grow along broad cohesive fronts to form an exophytic mass and are more associated with lymphatic or vascular invasion. These tumors occur more commonly in the elderly and male patients, and affect the antrum. The 2 subtypes are thought to progress through different carcinogenic pathways.

In 2010, the WHO system also created a histopathology classification system that was more detailed than the Lauren classification and based on morphologic characteristics, including 4 subtypes (papillary, tubular, mucinous, and poorly cohesive). However, the prognostic relevance of both classification systems has been controversial and insufficient to guide therapy. Using updated analytical techniques, the Cancer Genome Atlas Research Network has developed a new classification system based on comprehensive analysis of 295 primary gastric cancers: tumors positive for Epstein-Barr virus, microsatellite unstable tumors, genomically stable tumors, and tumors with chromosomal instability.[13] This classification system may be important for identifying possible therapeutic targets.

INHERITED CANCER SYNDROMES ASSOCIATED WITH GASTRIC CANCER

Several cancer predisposition genes are associated with an increased risk of gastric cancer. Original reports related to gastric cancer risks associated with various inherited cancer syndromes relied heavily on data derived largely from familial cancer registries worldwide. Earlier gastric cancer risk estimates may therefore be subject to ascertainment bias and overestimation, given that patients were often identified and selected for genetic testing based on young-onset gastric cancer and an increased number of gastric cancer cases among relatives. With advances in next-generation sequencing technologies, germline genetic testing has expanded to include the simultaneous testing of multiple cancer susceptibility genes, and additional genotype-phenotype correlations have been elucidated. As a result, the prevalence of inherited gastric cancer and its associated risk among numerous cancer syndromes have been redefined.

HEREDITARY DIFFUSE GASTRIC CANCER

Hereditary diffuse gastric cancer (HDGC) is an autosomal dominant inherited cancer syndrome in which affected patients across multiple generations develop poorly differentiated diffuse signet ring cell carcinoma at a young age, as well as lobular breast cancer in women.[14] HDGC is caused by inactivating germline mutations in *CDH1* (E-cadherin) where the most common cause of second *CDH1* allele inactivation is promoter methylation.

The clinical criteria to identify individuals at risk for HDGC has evolved over the last 20 years. Original clinical criteria were based on high burden of diffuse gastric cancer among multiple family members, often defined by young ages of cancer onset, or lobular breast cancer in a family with diffuse gastric cancer. However, less than 50% of individuals who fulfilled the original clinical criteria were identified as germline carriers of pathogenic variants in the *CDH1* gene.[15] Most recently, the International Gastric Cancer Linkage Consortium (IGCLC) revised recommendations based on individual and clinical criteria to determine eligibility for germline testing[16] (**Table 1**). In addition, genetic testing could be considered in patients with bilateral or familial lobular breast cancer diagnosed before the age of 50 years, patients with diffuse gastric cancer and cleft lip/palate, and those with precursor lesions for signet ring cell carcinoma.[3,17] One study using registry data from the Netherlands found that the addition of these criteria increased sensitivity to 89% in identifying patients with pathogenic germline *CDH1* mtuations.[18]

Genetic Alteration

A mutation in the gene for E-cadherin, a cell adhesion protein that normally acts as a tumor suppressor gene, was first described in 1998 in 3 Maori families from New Zealand.[19] Since then, this mutation has been well documented in multiple affected families from many different ethnic backgrounds.[20–23] A second germline truncating allele in *CTNNA1* has been described in families who meet the clinical testing criteria for diffuse gastric cancer but without obvious mutation in the *CDH1* gene.[24] The remaining allele was silenced in patients with cancer or signet ring cells. This gene encodes alpha-E-catenin, which functions in the same protein as E-cadherin.

Table 1
Hereditary diffuse gastric cancer testing criteria

Patients with a family history of:	• Two or more patients[a] with gastric cancer, at least 1 of whom has confirmed DGC • One or more cases of DGC at any age and 1 or more cases of lobular breast cancer in a patient <70 y old in different family members[a] • Two cases of LBC before age 50 y
Patient with personal history of:	• DGC diagnosed before age 50 y • DGC at any age in individuals of Maori ethnicity • DGC at any age in individuals with a personal or family history (first degree) of cleft lip/cleft palate • DGC and LBC, both diagnosed before age 70 y • Bilateral LBC, diagnosed before 70 y • Gastric in situ signet ring cells and/or pagetoid spread of signet ring cells in individuals <50 y old

Abbreviations: DGC, diffuse gastric cancer; LBC, lobular breast cancer.

[a] Patients and family members are first-degree or second-degree relatives of each other

Adapted from the International Gastric Cancer Linkage Consortium practice guidelines. Blair VR, et al. Hereditary diffuse gastric cancer: updated clinical practice guidelines. Lancet Oncol. 2020 Aug;21(8):e386-e397. doi: 10.1016/S1470-2045(20)30219-9. PMID: 32758476; PMCID: PMC7116190. Reprinted with permission of Elsevier, Inc.

Gastric Cancer Risks

With the advent of multigene panel testing and the increased uptake of this testing, particularly among women and families with breast cancer, the frequency of pathogenic variants in *CDH1* being detected has also increased, even among families without report of gastric cancer. A recent study describes the phenotype of *CDH1* mutation carriers in a cohort of 26,936 patients who had undergone germline genetic testing[25]; a total of 20 patients had mutations in *CDH1* detected, whereas 13 did not meet IGCLC clinical criteria for *CDH1* testing. Of those with pathogenic *CDH1* variants, 19 patients had a personal history of cancer, including breast cancer (both ductal and lobular), colon, and gastric cancers. Notably the 3 patients who underwent gastrectomy had evidence of diffuse gastric cancer on resection despite not meeting the diagnostic testing criteria.

The penetrance of gastric cancer and breast cancer is important when counseling affected patients. Earlier lifetime estimates of gastric cancer risk among *CDH1* carriers were as high as 67% for men and 83% for women but were derived from families that met the original, more stringent clinical criteria for HDGC and thereby were subject to ascertainment bias. Reported estimates among *CDH1* mutations were also subject to overestimation because of a common haplotype suggestive of a founder effect from Newfoundland, with an associated 40% risk of gastric cancer in affected men by age 75 years and 63% in women.[22]

In more recent studies where *CDH1* mutation carriers were identified through multigene panel testing, the lifetime risk of gastric cancer by age 80 years has been reported to be lower at 37.2% to 42%[26] in men and approximately 33% for women,[27] with as few as 33% of carriers meeting clinical criteria for HDGC.[27] With respect to the risk of lobular breast cancer among female carriers of pathogenic variants in the *CDH1* gene, a recent study reported a lifetime risk of 42% by the age of 80 years,[28] and, in a study of female carriers not ascertained based on fulfillment of clinical criteria for HDGC, the lifetime risk of lobular breast cancer was 55%.[27]

Endoscopic Surveillance and Surgical Management

Patients with pathogenic variants in the *CDH1* mutation and HDGC are advised to undergo prophylactic gastrectomy.[17] Patients who are symptomatic by the time diffuse gastric cancer is detected often have widely invasive disease and poor prognosis, with only 10% having possibly curable disease through surgical resection.[29] Many patients have microscopic foci of cancer on resected specimens; ideally, surgery should occur in the dormant period before the carcinoma proliferates and spreads.[30] Prophylactic gastrectomy is a morbid procedure that demands a significant lifestyle change, and the discussion and timing are individualized. In general, most patients are recommended to undergo this surgery by age 30 years or based on the family history of gastric cancer onset. Multiple studies of carriers who undergo prophylactic gastrectomies suggest they are very efficacious. One of the largest studies, of 41 patients with *CDH1* mutation who underwent prophylactic gastrectomy, found that 85% had 1 or more foci of signet cell gastric cancer.[31] Barriers to undergoing surgery included patient age, positive beliefs about endoscopic surveillance, close relatives who had negative surgical experiences, and fertility concerns and life stress. In contrast, facilitating factors included availability of social support, trust in health care providers, understanding associated risk, negative beliefs about surveillance and history of abnormal results, family-related factors, and positive attitude toward surgery.[32]

The diffuse nature of the disease, where there are no clear visual lesions to identify, limits endoscopic surveillance by esophagogastroduodenoscopy (EGD) and the identification of precursor or early-stage, treatable cancer.[33] In patients who opt to not undergo prophylactic gastrectomy, annual endoscopic surveillance is recommended at an expert center with multiple random biopsies following the Cambridge Protocol[3,17] in order to possibly identify microscopic foci of signet cells. Careful examination with extensive washing, inflation, and deflation to assess distensibility is recommended, as well as treatment of *H Pylori*, if detected. In addition to random biopsies, endoscopists should look for pale spots to biopsy because prior reports have correlated these areas to the presence of signet ring cell carcinoma.[34] Any suspicious findings, lesions, or abnormal biopsy results should prompt referral for gastrectomy. One study of patients who were undergoing surveillance found that 16 of 29 developed cancer and underwent gastrectomy within a median of 5 months.[35] Therefore, the primary recommendation is for prophylactic gastrectomy in identified *CDH1* carriers and strong consideration in individuals that meet clinical criteria for an HDGC kindred.[16,17] Endoscopy is reserved for those who refuse prophylactic gastrectomy or are physically unfit to undergo the surgery.[16,17,34]

INTESTINAL-TYPE ADENOCARCINOMA

Most hereditary syndromes associated with gastric adenocarcinoma are of the intestinal type. The lifetime risk of gastric cancer varies by syndrome and must be weighed against competing risk from other cancers (**Tables 2** and **3**). In addition, the gastric cancer risks may be underestimated in some syndromes, where ascertainment of cases may have been for other malignancies (ie, Lynch syndrome and familial adenomatous polyposis [FAP]).

LYNCH SYNDROME

Lynch syndrome is a prevalent hereditary cancer syndrome that affects 1 in 300 Americans, many of whom are unaware of their diagnosis.[6] The most common malignancy associated with Lynch syndrome is colorectal cancer; however, endometrial, ovarian, gastric, small bowel, ureter, and renal pelvic cancers are also Lynch-associated cancers.

Lynch syndrome has been associated with pathogenic variant in 1 of 4 DNA mismatch repair genes (*MLH1*, *MSH2*, *MSH6*, and *PMS2*), as well as *EPCAM*, which causes epigenetic silencing of the *MSH2* gene.[36,37] When a second mutation occurs in the normally functioning allele, the mismatch repair gene no longer repairs DNA and malignancies can occur, which are frequently associated with microsatellite instability. However, the penetrance and lifetime cancer risks vary by the specific mismatch repair gene mutation and it is well appreciated that pathogenic *MSH2* gene variants are more frequently associated with extracolonic malignancies.

Overall, Lynch syndrome is classically described as a colorectal cancer syndrome, reflecting the highest cumulative cancer risk for these patients. One large observational multicenter study of 3119 patients followed for a total of 24,475 years, including many cancer survivors, found that the lifetime risk of cancer varied by underlying mutation, with *MLH1* being highest risk followed by *MSH2* and *MSH6*, with *PMS2* mutations being significantly lower risk than the other mutations.[38] The cumulative risks for colorectal cancer were 46%, 43%, and 15% in *MLH1*, *MSH2*, and *MSH6* carriers; for endometrial cancer, 43%, 57%, and 46%; for ovarian cancer, 10%, 17%, and 13%; for upper gastrointestinal cancers, 21%, 10%, and 7%; for urinary tract cancers, 8%, 25%, and 11%; for prostate cancer, 17%, 32%, and 18%; and for brain tumors, 1%, 5%, and 1%, respectively.

Gastric Cancer Risks

Lynch syndrome carriers have up to a 10% lifetime risk of gastric cancer.[6,39,40] The burden of risk varies substantially by genotype, being near 10% for individuals with

Table 2
Genetic syndromes associated with gastric cancer

Gene	Syndrome	Predominant Cancers	Gene Function	Gastric Cancer Risk
CDH1, *CTNNA1*	HDGC	Gastric, female lobular breast	Tumor suppressor	33% women, 42% men, 37.2% overall[26,27] 67% men, 83% women by age 80 y in HDGC families[108]
MLH1	Lynch syndrome	Colorectal, endometrial, ovarian, urothelial, gastric, small bowel, biliary, brain	Mismatch repair	5%–7%[6,38,40,43]
MSH2	Lynch syndrome	Colorectal, endometrial, ovarian, urothelial, gastric, small bowel, biliary, brain	Mismatch repair	0.2%–9%[38,40,43,109]
MSH6	Lynch syndrome	Colorectal, endometrial, ovarian, urothelial, gastric, small bowel, biliary, brain	Mismatch repair	<1%–7.9%[6,42,109]
PMS2	Lynch syndrome	Colorectal, endometrial, ovarian	Mismatch repair	Inadequate data[6,109]
APC	Familial adenomatous polyposis	Colorectal	Tumor suppressor	1%–2%[56–58]
APC promoter 1B	Gastric adenomatous and proximal polyposis syndrome	Gastric, colorectal	Tumor suppressor	Inadequate data[110]
STK11	Peutz-Jeghers syndrome	Female breast, colorectal, stomach, small intestine, cervical, testicular, pancreatic	Tumor suppressor	29%[73,74]
TP53	Li-Fraumeni syndrome	Female breast, soft tissue sarcoma, osteosarcoma, colorectal, adrenocortical carcinoma, leukemia, brain and central nervous system tumors	Tumor suppressor	5%–10%[111]
SMAD4/ *BMPR1A*	Juvenile polyposis syndrome	Colorectal, small intestine	Tumor suppressor	21%[78,79,85]

Table 3
Inherited cancer syndrome and gastric cancer surveillance recommendations

Syndrome	Recommended Screening Modality	Age of Initiation (y)[a]	Interval
HDGC	EGD before prophylactic gastrectomy; continued if prophylactic gastrectomy is not pursued	30	Annual
Lynch syndrome	EGD + *H pylori* testing	30	Every 1–5 y
Familial adenomatous polyposis	EGD with dedicated ampullary examination and random sampling of fundic gland polyps	25–30	Pending ampullary examination and polyp pathology results
Gastric adenocarcinoma and proximal polyposis syndrome	EGD before prophylactic gastrectomy; continued if prophylactic gastrectomy is not pursued	Personalized based on affected family members' ages of polyp onset	Annual
Peutz-Jeghers syndrome	EGD	Once age 8 Restart age 18	If polyps present repeat every 3 y
Li-Fraumeni syndrome	EGD	25 or 5 y before the earliest known gastric cancer in the family	Every 2–5 y
Juvenile polyposis syndrome	EGD	12	Every 1–3 y
Familial intestinal gastric cancer	EGD	No recommendations	No recommendations

[a] Initiate 5 to 10 y before youngest age of gastric cancer diagnosis in family.
Derived from National Comprehensive Cancer Network guidelines, International Gastric Cancer Linkage Consortium, the American College of Gastroenterology, the United States Multi-Society Task Force, the European Society for Medical Oncology, the American Society for Clinical Oncology, and the Mallorca Group.

MLH1 and *MSH2* mutations, but may be similar to population level risk (~1% in the United States) for patients with *PMS2* mutations.[38,39,41–44] The average age of onset of gastric cancer for the former patients is usually in the early 50s. Most data for gastric cancer risk are derived from family cancer registries where most subjects were ascertained predominantly for their personal and/or family histories of colorectal cancer; history of gastric cancer may not have been reliably captured and could potentially be underestimated. In contrast, data on gastric cancer estimates from certain European family cancer registries may overestimate lifetime risk because there are particular founder mutations where gastric cancer is more consistently observed.[39]

Endoscopic Evaluation and Surveillance

Multiple societies have developed recommendations for gastric cancer screening for individuals with Lynch syndrome.[6,41,45–49] However, these recommendations are based on limited evidence and mostly on expert consensus. Most guidelines recommend esophagogastroduodenoscopy (EGD) and *H pylori* testing as the preferred modalities, with initiation at age 30 years, with the exception of the National Comprehensive Cancer Network (NCCN) guidelines, which recommend starting at age 40 years. Surveillance recommendations also vary from annually to every 5 years. For example, the NCCN guidelines recommend EGD every 3 to 5 years for patients at high risk.[6,48] Risk factors for these patients are similar to those for the general population, such as male sex, older age, first-degree relative with gastric cancer, Asian ethnicity, residing in or immigrating from countries with high incidence of gastric cancer, autoimmune gastritis, gastric intestinal metaplasia, and gastric adenomas. In 1 study of 73 individuals with Lynch syndrome–associated gene mutations and 32 family members without Lynch syndrome, there was no significant difference in occurrence of *H pylori*, intestinal metaplasia, or gastritis between the 2 groups.[50] Risk factors specific to Lynch syndrome carriers include carrying an *MLH1* or *MSH2* pathogenic variant.[6] More research is needed to determine the optimal age of initiation, surveillance technique, and intervals between examinations.

FAMILIAL ADENOMATOUS POLYPOSIS

FAP is an autosomal dominant hereditary polyposis syndrome caused by germline mutations in the adenomatous polyposis coli (*APC*) gene. The classic form of FAP is clinically defined by the presence of 100 or more synchronous colorectal adenomas. Attenuated FAP is a less severe entity, defined as the presence of fewer than 100 adenomatous polyps.[51]

FAP has been identified worldwide and is estimated to affect between 2.29 and 3.2 per 100,000 births.[45,52–54] FAP may be suspected either when the patient has a relative with the syndrome and mutation or in patients with the clinical phenotype. De novo cases of FAP account for approximately 25% of all newly diagnosed cases, where there is absence of family history. The carcinogenic pathway of FAP is shared with sporadic colon cancer where a loss of function in both *APC* alleles is highly penetrant and causes polyp development in childhood and colorectal cancer in young adulthood.[55] Patients with FAP have about 100% lifetime risk of colon cancer unless prevented either through endoscopic clearing of polyps or colectomy. Patients with FAP also have increased risk of duodenal or ampullary cancer, desmoid tumors, papillary thyroid cancer, adrenal adenomas, and osteomas of the bone.[45] Children are at risk of hepatoblastoma until about the age of 5 years, and screening with alpha-fetoprotein and ultrasonography is recommended until the age of 7 years. Other nonmalignant extraintestinal manifestations include congenital hypertrophy of the retinal pigmented epithelium and epidermoid cysts.

Gastric Cancer Risk, Endoscopic Evaluation, and Surveillance

The data on the risk of gastric cancer for individuals with FAP are evolving. The presence of benign fundic gland polyps is common and well documented, although adenomas in the stomach are rare. The incidence of gastric cancer in Western patients with FAP was thought to be about the same as the population risk, or 0.6%.[56,57] However a recent study of 767 patients with FAP who underwent upper endoscopy in a hereditary cancer clinic cohort reports a dramatic increase in gastric cancer.[58] Between 1979 and 2016, 10 patients were diagnosed with gastric adenocarcinoma, 9 of whom were diagnosed in the last 4 years of the study, and 8 of the 10 had low-grade or high-grade dysplasia on previous EGD. Given the difficulty in identifying carcinoma among dense polyposis, these investigators then developed a prospective study to identify endoscopic features that might predict cancer.[59] Using polyp color, pit pattern, surface architecture, and appearance under high-definition white light and narrow-band imaging, the endoscopists were able to identify high-risk polyps with sensitivity of 79% and specificity of 78.8%.

Current guidelines for endoscopic evaluation of the upper gastrointestinal tract have predominantly focused on surveillance of the duodenum for adenomatous polyposis, more so than for gastric adenomas. Endoscopic surveillance is recommended to begin at the age of 25 to 30 years and includes dedicated evaluation of the ampulla of Vater in the duodenum. Random sampling of fundic gland polyps is recommended when encountered and, for patients with cancer or high-grade dysplasia (not low grade), surgical consultation is recommended. The interval for endoscopic surveillance is otherwise recommended based on duodenal polyposis using the Spigelman criteria. However, if the risk of gastric cancer continues to increase among FAP carriers, recommendations for gastric cancer surveillance may need to be defined.

GASTRIC ADENOCARCINOMA AND PROXIMAL POLYPOSIS SYNDROME

Gastric adenocarcinoma and proximal polyposis syndrome (GAPPS) is a rare hereditary gastric cancer condition characterized by proximal gastric polyposis and increased risk of early-onset, intestinal-type adenocarcinoma, in the absence of colorectal polyposis. It is a novel, autosomal dominant condition that was first described in 2012,[60] with the associated variant elucidated in 2016,[61,62] which involves the promoter 1B region of the *APC* gene. Fundal gland polyps (FGPs) are the sentinel features of the GAPPS phenotype; however, a dysplasia- adenoma-adenocarcinoma sequence has been reported in the development of the malignant phenotype of GAPPS. A diagnosis of GAPPS is made by the presence of FGPs sparing the antrum and lesser curvature of the stomach, the absence of colonic and duodenal polyposis, an autosomal dominant inheritance pattern, and the exclusion of other gastric polyposis syndromes, as well as chronic use of PPIs.[63] The unique noninvolvement of the antrum in patients with GAPPS, coupled with the absence of a colonic polyposis phenotype, is an important clinical feature that distinguishes GAPPS and FAP. Family members at risk should undergo germline mutation testing for the presence of *APC* promotor 1B variants to initiate timely endoscopic evaluation and surveillance, in addition to other preventive strategies, including timing of risk-reducing surgery.

Gastric Cancer Risk, Endoscopic Evaluation, and Surveillance

The lifetime risk of gastric cancer in individuals with the GAPPS syndrome remains undefined because the natural history of GAPPS is not yet clearly defined. The rate of malignant transformation is unknown and endoscopic surveillance in carriers and family members with gastric polyposis and any grade of dysplasia on biopsy and polypectomy specimens may miss invasive cancer in other areas of the stomach. Heterogeneity in the impact of the individual primary promotor variants, along with differences in the frequency and type of second-hit events, and any underlying perturbations of the *APC* promotor 1A are likely drivers of the malignant phenotype, including rate of progression toward invasion and metastasis. The interindividual heterogeneity within GAPPS requires a personalized approach to family members at risk and affected by the phenotype. There are disconcerting reports that do not support prolonged endoscopic surveillance because it is common for individuals to present with disease by the third to fourth decade of life, and even as early as the late teens.[60,62,63] The endoscopic appearance can include confluent, carpetlike involvement with limited disruption of the mucosa, and presence of adenomatous lesions can be used to triage patients to undergo total gastrectomy, although data from larger case series for this rare condition are lacking. Nonetheless, the concerns of adequate sampling via endoscopic biopsies in the face of hundreds of heterogenous polypoid lesions, which may include FGPs with different degrees of dysplasia, adenomas, or mixed histology polyps, pose significant challenges and justify expedited referral to clinical genetics, surgery, and surgical oncology. Total gastrectomy should be considered in all patients with GAPPS with fundal gland polyposis and the presence of dysplasia on gastric biopsy or polypectomy specimens who are able to undergo major surgery.

Similar to gastric cancer, there is an incomplete understanding of other organs at risk for cancer. Colonic involvement in GAPPS has been described, and an increased incidence of colonic adenomas justifies inclusion of colonoscopic screening and surveillance into the routine work-up of patients with GAPPS.[64] However, the interval for surveillance is guided by the initial findings in carriers and may not be intensive for colorectal cancer prevention. It is thought that the mild colonic phenotype generally involves fewer than 20 total small, hyperplastic polyps or small adenomas in GAPPS carriers and is caused by an incomplete protection of *APC* promotor 1A activity.[62]

PEUTZ-JEGHERS SYNDROME

Peutz-Jeghers syndrome (PJS) is an autosomal dominant syndrome caused by germline mutations in *STK11* tumor suppressor gene. PJS is estimated to occur in between 1 in 50,000 and 1 in 200,000 live births.[65] It is characterized by early onset of gastrointestinal polyposis and cancers and mucocutaneous pigmentation, commonly at the vermilion border of the lips.[66,67] On histology, the polyps are hamartomatous polyps and occur most frequently in the stomach, small bowel, and colon, where 1 study estimated that 50% to 64% of patients had luminal tract polyps.[68] Patients may present at an early age with anemia, bleeding, obstruction, or intussusception caused by the polyps. One-third of patients have symptoms by age 10 years and 50% by age 20 years.[68]

PJS can be diagnosed clinically with if any of the following criteria are present[69,70]: 2 or more histologically confirmed Peutz-Jeghers (PJ) polyps; any number of PJ polyps in an individual who has a close relative with PJS; characteristic mucocutaneous pigmentation in an individual who has a family history of PJS in a close relative; or any number of PJ polyps in an individual who also has characteristic mucocutaneous pigmentation. In individuals who fulfill the aforementioned clinical criteria, 94% are found to carry the STK11 mutation.[66,70–72] PJS can also occur de novo in up to one-quarter of patients.[71]

Gastric Cancer, Endoscopic Evaluation, and Surveillance

The lifetime risk of gastric cancer in PJS is near 29%,[73,74] but may be overestimated because of ascertainment bias because most individuals and families with PJS were originally enrolled in family cancer registries for management of polyposis, and gastric cancer may not have been consistently reported. Several malignancies are associated with PJS and carriers have a high burden of cancer risk[75]; by age 70 years, PJS carriers have an 81% risk of developing cancer. A systematic review of multiple studies suggests the lifetime risks of cancer in PJS are 39% for colorectal, 29% for gastric,

13% for small bowel, 24% to 54% for breast, 21% for ovarian, 10% to 23% for cervical, 9% for uterine, 9% for testicular, 7% to 17% for lung, and 11% to 36% for pancreatic cancers.[76]

Several expert groups, including the American College of Gastroenterology (ACG), the NCCN, and the Mallorca group, have put forth recommendations for surveillance for these patients.[6,45,66] The Mallorca group and ACG recommend EGD, capsule endoscopy, and colonoscopy starting at age 8 years.[45,66] If polyps are found, surveillance should be continued every 3 years; if not, then repeat testing with all 3 modalities is recommended at age 18 years. Endoscopic management of polyps is recommended when feasible, with surgical consideration for advanced neoplasia and cancer, complications related to polyposis, or when disease burden is not amenable to endoscopic interventions.[65,77]

JUVENILE POLYPOSIS SYNDROME

Juvenile polyposis syndrome (JPS) is a rare autosomal dominant condition characterized by multiple hamartomatous polyps throughout the gastrointestinal tract, predominantly the colorectum (98% of cases), followed by the stomach (14%), jejunum and ileum (7%), and duodenum (7%). Its incidence is between 1 in 100,000 and 1 in 160,000 individuals[78] and it is associated with germline mutations in the *SMAD4* or bone morphogenetic protein receptor type-1A (*BMPR1A*) genes; both genes are related to the transforming growth factor-beta (TGF-beta) signaling pathway, involved with cell growth, differentiation, and apoptosis.[78,79] Clinical manifestations are typically seen by the third decade of life[79] and most often include gastrointestinal bleeding and anemia, and occasional abdominal pain, diarrhea, and prolapsed rectal polyps. *SMAD4*-related JPS has been linked to hereditary hemorrhagic telangiectasia; manifestations of this overlap syndrome include mucocutaneous telangiectasias, arteriovenous malformations, and epistaxis.[80]

A clinical diagnosis of JPS can be made if 1 of the following criteria are met more than 5 juvenile polyps of the colorectum, multiple juvenile polyps in other parts of the gastrointestinal tract, or any number of juvenile polyps in a person with a known family history of juvenile polyps. Germline mutations in either *SMAD4* or *BMPR1A* have been identified in approximately 40% to 60% of JPS cases, the remainder of which are thought to be caused by de novo mutations.[81] JPS is considered highly penetrant, with 1 study of 34 *SMAD4* mutation–positive individuals showing that 97% developed colorectal polyps and 68% developed gastric polyps.[82] Several genotype-phenotype correlations have been established. For example, individuals with recurrent 10q22q23 deletions affecting the *BMPR1A* gene have a more severe phenotype, with earlier onset of juvenile polyps and larger polyp burden.[83,84] In addition, individuals with *SMAD4* mutations are more likely to have significant polyposis of the upper gastrointestinal tract and a higher risk for gastric cancer.[85]

Gastric Cancer Risks

The gastrointestinal cancer risk in JPS is thought to arise from malignant transformation of the adenomatous components present in juvenile polyps.[78,79,86] Although generally limited by small sample sizes, studies have shown the incidence of gastric cancer in JPS to be between 11% and 29% in patients with gastric polyps.[78,79,85] In 1 study of 44 patients with clinical JPS from 30 kindreds, the average age of gastric cancer diagnosis was 56 years (range, 21–73 years); notably, all affected individuals had *SMAD4* mutations.[85] Similar findings were observed in another study of 80 unrelated patients with clinical or suspected JPS, which found that all 7 cases of gastric cancer were in families with *SMAD4* mutations.[87] Interestingly, although histologic analysis showed predominantly intestinal gastric cancer, 1 case of the diffuse subtype was identified, suggesting that the gastric cancer risk in JPS may not be exclusively related to malignant transformation of juvenile polyps.

Endoscopic Evaluation and Surveillance

Screening for gastric cancer involves upper endoscopy every 1 to 3 years beginning at age 12 years, or earlier if symptoms occur.[45] Surveillance should be repeated every 1 to 3 years, depending on polyp burden, and polyps 5 mm or larger should be removed. Although JPS is a hamartomatous polyposis syndrome, up to 75% of patients have mixed polyp types, including inflammatory, hyperplastic, and adenomatous polyps, the last of which is thought to predispose to malignant transformation.[88]

Complete or partial gastrectomy is indicated if cancer, high-grade dysplasia, or polyposis cannot be adequately controlled endoscopically. Given that upper gastrointestinal involvement tends to correspond with more severe disease in JPS, particularly in *SMAD4* mutation carriers, continued endoscopic monitoring for polyp recurrence postgastrectomy is likely needed, but clear surveillance recommendations are lacking.[89]

LI-FRAUMENI SYNDROME

Li-Fraumeni syndrome (LFS) is a rare autosomal dominant hereditary cancer syndrome associated with germline mutations in the tumor protein p53 gene (*TP53*). A wide spectrum of malignancies is seen in LFS, the most common being breast cancer (27%–31% of cases), followed by soft tissue sarcomas (17%–27%), osteosarcomas (3%–16%), brain tumors (9%–14%), adrenocortical carcinomas (6%–13%), and leukemias (2%–4%),[90–92] which are common in childhood or early adulthood. However, a variety of gastrointestinal malignancies are also associated with LFS, including gastric and colorectal cancers. In addition to the excess of early-onset cancers seen in LFS, carriers have a 40% to 49% risk of developing a second cancer, with a median onset of 10 years after the first cancer diagnosis. The 2 major classification systems used to identify patients who should undergo molecular testing for LFS are the classic LFS criteria and the Chompret criteria. Combined, these 2 approaches have been shown to confer a 95% sensitivity and 52% specificity in detecting patients with *TP53* mutations.[92]

Gastric Cancer Risk, Endoscopic Evaluation, and Surveillance

LFS is considered highly penetrant, with a 70% or higher lifetime risk of cancer in men and a 90% or higher lifetime risk of cancer in women.[93,94] Gastric cancer is an uncommon manifestation of LFS and lifetime risk estimates are not well established.[94–96] When observed in LFS, gastric cancer almost always presents at an earlier age than in the general population. Among 429 cancer-affected individuals from 62 *TP53* mutation–positive families, 21 (4.9%) patients from 14 families (22.6%) had a diagnosis of gastric cancer.[97] Notably, the mean and median ages at gastric cancer diagnosis were 43 and 36 years, respectively, which was significantly younger than the median age at diagnosis in the general population at 68 years. On pathology, both intestinal and diffuse gastric cancer were identified, with 50% of the tumors located in the proximal stomach.

With the goal of early tumor detection and reduction of cancer-related and treatment-related morbidity and mortality, proposals for clinical surveillance of *TP53* mutation carriers have been made by the NCCN and the American Association for

Cancer Research (AACR). For breast cancer, diagnostic screening with breast MRI is recommended annually starting at age 20 years; the addition of contrast-enhanced MRI and mammogram is still debated.[98] For colorectal cancer, diagnostic screening with colonoscopy is recommended every 2 to 5 years starting at age 25 years, or 5 to 10 years before the earliest known colorectal cancer in the family, whichever comes first. Whole-body MRI has been invoked as a useful surveillance tool with associated survival benefits in LFS patients; however, rates of false-positive findings that required further evaluation have been as high as 29.9%, indicating the need for controlled studies assessing relative risks and benefits.[98–100]

Screening for gastric cancer is recommended with upper endoscopy every 2 to 5 years starting at age 25 years, or 5 years before the earliest known gastric cancer in the family.[101] However, these recommendations are based on expert opinion because there is a paucity of data on the use and value of endoscopic evaluation for gastric cancer in LFS. A potential limitation in endoscopic screening may be related to the evaluation of diffuse-type gastric cancer because endoscopic findings are frequently normal in patients with this subtype, which is typically diagnosed on pathology following gastrectomy.[33]

FAMILIAL INTESTINAL GASTRIC CANCER

Familial gastric cancer describes families with intestinal-type gastric cancer in the absence of polyposis or a pathogenic germline mutation associated with this malignancy.[102,103] Although the rates of gastric cancer differ worldwide, it is clear that family history of gastric cancer is an independent risk factor, as supported by multiple case-control studies that report general risk ratios of 1.5 to 3.5.[104] Although the presence of first-degree relatives with intestinal-type gastric cancer is a strong and consistent risk factor for gastric cancer, the pathogenic mechanisms behind this familial aggregation are unclear. The possible causes for familial clustering include bacterial factors, environmental factors, or a combination thereof. Among individuals with a family history, current or past *H pylori* infection and having 2 or more first-degree affected relatives are associated with an increased risk of developing gastric cancer. *H pylori* eradication is an important preventive strategy in first-degree relatives of patients with gastric cancer, particularly those in their 20s and 30s, where early eradication could prevent the progression to intestinal metaplasia and reduce the synergistic risk in individuals with both *H pylori* infection and a family history.[105] In addition, no specific single nucleotide polymorphism has been shown to be associated with familial clustering of gastric cancer. Ongoing genome-wide association studies that incorporate environmental and modifiable risk factors may increase the understanding of the pathogenesis of gastric cancer among patients with family history.

In addition, familial intestinal gastric cancer (FIGC) has been defined as having a high burden of gastric cancer in the family. Clinically, patients meet criteria if there are 2 first-degree or second-degree relatives with gastric adenocarcinoma, where 1 had been diagnosed before age 50 years. Alternatively, 3 or more first-degree or second-degree relatives diagnosed at any age are included. In a single center study of 50 patients from FIGC kindreds, both germline and tumor testing was performed and compared with HDGC and sporadic cases to evaluate for genetic causes potentially underlying a monogenic or an oligogenic/polygenic inheritance pattern.[106] FIGC probands developed gastric cancer at least 10 years earlier, tumors more often displayed microsatellite instability, and there were significantly more somatic common variants than sporadic tumors. The investigators concluded that FIGC is likely a polygenic gastric cancer predisposing to disease and proposed that any family presenting

2 patients with gastric cancer, 1 confirmed on intestinal histology, independently of age, and with or without colorectal cancer, breast cancer, or gastric ulcers in other family members, could be considered FIGC.[106]

Although endoscopic surveillance is expected to benefit individuals with a family history of gastric cancer, further large-scale, prospective studies are warranted to evaluate the cost-effectiveness and optimal time point for endoscopy in individuals with FIGC. At present, there are no clear surveillance recommendations, and further studies are needed to better describe and understand families with this gastric cancer history.

GENETIC TESTING

Next-generation sequencing has led to the development of multigene panel tests, allowing providers to simultaneously test for multiple germline mutations associated with malignancy. For families with a history of multiple cancers, many of which overlap between known inherited cancer syndromes, multigene panel testing allows the increased identification of pathologic variants.[107] However, increased germline genetic testing for multiple cancer susceptibility genes also leads to the identification of more variants of unknown significance or pathogenic variants whose associated risks and clinical implications are not yet known. Genetic counseling is therefore necessary to determine which testing is appropriate and for interpreting testing results to guide patients and at-risk family members with cancer screening and preventive strategies, including risk-reducing, prophylactic surgeries. If a germline mutation is identified in an inherited cancer predisposition gene of which gastric cancer is but 1 manifestation, family members can benefit from earlier and enhanced screenings for gastric cancer, in addition to the other associated malignancies.

Referral for genetic counseling and testing is recommended for individuals diagnosed with gastric cancer who meet several clinical criteria related to personal and/

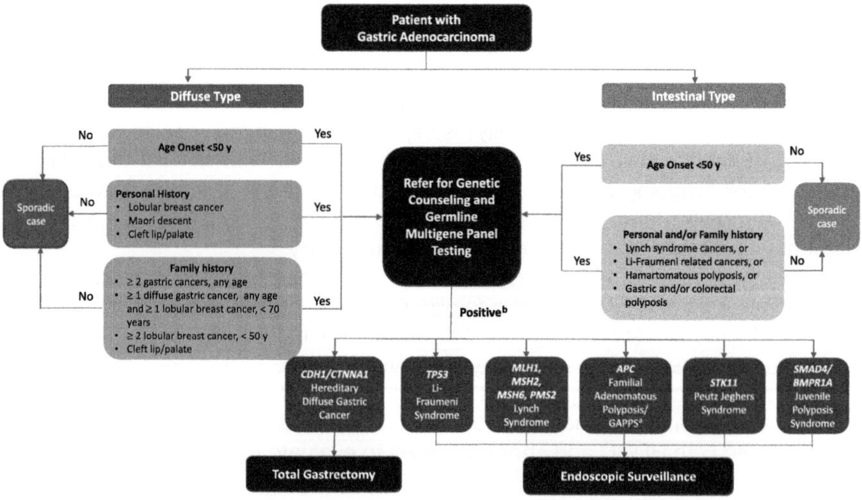

Fig. 1. Genetic risk assessment for individuals with gastric adenocarcinoma. [a]GAPPS caused by pathogenic variant in *APC* promoter 1B and prophylactic gastrectomy recommended. [b]Germline genetic testing for the newly identified pathogenic variant is recommended for all at-risk family members (cascade genetic testing).

or family cancer history (**Fig. 1**). Once a pathogenic variant is identified in the individuals with gastric cancer, at-risk family members benefit from genetic testing for the newly detected familial variant, a process referred to as cascade testing. This approach is cost-effective in identifying individuals unaffected by cancer but at highest risk of developing malignancy caused by a pathogenic germline variant and who can benefit the most from cancer prevention and early detection strategies.

SUMMARY

Appropriate assessment of familial and genetic risk for gastric cancer development may allow a personalized approach to gastric cancer prevention through screening and risk-reducing surgeries. The ability to better identify carriers with pathogenic genetic variants associated with gastric cancer *before* a diagnosis of cancer requires effective implementation of strategies for genetic risk assessment and testing, followed by optimal screening and surveillance recommendations to further reduce the morbidity and mortality.

CLINICS CARE POINTS

- Gastric cancer is associated with several germline pathogenic variants associated with inherited cancer syndromes.
- Patients with identified pathogenic variants in the *CDH1* gene should be considered for prophylactic gastrectomy, the timing of which can be as early as age 30 years and may vary based on presence or absence of family history of diffuse gastric cancer, burden of this cancer among multiple relatives, and/or abnormal findings detected on surveillance endoscopy.
- The management of *CDH1* carriers without family history of gastric cancer is evolving with respect to timing of prophylactic gastrectomy and the limitations of surveillance endoscopy.
- Patients with inherited cancer syndromes associated with intestinal-type gastric cancer benefit from gastric cancer screening by upper endoscopy, with age of initiation and interval recommendations tailored to the specific syndrome and/or pathogenic variant and its associated gastric cancer risk.
- The term FIGC may be used to describe those patients with a significant family history of gastric cancer who do not carry an associated pathogenic variant or meet clinical criteria for inherited cancer syndromes.
- Genetic testing and identification of germline pathogenic variants in select individuals with gastric cancer allows at-risk family members to undergo genetic testing with the benefit of cancer screening and preventive strategies for carriers of the familial variant.

DISCLOSURE

The authors have nothing to disclose.

REFERENCES

1. Thrift AP, El-Serag HB. Burden of gastric cancer. Clin Gastroenterol Hepatol 2020;18(3):534–42.
2. Siegel RL, Miller KD, Jemal A. Cancer statistics, 2020. CA Cancer J Clin 2020; 70(1):7–30.

3. Fitzgerald RC, Hardwick R, Huntsman D, et al. Hereditary diffuse gastric cancer: updated consensus guidelines for clinical management and directions for future research. J Med Genet 2010;47(7):436–44.
4. La Vecchia C, Negri E, Franceschi S, et al. Family history and the risk of stomach and colorectal cancer. Cancer 1992;70(1):50–5.
5. Corso G, Marrelli D, Roviello F. Familial gastric cancer: update for practice management. Fam Cancer 2011;10(2):391–6.
6. Gupta S, Provenzale D, Llor X, et al. NCCN guidelines insights: genetic/familial high-risk assessment: colorectal, version 2.2019. J Natl Compr Canc Netw 2019;17(9):1032–41.
7. Slavin TP, Weitzel JN, Neuhausen SL, et al. Genetics of gastric cancer: what do we know about the genetic risks? Transl Gastroenterol Hepatol 2019;4:55.
8. Assumpção P, Araújo T, Khayat A, et al. Hereditary gastric cancer: three rules to reduce missed diagnoses. World J Gastroenterol 2020;26(13):1382–93.
9. Choi IJ, Kim CG, Lee JY, et al. Family history of gastric cancer and Helicobacter pylori treatment. N Engl J Med 2020;382(5):427–36.
10. Canakis A, Pani E, Saumoy M, et al. Decision model analyses of upper endoscopy for gastric cancer screening and preneoplasia surveillance: a systematic review. Therap Adv Gastroenterol 2020;13. 1756284820941662.
11. Lauren P. The two histological main types of gastric carcinoma: diffuse and so-called intestinal-type carcinoma. an attempt at a histo-clinical classification. Acta Pathol Microbiol Scand 1965;64:31–49.
12. Ma J, Shen H, Kapesa L, et al. Lauren classification and individualized chemotherapy in gastric cancer. Oncol Lett 2016;11(5):2959–64.
13. Cancer Genome Atlas Research Network. Comprehensive molecular characterization of gastric adenocarcinoma. Nature 2014;513(7517):202–9.
14. Cisco RM, Ford JM, Norton JA. Hereditary diffuse gastric cancer: implications of genetic testing for screening and prophylactic surgery. Cancer 2008;113(7 Suppl):1850–6.
15. Petrovchich I, Ford JM. Genetic predisposition to gastric cancer. Semin Oncol 2016;43(5):554–9.
16. Blair VR, McLeod M, Carneiro F, et al. Hereditary diffuse gastric cancer: updated clinical practice guidelines. Lancet Oncol 2020;21(8):e386–97.
17. van der Post RS, Vogelaar IP, Carneiro F, et al. Hereditary diffuse gastric cancer: updated clinical guidelines with an emphasis on germline CDH1 mutation carriers. J Med Genet 2015;52(6):361–74.
18. van der Post RS, Vogelaar IP, Manders P, et al. Accuracy of hereditary diffuse gastric cancer testing criteria and outcomes in patients with a germline mutation in CDH1. Gastroenterology 2015;149(4):897–906.e9.
19. Guilford P, Hopkins J, Harraway J, et al. E-cadherin germline mutations in familial gastric cancer. Nature 1998;392(6674):402–5.
20. Brooks-Wilson AR, Kaurah P, Suriano G, et al. Germline E-cadherin mutations in hereditary diffuse gastric cancer: assessment of 42 new families and review of genetic screening criteria. J Med Genet 2004;41(7):508–17.
21. Dussaulx-Garin L, Blayau M, Pagenault M, et al. A new mutation of E-cadherin gene in familial gastric linitis plastica cancer with extra-digestive dissemination. Eur J Gastroenterol Hepatol 2001;13(6):711–5.
22. Kaurah P, MacMillan A, Boyd N, et al. Founder and recurrent CDH1 mutations in families with hereditary diffuse gastric cancer. JAMA 2007;297(21):2360–72.

23. Stone J, Bevan S, Cunningham D, et al. Low frequency of germline E-cadherin mutations in familial and nonfamilial gastric cancer. Br J Cancer 1999;79(11–12): 1935–7.
24. Majewski IJ, Kluijt I, Cats A, et al. An α-E-catenin (CTNNA1) mutation in hereditary diffuse gastric cancer. J Pathol 2013;229(4):621–9.
25. Lowstuter K, Espenschied CR, Sturgeon D, et al. Unexpected CDH1 mutations identified on multigene panels pose clinical management challenges. JCO Precis Oncol 2017;(1):1–12.
26. Xicola RM, Li S, Rodriguez N, et al. Clinical features and cancer risk in families with pathogenic CDH1 variants irrespective of clinical criteria. J Med Genet 2019;56(12):838–43.
27. Roberts ME, Ranola JMO, Marshall ML, et al. Comparison of CDH1 penetrance estimates in clinically ascertained families vs families ascertained for multiple gastric cancers. JAMA Oncol 2019;5(9):1325–31.
28. Hansford S, Kaurah P, Li-Chang H, et al. Hereditary diffuse gastric cancer syndrome: CDH1 mutations and beyond. JAMA Oncol 2015;1(1):23–32.
29. Koea JB, Karpeh MS, Brennan MF. Gastric cancer in young patients: demographic, clinicopathological, and prognostic factors in 92 patients. Ann Surg Oncol 2000;7(5):346–51.
30. Barber M, Murrell A, Ito Y, et al. Mechanisms and sequelae of E-cadherin silencing in hereditary diffuse gastric cancer. J Pathol 2008;216(3):295–306.
31. Strong VE, Gholami S, Shah MA, et al. Total gastrectomy for hereditary diffuse gastric cancer at a single center: postsurgical outcomes in 41 patients. Ann Surg 2017;266(6):1006–12.
32. McGarragle KM, Hart TL, Swallow C, et al. Barriers and facilitators to CDH1 carriers contemplating or undergoing prophylactic total gastrectomy. Fam Cancer 2020.
33. Jacobs MF, Dust H, Koeppe E, et al. Outcomes of endoscopic surveillance in individuals with genetic predisposition to hereditary diffuse gastric cancer. Gastroenterology 2019;157(1):87–96.
34. Iwaizumi M, Yamada H, Fukue M, et al. Two independent families with strongly suspected hereditary diffuse gastric cancer based on the probands' endoscopic findings. Clin J Gastroenterol 2020;13(5):754–8.
35. Lim YC, di Pietro M, O'Donovan M, et al. Prospective cohort study assessing outcomes of patients from families fulfilling criteria for hereditary diffuse gastric cancer undergoing endoscopic surveillance. Gastrointest Endosc 2014;80(1): 78–87.
36. Stoll J, Kupfer SS. Risk assessment and genetic testing for inherited gastrointestinal syndromes. Gastroenterol Hepatol (N Y) 2019;15(9):462–70.
37. Koornstra JJ, Mourits MJ, Sijmons RH, et al. Management of extracolonic tumours in patients with Lynch syndrome. Lancet Oncol 2009;10(4):400–8.
38. Møller P, Seppälä TT, Bernstein I, et al. Cancer risk and survival in path_MMR carriers by gene and gender up to 75 years of age: a report from the Prospective Lynch Syndrome Database. Gut 2018;67(7):1306–16.
39. Kim J, Braun D, Ukaegbu C, et al. Clinical factors associated with gastric cancer in individuals with lynch syndrome. Clin Gastroenterol Hepatol 2020;18(4): 830–7.e1.
40. Capelle LG, Van Grieken NC, Lingsma HF, et al. Risk and epidemiological time trends of gastric cancer in Lynch syndrome carriers in the Netherlands. Gastroenterology 2010;138(2):487–92.

41. Vasen HF, Blanco I, Aktan-Collan K, et al. Revised guidelines for the clinical management of Lynch syndrome (HNPCC): recommendations by a group of European experts. Gut 2013;62(6):812–23.
42. Bonadona V, Bonaiti B, Olschwang S, et al. Cancer risks associated with germline mutations in MLH1, MSH2, and MSH6 genes in Lynch syndrome. JAMA 2011;305(22):2304–10.
43. Engel C, Loeffler M, Steinke V, et al. Risks of less common cancers in proven mutation carriers with lynch syndrome. J Clin Oncol 2012;30(35):4409–15.
44. Watson P, Vasen HFA, Mecklin JP, et al. The risk of extra-colonic, extra-endometrial cancer in the Lynch syndrome. Int J Cancer 2008;123(2):444–9.
45. Syngal S, Brand RE, Church JM, et al. ACG clinical guideline: genetic testing and management of hereditary gastrointestinal cancer syndromes. Am J Gastroenterol 2015;110(2):223–62 [quiz: 263].
46. Giardiello FM, Allen JI, Axilbund JE, et al. Guidelines on genetic evaluation and management of Lynch syndrome: a consensus statement by the US Multi-Society Task Force on colorectal cancer. Gastroenterology 2014;147(2):502–26.
47. Balmaña J, Balaguer F, Cervantes A, et al. Familial risk-colorectal cancer: ESMO clinical practice guidelines. Ann Oncol 2013;24(Suppl 6):vi73–80.
48. Stoffel EM, Mangu PB, Gruber SB, et al. Hereditary colorectal cancer syndromes: American Society of Clinical Oncology Clinical Practice Guideline endorsement of the familial risk-colorectal cancer: European Society for Medical Oncology Clinical Practice Guidelines. J Clin Oncol 2015;33(2):209–17.
49. Vangala DB, Cauchin E, Balmaña J, et al. Screening and surveillance in hereditary gastrointestinal cancers: recommendations from the European Society of Digestive Oncology (ESDO) expert discussion at the 20th European Society for Medical Oncology (ESMO)/World Congress on Gastrointestinal Cancer, Barcelona, June 2018. Eur J Cancer 2018;104:91–103.
50. Renkonen-Sinisalo L, Sipponen P, Aarnio M, et al. No support for endoscopic surveillance for gastric cancer in hereditary non-polyposis colorectal cancer. Scand J Gastroenterol 2002;37(5):574–7.
51. Hernegger GS, Moore HG, Guillem JG. Attenuated familial adenomatous polyposis: an evolving and poorly understood entity. Dis Colon Rectum 2002;45(1):127–34 [discussion: 134–26].
52. Bülow S. Results of national registration of familial adenomatous polyposis. Gut 2003;52(5):742–6.
53. Iwama T, Tamura K, Morita T, et al. A clinical overview of familial adenomatous polyposis derived from the database of the Polyposis Registry of Japan. Int J Clin Oncol 2004;9(4):308–16.
54. Järvinen HJ. Epidemiology of familial adenomatous polyposis in Finland: impact of family screening on the colorectal cancer rate and survival. Gut 1992;33(3):357–60.
55. Perchiniak EM, Groden J. Mechanisms regulating microtubule binding, DNA replication, and apoptosis are controlled by the intestinal tumor suppressor APC. Curr Colorectal Cancer Rep 2011;7(2):145–51.
56. Jagelman DG, DeCosse JJ, Bussey HJ. Upper gastrointestinal cancer in familial adenomatous polyposis. Lancet 1988;1(8595):1149–51.
57. Bianchi LK, Burke CA, Bennett AE, et al. Fundic gland polyp dysplasia is common in familial adenomatous polyposis. Clin Gastroenterol Hepatol 2008;6(2):180–5.
58. Mankaney G, Leone P, Cruise M, et al. Gastric cancer in FAP: a concerning rise in incidence. Fam Cancer 2017;16(3):371–6.

59. Mankaney GN, Cruise M, Sarvepalli S, et al. Surveillance for pathology associated with cancer on endoscopy (SPACE): criteria to identify high-risk gastric polyps in familial adenomatous polyposis. Gastrointest Endosc 2020;92(3): 755–62.
60. Worthley DL, Phillips KD, Wayte N, et al. Gastric adenocarcinoma and proximal polyposis of the stomach (GAPPS): a new autosomal dominant syndrome. Gut 2012;61(5):774–9.
61. Repak R, Kohoutova D, Podhola M, et al. The first European family with gastric adenocarcinoma and proximal polyposis of the stomach: case report and review of the literature. Gastrointest Endosc 2016;84(4):718–25.
62. Li J, Woods SL, Healey S, et al. Point mutations in exon 1B of APC reveal gastric adenocarcinoma and proximal polyposis of the stomach as a familial adenomatous polyposis variant. Am J Hum Genet 2016;98(5):830–42.
63. Rudloff U. Gastric adenocarcinoma and proximal polyposis of the stomach: diagnosis and clinical perspectives. Clin Exp Gastroenterol 2018;11:447–59.
64. McDuffie LA, Sabesan A, Allgäeuer M, et al. β-Catenin activation in fundic gland polyps, gastric cancer and colonic polyps in families afflicted by 'gastric adenocarcinoma and proximal polyposis of the stomach' (GAPPS). J Clin Pathol 2016; 69(9):826–33.
65. Giardiello FM, Trimbath JD. Peutz-Jeghers syndrome and management recommendations. Clin Gastroenterol Hepatol 2006;4(4):408–15.
66. Beggs AD, Latchford AR, Vasen HF, et al. Peutz-Jeghers syndrome: a systematic review and recommendations for management. Gut 2010;59(7):975–86.
67. Jeghers H, Mc KV, Katz KH. Generalized intestinal polyposis and melanin spots of the oral mucosa, lips and digits; a syndrome of diagnostic significance. N Engl J Med 1949;241(25):993, illust; passim.
68. Utsunomiya J, Gocho H, Miyanaga T, et al. Peutz-Jeghers syndrome: its natural course and management. Johns Hopkins Med J 1975;136(2):71–82.
69. Aaltonen LA. Hereditary intestinal cancer. Semin Cancer Biol 2000;10(4): 289–98.
70. Aretz S, Stienen D, Uhlhaas S, et al. High proportion of large genomic STK11 deletions in Peutz-Jeghers syndrome. Hum Mutat 2005;26(6):513–9.
71. Schreibman IR, Baker M, Amos C, et al. The hamartomatous polyposis syndromes: a clinical and molecular review. Am J Gastroenterol 2005;100(2): 476–90.
72. Volikos E, Robinson J, Aittomäki K, et al. LKB1 exonic and whole gene deletions are a common cause of Peutz-Jeghers syndrome. J Med Genet 2006;43(5):e18.
73. Lindor NM, McMaster ML, Lindor CJ, et al. Concise handbook of familial cancer susceptibility syndromes - second edition. J Natl Cancer Inst Monogr 2008;(38):1–93.
74. Giardiello FM, Brensinger JD, Tersmette AC, et al. Very high risk of cancer in familial Peutz-Jeghers syndrome. Gastroenterology 2000;119(6):1447–53.
75. Lim W, Olschwang S, Keller JJ, et al. Relative frequency and morphology of cancers in STK11 mutation carriers. Gastroenterology 2004;126(7):1788–94.
76. van Lier MG, Wagner A, Mathus-Vliegen EM, et al. High cancer risk in Peutz-Jeghers syndrome: a systematic review and surveillance recommendations. Am J Gastroenterol 2010;105(6):1258–64 [author reply: 1265].
77. Amaro R, Diaz G, Schneider J, et al. Peutz-Jeghers syndrome managed with a complete intraoperative endoscopy and extensive polypectomy. Gastrointest Endosc 2000;52(4):552–4.

78. Latchford AR, Neale K, Phillips RKS, et al. Juvenile Polyposis syndrome: a study of genotype, phenotype, and long-term outcome. Dis Colon Rectum 2012; 55(10):1038–43.
79. Chow E, Macrae F. A review of juvenile polyposis syndrome. J Gastroenterol Hepatol 2005;20(11):1634–40.
80. Gallione CJ, Repetto GM, Legius E, et al. A combined syndrome of juvenile polyposis and hereditary haemorrhagic telangiectasia associated with mutations in MADH4 (SMAD4). Lancet 2004;363(9412):852–9.
81. Fogt F, Brown CA, Badizadegan K, et al. Low prevalence of loss of heterozygosity and SMAD4 mutations in sporadic and familial juvenile polyposis syndrome-associated juvenile polyps. Am J Gastroenterol 2004;99(10):2025–31.
82. Wain KE, Ellingson MS, McDonald J, et al. Appreciating the broad clinical features of SMAD4 mutation carriers: a multicenter chart review. Genet Med 2014; 16(8):588–93.
83. Sayed MG, Ahmed AF, Ringold JR, et al. Germline SMAD4 or BMPRIA mutations and phenotype of juvenile polyposis. Ann Surg Oncol 2002;9(9):901–6.
84. Dahdaleh F, Carr J, Calva D, et al. Juvenile polyposis and other intestinal polyposis syndromes with microdeletions of chromosome 10q22–23. Clin Genet 2012;81(2):110–6.
85. Aytac E, Sulu B, Heald B, et al. Genotype-defined cancer risk in juvenile polyposis syndrome. Br J Surg 2015;102(1):114–8.
86. Brosens LA, van Hattem A, Hylind LM, et al. Risk of colorectal cancer in juvenile polyposis. Gut 2007;56(7):965–7.
87. Aretz S, Stienen D, Uhlhaas S, et al. High proportion of large genomic deletions and a genotype phenotype update in 80 unrelated families with juvenile polyposis syndrome. J Med Genet 2007;44(11):702–9.
88. Gilad O, Rosner G, Fliss-Isakov N, et al. Clinical and histologic overlap and distinction among various hamartomatous polyposis syndromes. Clin Transl Gastroenterol 2019;10(5):1–9.
89. Oncel M, Church JM, Remzi FH, et al. Colonic surgery in patients with juvenile polyposis syndrome: a case series. Dis Colon Rectum 2005;48(1):49–56.
90. Malkin D. Li-Fraumeni syndrome. Genes Cancer 2011;2(4):475–84.
91. Bougeard G, Renaux-Petel M, Flaman J-M, et al. Revisiting Li-Fraumeni syndrome from TP53 mutation carriers. J Clin Oncol 2015;33(21):2345–52.
92. Gonzalez KD, Noltner KA, Buzin CH, et al. Beyond Li Fraumeni syndrome: clinical characteristics of families with p53 germline mutations. J Clin Oncol 2009; 27(8):1250–6.
93. Guha T, Malkin D. Inherited TP53 mutations and the Li-Fraumeni syndrome. Cold Spring Harb Perspect Med 2017;7(4):a026187.
94. Mai PL, Best AF, Peters JA, et al. Risks of first and subsequent cancers among TP53 mutation carriers in the National Cancer Institute Li-Fraumeni syndrome cohort. Cancer 2016;122(23):3673–81.
95. Li F, Fraumeni J, Mulvihill J, et al. A cancer family syndrome in twenty-four kindreds. Cancer Res 1988;48:5358–62.
96. Chompret A, Brugieres L, Ronsin M, et al. P53 germline mutations in childhood cancers and cancer risk for carrier individuals. Br J Cancer 2000;82(12):1932–7.
97. Masciari S, Dewanwala A, Stoffel EM, et al. Gastric cancer in individuals with Li-Fraumeni syndrome. Genet Med 2011;13(7):651–7.
98. Kratz CP, Achatz MI, Brugieres L, et al. Cancer screening recommendations for Individuals with Li-Fraumeni syndrome. Clin Cancer Res 2017;23(11):e38–45.

99. Villani A, Tabori U, Schiffman J, et al. Biochemical and imaging surveillance in germline TP53 mutation carriers with Li-Fraumeni syndrome: a prospective observational study. Lancet Oncol 2011;12(6):559–67.
100. Ballinger ML, Best A, Mai PL, et al. Baseline surveillance in Li-Fraumeni syndrome using whole-body magnetic resonance imaging: a meta-analysis. JAMA Oncol 2017;3(12):1634–9.
101. Network NCC. NCCN Clinical Practice Guidelines in Oncology-v3.2019: Genetic/Familial High-Risk Assessment: Li-Fraumeni Syndrome.
102. Oliveira C, Pinheiro H, Figueiredo J, et al. Familial gastric cancer: genetic susceptibility, pathology, and implications for management. Lancet Oncol 2015; 16(2):e60–70.
103. Corso G, Roncalli F, Marrelli D, et al. History, pathogenesis, and management of familial gastric cancer: original study of John XXIII's family. Biomed Res Int 2013; 2013:385132.
104. Choi YJ, Kim N. Gastric cancer and family history. Korean J Intern Med 2016; 31(6):1042–53.
105. Shin CM, Kim N, Lee HS, et al. Intrafamilial aggregation of gastric cancer: a comprehensive approach including environmental factors, Helicobacter pylori virulence, and genetic susceptibility. Eur J Gastroenterol Hepatol 2011;23(5): 411–7.
106. Carvalho J, Oliveira P, Senz J, et al. Redefinition of familial intestinal gastric cancer: clinical and genetic perspectives. J Med Genet 2021;58(1):1–11.
107. Kastrinos F, Samadder NJ, Burt RW. Use of family history and genetic testing to determine risk of colorectal cancer. Gastroenterology 2020;158(2):389–403.
108. Pharoah PD, Guilford P, Caldas C. Incidence of gastric cancer and breast cancer in CDH1 (E-cadherin) mutation carriers from hereditary diffuse gastric cancer families. Gastroenterology 2001;121(6):1348–53.
109. Gupta S, Weiss J, Axell L, et al. Genetic/familial high-risk assessment: colorectal. NCCN Clinical Practice Guidelines. 2020.
110. Foretová L, Navrátilová M, Svoboda M, et al. GAPPS - gastric adenocarcinoma and proximal polyposis of the stomach syndrome in 8 families tested at Masaryk Memorial Cancer Institute - Prevention and Prophylactic Gastrectomies. Klin Onkol 2019;32(Supplementum2):109–17.
111. Daly M, Pal T, Berry M, et al. Genetic/familial high-risk assessment: breast, ovarian, and pancreatic NCCN Clinical Practice Guidelines in Oncology. 2020.

Endoscopic Screening and Surveillance for Gastric Cancer

Bokyung Kim, MD, Soo-Jeong Cho, MD, PhD*

KEYWORDS

• Screening • Surveillance • Gastric cancer • Upper gastrointestinal endoscopy

KEY POINTS

- The value of screening asymptomatic individuals for gastric cancer depends on the incidence, screening methods, and management of gastric cancer.
- Upper gastrointestinal endoscopy is increasingly preferred as a screening method for gastric cancer.
- Population-based nationwide endoscopic screening of gastric cancer decreased gastric cancer mortality in countries with high incidence rates, such as South Korea and Japan.
- Endoscopic surveillance is targeted to high-risk individuals with gastric premalignant lesions, family history of gastric cancer, and previous history of gastric cancer, but no standardized recommendations have been established.

INTRODUCTION

Gastric cancer is one of the most common cancers worldwide.[1,2] The incidence of gastric cancer varies widely by geographic region, with half of new cases occurring in East Asia.[3] The value of screening asymptomatic individuals for gastric cancer depends on the incidence, screening methods, and management of gastric cancer.[4] Population-based national screening for gastric cancer has been implemented in some countries with a high incidence of gastric cancer, such as South Korea and Japan.[5] Two main modalities for gastric cancer screening are upper gastrointestinal endoscopy and upper gastrointestinal series (UGIS). Several studies have reported higher detection rates of gastric cancer with upper intestinal endoscopy compared with UGIS, and gastrointestinal endoscopy has been increasingly used in screening for gastric cancer in recent years.[4,6–8] Some observational studies suggest that gastric cancer screening has contributed to detection of cancer in early stages and an overall decline in gastric cancer mortality.[9–17] In terms of surveillance, endoscopic

Department of Internal Medicine and Liver Research Institute, Seoul National University College of Medicine, 103 Daehak-ro, Jongno-gu, Seoul 03080, Korea
* Corresponding author.
E-mail address: crystal522@daum.net

Gastrointest Endoscopy Clin N Am 31 (2021) 489–501
https://doi.org/10.1016/j.giec.2021.03.004
giendo.theclinics.com

surveillance in high-risk subgroups such as individuals with gastric premalignant lesions or family history of gastric cancer is expected to be beneficial but standard surveillance strategies are lacking.[18–26] This review aims to discuss current evidence and strategies for endoscopic screening and surveillance for gastric cancer.

GASTRIC CANCER INCIDENCE AND MORTALITY

Every year, approximately one million people are diagnosed with gastric cancer worldwide.[1,2] It is one of the most common cancers, and the incidence is highly geographically heterogeneous. Incidence rates are the highest in East Asia, Central Asia, Eastern Europe, and South America, whereas the lowest rates are in North America, North Africa, and East Africa.[1–3] Although the incidence and mortality of gastric cancer has decreased over a few decades, it remains the fifth most commonly diagnosed cancer and third leading cause of cancer mortality.[2,27–29] The decline of the incidence and mortality of gastric cancer is likely attributable to reduction of *Helicobacter pylori* infection, changes in food preservation, and better diagnostic and treatment options.[30–32] Notably, the 5-year survival rates are exceptionally high in South Korea and Japan, reported as 60.3% to 76.5%, compared with the worldwide range of around 20% to 40%.[33–36] One of the most important factors that can explain these differences is the implementation of population-based national screening program for detection of gastric cancer in the 2 countries.

SCREENING AND SURVEILLANCE MODALITY

The ideal modality for gastric cancer screening should be safe, simple, validated, and cost-effective. Several modalities including upper gastrointestinal endoscopy, UGIS, and blood tests such as *H pylori* serology, pepsinogen (PG), microRNA, and serum trefoil factor have been proposed for screening methods.[7,37–43] The 2 main modalities for gastric cancer screening are upper gastrointestinal endoscopy and UGIS, as they enable visualization of the gastrointestinal tract.

Upper gastrointestinal endoscopy allows direct visualization of the gastric mucosa, and biopsy can be performed at suspicious sites for the diagnosis of premalignant lesions as well as gastric cancer. Recently, advanced endoscopic imaging techniques such as narrow band imaging, autofluorescence imaging, magnification endoscopy, and confocal laser endomicroscopy have been increasingly used for diagnosis.[44–47] UGIS, also known as barium meal, allows identification of malignant gastric ulcers and infiltrating lesions including some early gastric cancers. It was used as the initial tool for gastric cancer screening from the early 1960s in Japan and showed reduction in gastric cancer mortality by 40% to 60% in case-control studies.[13,48] Recent studies have reported higher sensitivity in cancer detection with upper gastrointestinal endoscopy compared with UGIS. A study from Japan reported the detection rate of gastric cancer by upper gastrointestinal endoscopy to be 2.7- to 4.6-fold higher than that of UGIS.[4,7] Two Korean studies showed the probability of detecting gastric cancer with upper gastrointestinal endoscopy was 2.9- to 3.8-fold higher than that of UGIS.[6,8] In recent years, upper gastrointestinal endoscopy has been increasingly used for gastric cancer screening and has become the primary modality for screening in South Korea and Japan.[42,49] The reported sensitivities and specificities of upper gastrointestinal endoscopy and UGIS in the National Cancer Screening Program of South Korea and Japan are summarized in **Table 1**.[6,8,52,53]

However, it should be noted that the cost of upper gastrointestinal endoscopy is quite low in these countries (approximately 40 US dollars in South Korea). In most other countries, upper gastrointestinal endoscopy is an expensive procedure, which

Table 1
Sensitivity and specificity of upper gastrointestinal endoscopy and upper gastrointestinal series in the National Cancer Screening Program of South Korea and Japan

		Upper Gastrointestinal Endoscopy			UGIS		
Author	Follow-up Period (y)	Sensitivity (%)	Specificity (%)	Positive Predictive Value (%)	Sensitivity (%)	Specificity (%)	Positive Predictive Value (%)
Lee et al,[8] 2010	1	59.0	96.3	6.1	42.1	89.8	0.8
Choi et al,[6] 2012	1	69.0	96.0	6.2	36.7	96.1	1.7
Hamashima et al.,[52] 2013	1	88.6	85.1	-	83.1	85.6	-

Data from Refs.[6,8,50,51]

makes the implementation of national screening program difficult, along with the need for additional experienced endoscopists and potential complications.[52,53]

NATIONAL SCREENING PROGRAM OF GASTRIC CANCER

Screening for gastric cancer has been introduced in several East Asian countries with a high incidence of gastric cancer. At present, Korea and Japan are the only countries that have implemented population-based nationwide gastric cancer screening program. In Singapore and Taiwan, screening program is mainly targeted at high-risk populations.[4] Many other countries do not have nationwide screening programs for gastric cancer, especially in areas with low incidence rates of gastric cancer including United States and most Europe countries.

South Korea

South Korea has the highest incidence of gastric cancer in the world.[2] It was the first country to introduce upper gastrointestinal endoscopy as a nationwide gastric cancer screening method. The National Cancer Screening Program (NCSP) was launched in 1999 by the Ministry of Health and Welfare in South Korea. NCSP has provided biennial screening for gastric cancer with upper gastrointestinal endoscopy or UGIS for individuals aged 40 years and older.[54] The participation rates for gastric cancer screening increased from 7.40% in 2002 to 45.40% in 2011. In terms of screening modality, upper gastrointestinal endoscopy has been increasingly used compared with UGIS, from 31.15% in 2002 to 72.55% in 2011.[49] In addition, quality assurance is required based on the law, and the screening results are collected to the national cancer registry.

Since the NCSP began, the risk of death from gastric cancer has decreased by 47% with upper gastrointestinal endoscopy.[10] In South Korea, cost of upper gastrointestinal endoscopy is similar to that of UGIS. Considering the low cost of upper gastrointestinal endoscopy, the high incidence of gastric cancer, and the effect in reducing gastric cancer mortality, upper gastrointestinal endoscopy seems to be the most cost-effective modality of gastric cancer screening in South Korea.[8,42]

Japan

Japan was the first country to introduce nationwide gastric cancer screening program. It was initially introduced in Miyagi Prefecture with UGIS in 1960. In 1983, nationwide gastric cancer screening program with UGIS was adopted for individuals aged 40 years and older.[38] In 2015, upper gastrointestinal endoscopy was added to the Japanese guideline for gastric cancer screening.[55] In the updated guideline released in 2018, population-based nationwide screening is recommended for individuals aged 50 years and older with upper gastrointestinal endoscopy or UGIS.[56,57] The participation rate of gastric cancer screening in Japan differs largely among the municipalities and has been reported to increase from 20.7% to 26.7% after the introduction of upper gastrointestinal endoscopy as a screening method.[57,58] The cost for upper gastrointestinal endoscopy in Japan is around $112 US dollars. As in South Korea, upper gastrointestinal endoscopy is increasingly preferred as screening modality compared with UGIS in Japan.[57,59] The Japanese government collects the results of cancer screening and publishes a summary every year.

Other Countries

In Taiwan, gastric cancer screening program has been implemented in Matsu Island, where gastric cancer incidence is relatively high. In 1995, screening program with upper gastrointestinal endoscopy was recommended to individuals with low serum level of PG (<30 ng/mL).[60] In 2004, Taiwanese Ministry of Health initiated population-based *H pylori* eradication program, which provided upper gastrointestinal endoscopy and *H pylori* eradication for individuals who were tested positive for C-urea breath test.[61]

In Singapore, gastric cancer screening is targeted at high-risk groups rather than population-based nationwide screening. A cost-benefit study of endoscopic screening for gastric cancer in Singapore concluded that endoscopic screening was cost-effective in moderate- to high-risk groups such as Chinese men aged 50 to 70 years.[4,62]

China has no nationwide screening program but has adopted gastric cancer screening for high-risk groups in some regions with high incidence of gastric cancer. In 2008, two-step screening program including upper gastrointestinal endoscopy was adopted in high-risk regions in China, including Wuwei, Linqu and Zhuanghe, by the Central Financial Transfer Payment Projects.[63,64]

EFFECTIVENESS OF SCREENING PROGRAM OF GASTRIC CANCER: MORTALITY REDUCTION

To date, no randomized controlled trial has been conducted regarding the effect of gastric cancer screening on mortality and is difficult to conduct. Several case-control studies and cohort studies were performed in Japan, South Korea, and China.[10,65–74] In a recent meta-analysis including 4 case-control studies and 6 cohort studies in Asia, which comprised about 34,000 individuals, endoscopic screening for gastric cancer was associated with 40% reduction of gastric cancer mortality (**Fig. 1**). There was no association between endoscopic screening and the incidence of gastric cancer.[74] Although significant heterogeneity between the included studies and possible confounding effect by *H pylori*, the investigators concluded that upper gastrointestinal endoscopy for gastric cancer screening may reduce the risk of gastric cancer mortality in Asian countries.[74] Several case-control studies and cohort studies conducted in Japan reported a 31%–79% reduction in mortality of gastric cancer in individuals screened with upper gastrointestinal endoscopy.[65,66,68,69,71,72] The largest study was conducted in South Korea as a nested case-control study with 27,290

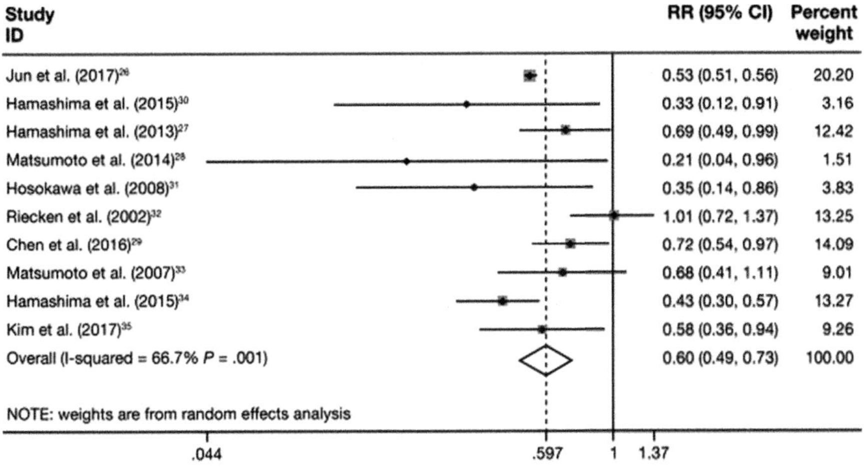

Fig. 1. Forest plot of reduction of gastric cancer morality after endoscopic screening. ID, identification. (*From* Zhang X, Li M, Chen S, et al. Endoscopic Screening in Asian Countries Is Associated With Reduced Gastric Cancer Mortality: A Meta-analysis and Systematic Review. *Gastroenterology.* 2018;155(2):347 to 354 e349; with permission.)

individuals aged 40 years or older.[10] The study analyzed the effect of NCSP with upper gastrointestinal endoscopy and UGIS on gastric cancer mortality and compared the effect between 2 different screening modalities. The risk for gastric cancer mortality was reduced by 47% for ever-screened individuals with upper gastrointestinal endoscopy compared with individuals who were never screened. Interestingly, endoscopic screening showed a dose-dependent effect in gastric cancer mortality. In individuals who underwent endoscopy twice, gastric cancer mortality was reduced by 68% and in individuals who underwent endoscopy 3 times or more, gastric cancer mortality was reduced by 81%. Also, analysis of time interval from the last screening date to the diagnosis date of gastric cancer showed the effect in mortality reduction remained significant even in intervals of 48 months or more. Individuals who were ever screened with UGIS only did not show significant reduction in gastric cancer mortality.

ISSUES AND CONCERNS OF SCREENING PROGRAM

Screening Interval

The interval of gastric cancer screening is important in the aspect of medical cost and the risk of gastric cancer progression. Short intervals may warrant early detection, but problems such as patient compliance, medical cost, and lack of facilities arise. Long screening intervals may be economical, but risk of gastric cancers detected in advanced stage cannot be excluded. A study of 2362 patients that aimed to evaluate the effect of endoscopic screening interval on overall survival of patients with gastric cancer concluded that endoscopic evaluation with 1 to 3 years interval before gastric cancer diagnosis reduced overall mortality of patients with gastric cancer.[75] The study also conducted a spline analysis and confirmed a U-shaped relationship between the endoscopic screening interval and the mortality risk and concluded that screening interval of 32 months seems to be associated with the lowest overall mortality (hazard ratio, 0.65; 95% confidence interval 0.52–0.81).[75]

Cost-effectiveness

Cost-effectiveness analysis was conducted in several countries including United States. In United States, one study evaluated the incremental cost-effectiveness ratio (ICER) of one-time screening of gastric cancer at the age of 50 years and concluded that the ICER for screening remained high.[76] Another study reported that endoscopic screening is cost-effective for Asian Americans, especially for Japanese, Korean, and Chinese Americans aged 50 years or older in the United States.[77]

In South Korea, several studies regarding cost-effectiveness were conducted, as the Korean government requires such studies as a report of the NCSP program. Until now, 3 studies reported the screening program to be cost-effective, and endoscopic screening was a more cost-effective strategy compared with UGIS.[8,42,78] One study using time-dependent Markov model comparing different screening methods and intervals concluded that annual endoscopy was most cost-effective in men aged 50–80 years and biennial endoscopy was most cost-effective in women aged 50–80 years.[8] Similarly, one Japanese study reported upper gastrointestinal endoscopy to be the best method for detecting early gastric cancer and the most cost-effective strategy compared with other screening methods including UGIS.[7]

Missed Cancers and Endoscopic Quality

Missed cancer rates vary by country, with 2% to 10% in Western populations and 20% to 40% in Eastern Asia. Differences in gastric cancer incidence, indication, and adoption of screening programs may have contributed to the discrepancy.[79] A recent Japanese study reported that an endoscopist with experience in less than 500 cases of upper gastrointestinal endoscopy was associated with 3-fold increased risk of missed gastric cancer.[80] A recent Korean study reported that observation time of longer than 3 minutes or more increased the detection rate of early gastric cancer and gastric dysplasia compared with observation time of less than 3 minutes.[81] The European Society of Gastrointestinal Endoscopy (ESGE) quality improvement initiative recommended several performance measures including procedure time of minimum 7 minutes for the first diagnostic upper gastrointestinal endoscopy.[82]

SURVEILLANCE IN HIGH-RISK POPULATION

Although screening programs in South Korea and Japan are known to be effective in reducing mortality and are cost-effective, it should be noted that the cost of upper gastrointestinal endoscopy is low and the incidence of gastric cancer is high in these countries. Such nationwide population-based screening programs would be difficult to apply in others countries with low incidence of gastric cancer or with limited medical resources. Therefore, in many other countries, upper gastrointestinal endoscopy is targeted to high-risk population as a surveillance strategy. Currently, however, no standardized international recommendations have been established.

Atrophic Gastritis, Intestinal Metaplasia, and Gastric Dysplasia

Atrophic gastritis and intestinal metaplasia are well known as the precursor lesions of gastric cancer.[83] Chronic inflammation of gastric mucosa is known to trigger a sequence of chronic active gastritis, atrophic gastritis, intestinal metaplasia, dysplasia, and gastric adenocarcinoma.[84] Thus, surveillance of gastric cancer is considered to be important in patients with gastric atrophy, intestinal metaplasia, and dysplasia.

A multidisciplinary group in Europe including the ESGE published management guidelines for precancerous conditions and lesions in the stomach (MAPS) in 2012.

The guidelines emphasize surveillance in high-risk groups with gastric atrophy, intestinal metaplasia, and dysplasia. Suggested surveillance interval varies according to the degree and extent of atrophy and intestinal metaplasia and grade of dysplasia, which ranges from 6 months to 3 years. However, this guideline does not address screening methodologies in general populations.[85]

On the contrary, a recent guideline on management of gastric intestinal metaplasia published by the American Gastroenterological Association suggests against routine use of endoscopic surveillance in patients with gastric intestinal metaplasia. The guideline suggested patients with gastric intestinal metaplasia at higher risk for gastric cancers, such as patients with family history of gastric cancer, ethnic minorities, or patients with extensive gastric intestinal metaplasia, may elect for surveillance.[19]

In Japan, a recent recommendation suggested 1- to 2-year surveillance in patients with gastric atrophy.[86] Another study reported the usefulness of surveillance using risk stratification by *H pylori* serology in combination with PG test results and recommended 1-year surveillance for *H pylori*-negative and PG-positive cases.[40]

Family History

Individuals with family history of gastric cancer are associated with higher risk of gastric cancer with odds ratio ranging from 2 to 10.[87] However, there was no definite endoscopic surveillance guidelines of family members of patients with sporadic gastric cancer. A small portion of gastric cancer is related to hereditary syndromes. In family members of hereditary diffuse gastric cancer, annual endoscopic surveillance with high-definition endoscope is recommended in individuals who did not receive gastrectomy.[88]

Surveillance for Metachronous Gastric Cancer

Patients with history of gastric cancer treated with surgery or endoscopic resection have a risk for cancer development in the remnant stomach. Previous studies have reported the incidence of metachronous gastric cancer of about 3% to 4% per year.[80,89,90] In a Japanese guideline, the interval of endoscopic surveillance after endoscopic resection of gastric cancer was recommended to be annual or biannual.[91] Several other studies recommend the endoscopic follow-up interval to be within 3 months for the initial follow-up, 6 months, and then 12 months.[80,92]

SUMMARY

Gastric cancer is one of the most common cancers worldwide. The incidence varies widely by geographic region, with half of new cases occurring in East Asia. Population-based nationwide screening for gastric cancer is implemented in some Eastern Asian countries with high incidence of gastric cancer including South Korea and Japan. Upper gastrointestinal endoscopy is increasingly preferred as a screening method. Endoscopic screening for gastric cancer decreased the mortality of gastric cancer and the effect on mortality reduction was superior to UGIS. Endoscopic screening is a cost-effective screening modality in countries with high incidence of gastric cancer and an interval of 1 to 3 years seems optimal. To reduce missed cancers and improve screening quality, sufficient procedure time and endoscopic experience should be achieved. In countries with low incidence of gastric cancer, surveillance targeted to high-risk population such as individuals with atrophy, intestinal metaplasia, gastric dysplasia, family history of gastric cancer, and previous history of gastric cancer should be considered.

CLINICS CARE POINTS

- Population-based endoscopic screening of gastric cancer decreased gastric cancer mortality in countries with high incidence of gastric cancer such as South Korea and Japan. In these countries, endoscopic screening is a cost-effective modality. However, the benefit and cost-effectiveness of population-based screening is uncertain in countries with low incidence of gastric cancer.
- Sufficient procedure time and endoscopic experience should be achieved to reduce missed cancers and improve screening quality.
- In countries with low incidence of gastric cancer, surveillance targeted to high-risk population such as individuals with atrophy, intestinal metaplasia, gastric dysplasia, family history of gastric cancer, and previous history of gastric cancer should be considered.

DISCLOSURE

This study was supported by grants from the National Research Foundation of Korea (#NRF-2019R1A2C1009923), the Korean College of Helicobacter and Upper Gastrointestinal Research Foundation (#KCHUGR - 202002001), and the SNUH research fund (#03-2020-0370).

REFERENCES

1. Torre LA, Bray F, Siegel RL, et al. Global cancer statistics, 2012. CA Cancer J Clin 2015;65(2):87–108.
2. Bray F, Ferlay J, Soerjomataram I, et al. Global cancer statistics 2018: GLOBOCAN estimates of incidence and mortality worldwide for 36 cancers in 185 countries. CA Cancer J Clin 2018;68(6):394–424.
3. Ferlay J, Shin HR, Bray F, et al. Estimates of worldwide burden of cancer in 2008: GLOBOCAN 2008. Int J Cancer 2010;127(12):2893–917.
4. Leung WK, Wu MS, Kakugawa Y, et al. Screening for gastric cancer in Asia: current evidence and practice. Lancet Oncol 2008;9(3):279–87.
5. Fock KM, Talley N, Moayyedi P, et al. Asia-Pacific consensus guidelines on gastric cancer prevention. J Gastroenterol Hepatol 2008;23(3):351–65.
6. Choi KS, Jun JK, Park EC, et al. Performance of different gastric cancer screening methods in Korea: a population-based study. PLoS One 2012;7(11):e50041.
7. Tashiro A, Sano M, Kinameri K, et al. Comparing mass screening techniques for gastric cancer in Japan. World J Gastroenterol 2006;12(30):4873–4.
8. Lee HY, Park EC, Jun JK, et al. Comparing upper gastrointestinal X-ray and endoscopy for gastric cancer diagnosis in Korea. World J Gastroenterol 2010;16(2):245–50.
9. Hisamichi S, Sugawara N, Fukao A. Effectiveness of gastric mass screening in Japan. Cancer Detect Prev 1988;11(3–6):323–9.
10. Jun JK, Choi KS, Lee HY, et al. Effectiveness of the Korean National Cancer screening program in reducing gastric cancer mortality. Gastroenterology 2017;152(6):1319–+.
11. Murakami R, Tsukuma H, Ubukata T, et al. Estimation of validity of mass-screening program for gastric-cancer in Osaka, Japan. Cancer 1990;65(5):1255–60.

12. Oshima A, Hirata N, Ubukata T, et al. Evaluation of a mass-screening program for stomach-cancer with a case-control study design. Int J Cancer 1986;38(6): 829–33.
13. Inaba S, Hirayama H, Nagata C, et al. Evaluation of a screening program on reduction of gastric cancer mortality in Japan: Preliminary results from a cohort study. Prev Med 1999;29(2):102–6.
14. Kunisaki C, Ishino J, Nakajima S, et al. Outcomes of mass screening for gastric carcinoma. Ann Surg Oncol 2006;13(2):221–8.
15. Mizoue T, Yoshimura T, Tokui N, et al. Prospective study of screening for stomach cancer in Japan. Int J Cancer 2003;106(1):103–7.
16. Choi KS, Jun JK, Suh M, et al. Effect of endoscopy screening on stage at gastric cancer diagnosis: results of the National Cancer Screening Programme in Korea. Br J Cancer 2015;112(3):608–12.
17. Zhang X, Li M, Chen S, et al. Endoscopic screening in asian countries is associated with reduced gastric cancer mortality: a meta-analysis and systematic review. Gastroenterology 2018;155(2):347–354 e9.
18. Pimentel-Nunes P, Libanio D, Marcos-Pinto R, et al. Management of epithelial precancerous conditions and lesions in the stomach (MAPS II): European Society of Gastrointestinal Endoscopy (ESGE), European Helicobacter and Microbiota Study Group (EHMSG), European Society of Pathology (ESP), and Sociedade Portuguesa de Endoscopia Digestiva (SPED) guideline update 2019. Endoscopy 2019;51(4):365–88.
19. Gupta S, Li D, El Serag HB, et al. AGA clinical practice guidelines on management of gastric intestinal Metaplasia. Gastroenterology 2020;158(3):693–702.
20. Areia M, Carvalho R, Cadime AT, et al. Screening for gastric cancer and surveillance of premalignant lesions: a systematic review of cost-effectiveness studies. Helicobacter 2013;18(5):325–37.
21. Busuttil RA, Boussioutas A. Intestinal metaplasia: a premalignant lesion involved in gastric carcinogenesis. J Gastroenterol Hepatol 2009;24(2):193–201.
22. Tava F, Luinetti O, Ghigna MR, et al. Type or extension of intestinal metaplasia and immature/atypical "indefinite-for-dysplasia" lesions as predictors of gastric neoplasia. Hum Pathol 2006;37(11):1489–97.
23. Whiting JL, Sigurdsson A, Rowlands DC, et al. The long term results of endoscopic surveillance of premalignant gastric lesions. Gut 2002;50(3):378–81.
24. Zullo A, Hassan C, Romiti A, et al. Follow-up of intestinal metaplasia in the stomach: When, how and why. World J Gastrointest Oncol 2012;4(3):30–6.
25. Chung SJ, Park MJ, Kang SJ, et al. Effect of annual endoscopic screening on clinicopathologic characteristics and treatment modality of gastric cancer in a high-incidence region of Korea. Int J Cancer 2012;131(10):2376–84.
26. Yoon H, Kim N, Lee HS, et al. Effect of endoscopic screening at 1-year intervals on the clinicopathologic characteristics and treatment of gastric cancer in South Korea. J Gastroenterol Hepatol 2012;27(5):928–34.
27. Luo G, Zhang Y, Guo P, et al. Global patterns and trends in stomach cancer incidence: age, period and birth cohort analysis. Int J Cancer 2017;141(7):1333–44.
28. Jemal A, Siegel R, Xu J, et al. Cancer statistics, 2010. CA Cancer J Clin 2010; 60(5):277–300.
29. Katanoda K, Yako-Suketomo H. Comparison of time trends in stomach cancer incidence (1973-2002) in Asia, from Cancer Incidence in Five Continents, Vols IV-IX. Jpn J Clin Oncol 2009;39(1):71–2.
30. Balakrishnan M, George R, Sharma A, et al. Changing Trends in Stomach Cancer Throughout the World. Curr Gastroenterol Rep 2017;19(8):36.

31. Rawla P, Barsouk A. Epidemiology of gastric cancer: global trends, risk factors and prevention. Prz Gastroenterol 2019;14(1):26–38.
32. Sitarz R, Skierucha M, Mielko J, et al. Gastric cancer: epidemiology, prevention, classification, and treatment. Cancer Manag Res 2018;10:239–48.
33. Allemani C, Matsuda T, Di Carlo V, et al. Global surveillance of trends in cancer survival 2000-14 (CONCORD-3): analysis of individual records for 37 513 025 patients diagnosed with one of 18 cancers from 322 population-based registries in 71 countries. Lancet 2018;391(10125):1023–75.
34. Hong S, Won YJ, Park YR, et al. Cancer Statistics in Korea: incidence, mortality, survival, and prevalence in 2017. Cancer Res Treat 2020;52(2):335–50.
35. Matsuda T, Ajiki W, Marugame T, et al. Population-based survival of cancer patients diagnosed between 1993 and 1999 in Japan: a chronological and international comparative study. Jpn J Clin Oncol 2011;41(1):40–51.
36. Collaborators GBDSC. The global, regional, and national burden of stomach cancer in 195 countries, 1990-2017: a systematic analysis for the Global Burden of Disease study 2017. Lancet Gastroenterol Hepatol 2020;5(1):42–54.
37. Aikou S, Ohmoto Y, Gunji T, et al. Tests for serum levels of trefoil factor family proteins can improve gastric cancer screening. Gastroenterology 2011;141(3):837.
38. Hamashima C, Shibuya D, Yamazaki H, et al. The Japanese guidelines for gastric cancer screening. Jpn J Clin Oncol 2008;38(4):259–67.
39. Miki K, Morita M, Sasajima M, et al. Gastric cancer screening using the serum pepsinogen test method. Am J Gastroenterol 2002;97(9):S46.
40. Watabe H, Mitsushima T, Yamaji Y, et al. Predicting the development of gastric cancer from combining Helicobacter pylori antibodies and serum pepsinogen status: a prospective endoscopic cohort study. Gut 2005;54(6):764–8.
41. Yoshihara M, Hiyama T, Yoshida S, et al. Reduction in gastric cancer mortality by screening based on serum pepsinogen concentration: a case-control study. Scand J Gastroentero 2007;42(6):760–4.
42. Cho E, Kang MH, Choi KS, et al. Cost-effectiveness outcomes of the national gastric cancer screening program in South Korea. Asian Pac J Cancer Prev 2013;14(4):2533–40.
43. Cui L, Lou YR, Zhang XJ, et al. Detection of circulating tumor cells in peripheral blood from patients with gastric cancer using piRNAs as markers. Clin Biochem 2011;44(13):1050–7.
44. Lim LG, Yeoh KG, Salto-Tellez M, et al. Experienced versus inexperienced confocal endoscopists in the diagnosis of gastric adenocarcinoma and intestinal metaplasia on confocal images. Gastrointest Endosc 2011;73(6):1141–7.
45. Shaw D, Blair V, Framp A, et al. Chromoendoscopic surveillance in hereditary diffuse gastric cancer: an alternative to prophylactic gastrectomy? Gut 2005; 54(4):461–8.
46. Mayinger B, Jordan M, Horbach T, et al. Evaluation of in vivo endoscopic autofluorescence spectroscopy in gastric cancer. Gastrointest Endosc 2004;59(2): 191–8.
47. Tajiri H, Doi T, Endo H, et al. Routine endoscopy using a magnifying endoscope for gastric cancer diagnosis. Endoscopy 2002;34(10):772–7.
48. Fukao A, Tsubono Y, Tsuji I, et al. The evaluation of screening for gastric cancer in Miyagi Prefecture, Japan: a population-based case-control study. Int J Cancer 1995;60(1):45–8.
49. Lee S, Jun JK, Suh M, et al. Gastric cancer screening uptake trends in Korea: results for the National Cancer Screening Program from 2002 to 2011: a prospective cross-sectional study. Medicine (Baltimore) 2015;94(8):e533.

50. Hamashima C, Okamoto M, Shabana M, et al. Sensitivity of endoscopic screening for gastric cancer by the incidence method. Int J Cancer 2013; 133(3):653–9.
51. Choi KS, Suh M. Screening for gastric cancer: the usefulness of endoscopy. Clin Endosc 2014;47(6):490–6.
52. Kim GH, Liang PS, Bang SJ, et al. Screening and surveillance for gastric cancer in the United States: is it needed? Gastrointest Endosc 2016;84(1):18–28.
53. Kato M, Asaka M. Recent development of gastric cancer prevention. Jpn J Clin Oncol 2012;42(11):987–94.
54. Yoo KY. Cancer control activities in the Republic of Korea. Jpn J Clin Oncol 2008; 38(5):327–33.
55. Sugano K. Screening of gastric cancer in Asia. Best Pract Res Clin Gastroenterol 2015;29(6):895–905.
56. Hamashima C, Kim Y, Choi KS. Comparison of guidelines and management for gastric cancer screening between Korea and Japan. Value Health 2015;18(3): A272–.
57. Hamashima C. Systematic Review G, Guideline Development Group for Gastric Cancer Screening G. Update version of the Japanese Guidelines for Gastric Cancer Screening. Jpn J Clin Oncol 2018;48(7):673–83.
58. Shabana M, Hamashima C, Nishida M, et al. Current status and evaluation of endoscopic screening for gastric cancer. Jpn J Cancer Detect Diagn 2010;17: 229–35 [In Japanese].
59. Hamashima C, Goto R. Potential capacity of endoscopic screening for gastric cancer in Japan. Cancer Sci 2017;108(1):101–7.
60. Liu CY, Wu CY, Lin JT, et al. Multistate and multifactorial progression of gastric cancer: results from community-based mass screening for gastric cancer. J Med Screen 2006;13(Suppl 1):S2–5.
61. Lee YC, Wu HM, Chen TH, et al. A community-based study of Helicobacter pylori therapy using the strategy of test, treat, retest, and re-treat initial treatment failures. Helicobacter 2006;11(5):418–24.
62. Dan YY, So JB, Yeoh KG. Endoscopic screening for gastric cancer. Clin Gastroenterol Hepatol 2006;4(6):709–16.
63. WC Y. Progress in early detection and treatment for gastric cancer. Zhongguo Zhong Liu 2009;18:695–9.
64. Yuan Y. Population-based gastric cancer screening in Zhuanghe, Liaoning, from 1997 to 2011. Zhonghua Zhong Liu Za Zhi 2012;34(7):538–42.
65. Hamashima C, Ogoshi K, Okamoto M, et al. A community-based, case-control study evaluating mortality reduction from gastric cancer by endoscopic screening in Japan. PLoS One 2013;8(11):e79088.
66. Matsumoto S, Yoshida Y. Efficacy of endoscopic screening in an isolated island: a case-control study. Indian J Gastroenterol 2014;33(1):46–9.
67. Chen Q, Yu L, Hao CQ, et al. Effectiveness of endoscopic gastric cancer screening in a rural area of Linzhou, China: results from a case-control study. Cancer Med 2016;5(9):2615–22.
68. Hamashima C, Shabana M, Okada K, et al. Mortality reduction from gastric cancer by endoscopic and radiographic screening. Cancer Sci 2015;106(12): 1744–9.
69. Hosokawa O, Miyanaga T, Kaizaki Y, et al. Decreased death from gastric cancer by endoscopic screening: association with a population-based cancer registry. Scand J Gastroenterol 2008;43(9):1112–5.

70. Riecken B, Pfeiffer R, Ma JL, et al. No impact of repeated endoscopic screens on gastric cancer mortality in a prospectively followed Chinese population at high risk. Prev Med 2002;34(1):22–8.
71. Matsumoto S, Yamasaki K, Tsuji K, et al. Results of mass endoscopic examination for gastric cancer in Kamigoto Hospital, Nagasaki Prefecture. World J Gastroenterol 2007;13(32):4316–20.
72. Hamashima C, Ogoshi K, Narisawa R, et al. Impact of endoscopic screening on mortality reduction from gastric cancer. World J Gastroenterol 2015;21(8): 2460–6.
73. Kim H, Hwang Y, Sung H, et al. Effectiveness of gastric cancer screening on gastric cancer incidence and mortality in a community-based prospective cohort. Cancer Res Treat 2018;50(2):582–9.
74. Zhang X, Li M, Chen ST, et al. EndoscopiC SCreening in Asian Countries is associated with reduced gastric cancer mortality: a meta-analysis and systematic review. Gastroenterology 2018;155(2):347–54.
75. Choi SI, Park B, Joo J, et al. Three-year interval for endoscopic screening may reduce the mortality in patients with gastric cancer. Surg Endosc Other Interv Tech 2019;33(3):861–9.
76. Gupta N, Bansal A, Wani SB, et al. Endoscopy for upper GI cancer screening in the general population: a cost-utility analysis. Gastrointest Endosc 2011;74(3): 610–24.e2.
77. Shah SC, Canakis A, Peek RM Jr, et al. Endoscopy for Gastric Cancer Screening Is Cost Effective for Asian Americans in the United States. Clin Gastroenterol Hepatol 2020;18(13):3026–39.
78. Chang HS, Park EC, Chung W, et al. Comparing endoscopy and upper gastrointestinal X-ray for gastric cancer screening in South Korea: a cost-utility analysis. Asian Pac J Cancer Prev 2012;13(6):2721–8.
79. Veitch AM, Uedo N, Yao K, et al. Optimizing early upper gastrointestinal cancer detection at endoscopy. Nat Rev Gastroenterol Hepatol 2015;12(11):660–7.
80. Kato M, Nishida T, Yamamoto K, et al. Scheduled endoscopic surveillance controls secondary cancer after curative endoscopic resection for early gastric cancer: a multicentre retrospective cohort study by Osaka University ESD study group. Gut 2013;62(10):1425–32.
81. Park JM, Huo SM, Lee HH, et al. Longer observation time increases proportion of neoplasms detected by esophagogastroduodenoscopy. Gastroenterology 2017; 153(2):460–469 e1.
82. Bisschops R, Areia M, Coron E, et al. Performance measures for upper gastrointestinal endoscopy: a European Society of Gastrointestinal Endoscopy (ESGE) Quality Improvement Initiative. Endoscopy 2016;48(9):843–64.
83. Uemura N, Okamoto S, Yamamoto S, et al. Helicobacter pylori infection and the development of gastric cancer. N Engl J Med 2001;345(11):784–9.
84. Correa P. Human gastric carcinogenesis: a multistep and multifactorial process–First American Cancer Society Award Lecture on Cancer Epidemiology and Prevention. Cancer Res 1992;52(24):6735–40.
85. Dinis-Ribeiro M, Areia M, de Vries AC, et al. Management of precancerous conditions and lesions in the stomach (MAPS): guideline from the European Society of Gastrointestinal Endoscopy (ESGE), European Helicobacter Study Group (EHSG), European Society of Pathology (ESP), and the Sociedade Portuguesa de Endoscopia Digestiva (SPED). Endoscopy 2012;44(1):74–94.
86. Asaka M. A new approach for elimination of gastric cancer deaths in Japan. Int J Cancer 2013;132(6):1272–6.

87. Yaghoobi M, Bijarchi R, Narod SA. Family history and the risk of gastric cancer. Br J Cancer 2010;102(2):237–42.
88. Kluijt I, Sijmons RH, Hoogerbrugge N, et al. Familial gastric cancer: guidelines for diagnosis, treatment and periodic surveillance. Fam Cancer 2012;11(3):363–9.
89. Nasu J, Doi T, Endo H, et al. Characteristics of metachronous multiple early gastric cancers after endoscopic mucosal resection. Endoscopy 2005;37(10): 990–3.
90. Jang MY, Cho JW, Oh WG, et al. Clinicopathological characteristics of synchronous and metachronous gastric neoplasms after endoscopic submucosal dissection. Korean J Intern Med 2013;28(6):687–93.
91. Japanese Gastric Cancer A. Japanese gastric cancer treatment guidelines 2014 (ver. 4). Gastric Cancer 2017;20(1):1–19.
92. Nakajima T, Oda I, Gotoda T, et al. Metachronous gastric cancers after endoscopic resection: how effective is annual endoscopic surveillance? Gastric Cancer 2006;9(2):93–8.

Improving the Early Diagnosis of Gastric Cancer

Robert J. Huang, MD, MS*, Joo Ha Hwang, MD, PhD

KEYWORDS

- *Helicobacter pylori* • Intestinal metaplasia • Endoscopic screening • Early detection
- Cancer stage • East Asia

KEY POINTS

- Patients are diagnosed with gastric cancer at more advanced stages and have overall lower survival in the United States compared with East Asia.
- Observational data from Japan and South Korea, nations with national gastric cancer screening programs, show that endoscopic screening may improve gastric cancer mortality.
- In the United States high-risk racial/ethnic groups (Alaskan Natives, American Indians, Asians, Blacks, Hispanics), first-generation immigrants form high-incidence regions, and individuals with a family history may benefit from screening.
- Individuals with intestinal metaplasia, particularly extensive or histologically severe disease, may benefit from endoscopic surveillance.
- A video of use of chromoendoscopy to enhance detection of gastric intestinal metaplasia accompanies this article.

Video content accompanies this article at http://www.giendo.theclinics.com.

INTRODUCTION

Every year 1.2 million persons are diagnosed with and 860,000 persons die from gastric cancer (GC) worldwide,[1] making GC the fifth leading cause of cancer incidence and third leading cause of cancer mortality, respectively.[2] Outcomes from GC in most of the world remain poor, including in the United States (US). In the US, GC afflicts 27,000 each year[3] and carries a dismal prognosis (5-year survival of 27%).[4] These statistics reflect the fact that most of the GCs in the US are diagnosed at advanced stages,[4] where curative resection is unlikely. Strategies to improve the early diagnosis of GC are therefore crucial to improving survival.

Division of Gastroenterology and Hepatology, Stanford University, 300 Pasteur Drive, Alway Building M211, Stanford, CA 94305, USA
* Corresponding author.
E-mail address: rjhuang@stanford.edu

Gastrointest Endoscopy Clin N Am 31 (2021) 503–517
https://doi.org/10.1016/j.giec.2021.03.005

GCs are classified as cardia or noncardia based on the anatomic location of origin within the stomach. Cardia GCs, which share risk factors and natural history with esophageal adenocarcinomas, constitute approximately one-quarter of GCs worldwide.[5] Noncardia GCs constitute three-quarters of GCs worldwide, have witnessed improvements in outcomes following adoption of screening programs in nations of East Asia,[6,7] and are the focus of this review.

HELICOBACTER PYLORI AND CORREA'S CASCADE

Development of noncardia GC has been linked, in multiple epidemiologic studies, with infection with the gram-negative, microaerophilic organism *H pylori* (Hp).[8,9] Worldwide Hp prevalence rates range from less than 40% in industrialized nations of Western Europe and North America to greater than 70% in areas of South America, Africa, Eastern Europe, and East Asia.[10] Hp infection is associated with a 3-fold increase in lifetime odds of development of noncardia GC; moreover, Hp is believed responsible for 75% to 95% of all GC cases worldwide.[11,12] Colonization with Hp induces a state of chronic inflammatory insult that leads to a cascade of mucosa perturbations, termed Correa's cascade (**Fig. 1**).[13] In Correa's cascade, chronic gastritis is followed by progressive atrophy of the oxyntic or antral gastric mucosa and then eventual replacement by intestinal mucosa consisting of Paneth, goblet, and absorptive cells. Intestinal metaplasia (IM) of the stomach is an important precursor lesion in the pathway to GC,[14–17] and regional prevalence of IM correlates closely with incidence of GC worldwide.[18] Even with decreasing prevalence of Hp, with the secular aging of the global population GC cases and deaths are expected to climb well into the twenty-first century.[19,20]

GASTRIC CANCER SCREENING AND OUTCOMES IN EAST ASIA

The incidence of GC is significantly higher in nations of East Asia compared with the US. Although the incidence of GC is roughly 6 per 100,000 in the US, it is approximately 28 per 100,000 in Japan and 34 per 100,000 in South Korea. Yet although incidence of GC is much higher in these countries, survival from GC is also higher compared with the US or Western Europe (**Fig. 2**). Five-year observed survival from GC exceeds 60% in both South Korea and Japan, compared with less than 30% for the US and Western Europe.[21,22] These differences in survival are due in large part to differences in stage of diagnosis. Although nearly 60% of GCs are diagnosed at a surgically or endoscopically curable stage in South Korea and Japan, fewer than a quarter of GCs are diagnosed at such stages in the West.[4,23–25]

In Japan, a national screening program for GC was first introduced in 1983. This program consisted of radiography-based screening of all adults older than or equal to 40 years, with endoscopic examination performed on individuals with abnormal radiographic results.[26] Based on the results of several rigorous observational studies, the national screening program was amended in 2016 to allow for either endoscopic or radiographic screening for adults older than or equal to 50 years on a biennial basis.[26]

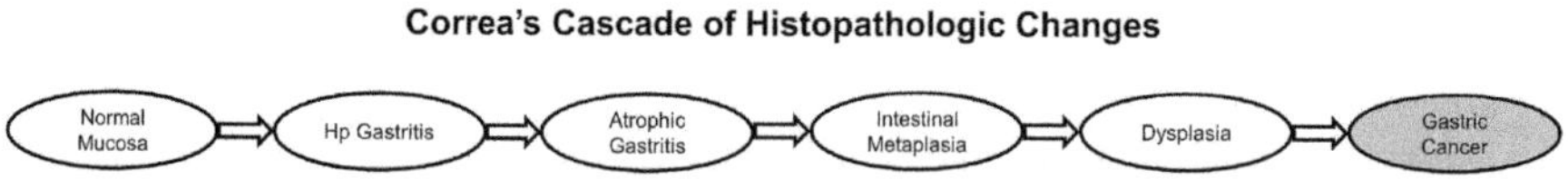

Fig. 1. Proposed carcinogenic cascade induced by *Helicobacter pylori* (Hp) and other environmental insult. Patients with atrophic gastritis, intestinal metaplasia, and dysplasia remain at increased risk for gastric cancer even following Hp eradication.

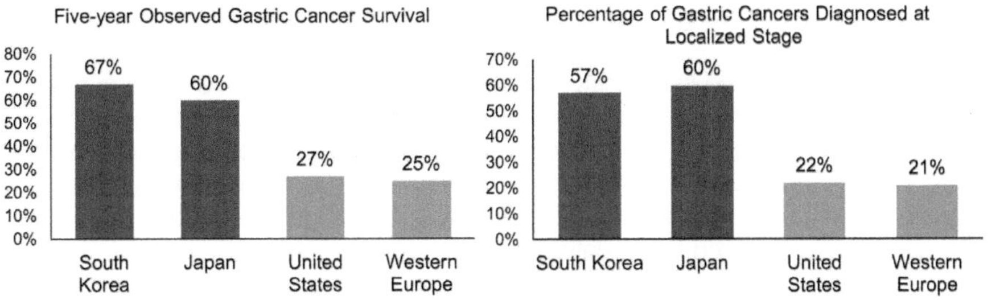

Fig. 2. Left panel depicts 5-year observed survival following gastric cancer diagnosis in East Asia (South Korea, Japan) and Western nations (United States and Europe). Right panel depicts the proportion of all gastric cancers diagnosed at localized stage based on United States National Cancer Institute summary staging. (*Data from* Refs.[4,23–25])

Although endoscopic screening is rapidly being adopted throughout Japan, radiographic screening is still the predominant screening modality in most prefectures.[27]

South Korea initiated a biennial screening program consisting of either endoscopic or radiographic screening for adults older than or equal to 40 years in 2002.[28] In practice, endoscopic screening has been the predominant modality practiced in South Korea due to patient preference. Since the initiation of the national screening program, the proportion of GCs diagnosed as early GC (defined as tumor with invasion limited to mucosa or submucosa) has increased from 39% in 2001 to 73% in 2016.[29] Moreover, observed 5-year survival has increased from 46% to 75%.[29]

EFFICACY AND SAFETY OF SCREENING MODALITIES

Radiographic Screening

Radiographic screening involves the ingestion of a contrast agent (often barium) and subsequent fluoroscopic imaging of the gastric lumen. Contrast radiography allows for the detection of luminal pathology including ulcers, polyps, and masses. However, compared with modern endoscopy, radiography has both limited sensitivity and specificity.[30] Cancer registry data suggest that the sensitivity of radiographic screening ranges from 60% to 80% and specificity from 80% to 90%.[6] It should also be noted that for early GC (where a luminal prominence or depression may be minimal), the sensitivity of radiography has been reported to be significantly lower (14%–36%).[31,32]

The efficacy of radiographic screening has been assessed in several observational studies, including both cohort and case-control studies,[26] although notably no randomized controlled trial has been conducted comparing radiographic screening with standard of care. From cohort studies from Japan[33,34] comparing radiographic screening with no screening over long-term follow-up (11–13 years), receiving radiographic screening was associated with both reductions in GC-specific mortality (relative risk 0.52–0.54) as well as all-cause mortality (relative risk 0.71–0.83). However, during the period of these studies radiography was also a standard test for assessment of gastrointestinal symptoms, introducing the possibility of confounding by indication. Moreover, receipt of subsequent screening (such as by endoscopy) in the follow-up period was not ascertained possibly causing overestimation of the effect size. The safety profile of radiographic screening is generally favorable, with mild risk of constipation or ileus and rare cases of aspiration pneumonia.[6] In a report of more than 3 million radiographic screening procedures performed, only a single death was attributed to an adverse event related to screening.[26] Radiation exposure from photofluorographic screening is in the range of 0.6 mSv (by comparison a standard chest radiograph exposure is approximately 0.1 mSv).

As a relatively safe and inexpensive modality, radiography may continue to serve a role for GC screening in resource-limited settings. However, as the primary motivation for screening is to improve the detection of early stage cancers, radiography has limited utility compared with modern, high-resolution gastrointestinal endoscopy. Moreover, when an abnormality is detected through radiography, a confirmatory upper endoscopy is required for visualization and tissue acquisition.

Endoscopic Screening

Since 2001 in South Korea and 2016 in Japan,[29] endoscopic screening has been offered as an alternative modality to radiographic screening. Endoscopic screening offers several advantages to radiographic screening, including the ability to directly visualize the gastric mucosa and tissue sampling of abnormal-appearing tissue or visible lesions. Compared with radiographic screening, endoscopic screening demonstrates both better sensitivity and specificity.[26,35] This increased sensitivity is especially important for early GCs that demonstrate only subtle mucosal changes and that may not have an elevated or depressed component visible on contrast radiography. Techniques to enhance mucosal contrast have been developed to improve detection of subtle lesions, such as narrow-band imaging and chromoendoscopy (Video 1). In narrow-band imaging, conventional white light is filtered into defined wavelengths in order to maximize absorption by hemoglobin, as well as limit penetration of light beyond the mucosal surface. Given this shorter wavelength, the resulting "blue" light penetrates less deeply than conventional white light and may improve contrast of the mucosal surface. Chromoendoscopy also serves to amplify contrast of mucosal lesions through the use of dye-based staining of the gastric mucosa with biologically compatible agents such as acetic acid or methylene blue.[36,37] Application of dilute acetic acid can modify the optical properties of the epithelium by slightly altering the pH or by reversibly altering the structure of cellular proteins to reflect white light. Methylene blue is actively absorbed by small intestinal epithelium but not normal gastric epithelium, enhancing contrast between metaplastic and normal gastric epithelium. Chromoendoscopy may improve the delineation of surface irregularities, which in turn may improve the diagnosis and staging of early GCs.[38] Early GC detection may allow for opportunities for endoscopic resection through endoscopic submucosal dissection (ESD, **Fig. 3**). For GCs confined to the mucosa or proximal submucosa (with invasion depth of <500 microns) and without lymph node involvement, ESD offers similar cure rate and fewer rates of adverse events compared with surgical gastrectomy based on retrospective series from East Asia.[39,40]

The efficacy of endoscopic screening in decreasing cancer-specific mortality has been evaluated in observational studies form East Asia. A systematic review and meta-analysis of the protective effect of endoscopic screening on cancer-specific mortality identified 10 studies (6 cohort studies and 4 case-control studies) from South Korea, Japan, and China.[41] Receipt of endoscopic screening was associated with an approximate 40% reduction in risk for GC-specific mortality in the pooled estimate, with a robust protective effect found compared both against no-screening and radiographic screening controls.[41] When reviewing the existing evidence in support of endoscopic screening, the Japanese Guideline Development Group initially found inadequate observational data to justify population-level endoscopic screening in 2008.[6,42] However, based on the results of numerous high-quality observational studies published after 2008, the Japanese guidelines were amended to favor endoscopic screening in 2018 with an evidence score of 2+ (moderate-quality case-control

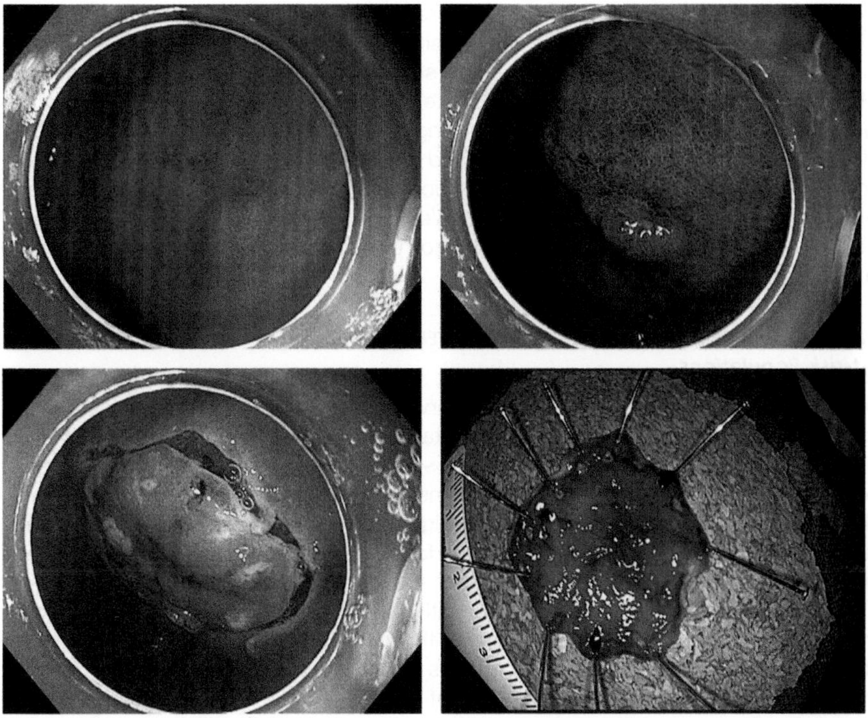

Fig. 3. Top left panel depicts a subtle, flat, erythematous lesion, which was biopsied to be gastric adenocarcinoma. Use of narrow-band imaging (*top right*) enhances visualization and delineation of the lesion. This lesion was staged as an early gastric cancer (tumor invasive to no deeper than mucosa or submucosa) and removed by endoscopic submucosal dissection (*bottom left*). *En bloc* resection specimen (*bottom right*) confirmed tumor confined to mucosal layer, without lymphovascular invasion and with negative lateral and deep margins consistent with curative resection.

and cohort studies with a low risk for bias, confounding or chance, and a moderate probability that the relation is causal).[26] Notably, the primary endpoint of these studies has been GC-specific mortality (as opposed to overall mortality). Currently no randomized controlled trial data exist for the benefits of endoscopic screening.

In the US and Europe most upper endoscopies are performed under sedation (either moderate or deep). The risk of cardiopulmonary events related to sedation has been estimated to be between 1 in 170 and 1 in 10,000, with the higher range of estimates incorporating minor events (such as changes in oxygen saturation or heart rate).[43] The Japanese Association of Gastroenterological Cancer Screening has found an overall rate of complications of 87 per 100,000 for endoscopic screening and 43 per 100,000 for radiographic screening.[26]

Serologic Screening

Hp-induced inflammation begins in the antrum and proceeds upward to the corpus with chronic infection. Human pepsinogens are classified into 2 biologically distinct types, pepsinogen I and pepsinogen II. As inflammation proceeds toward the corpus with chronic Hp infection, levels of pepsinogen I (produced by chief cells in the corpus) decrease, whereas levels of pepsinogen II remain more constant.[44] As such, a decreased level of pepsinogen I and decreased pepsinogen I/II ratio may indicate advanced atrophic gastritis.[44] Serum pepsinogens in combination with Hp IgG antibody have been evaluated as noninvasive screening tools in East Asian cohorts.[45–47] However, use of these markers demonstrate significant limitations including a high degree of heterogeneity in reported testing characteristics between populations, differing cutoff points, and variability based on proton pump inhibitor use.[48,49] These methods are not currently used for population-level screening in either South Korea or Japan. Their use may also be limited in Western populations, which differ in prevalence of Hp infection, proton pump inhibitor therapy use, and rates of autoimmune atrophic gastritis.[49,50]

GASTRIC CANCER SCREENING IN THE UNITED STATES

At-risk Populations

In the US, GC survival is poor (5-year observed survival of 27%) and most of the cancers are diagnosed at regional or distant stages.[4] Although overall incidence of GC is modest among the general population (~6 per 100,000), certain high-risk racial (Asians, Alaskan Indians, American Indians, Blacks/African Americans) and ethnic (Hispanics) groups may face significantly higher risk (**Fig. 4**). Very high-risk subgroups such as Japanese and Korean Americans face an incidence 6- to 8-fold higher than non-Hispanic Whites.[51] Beyond race and ethnicity, Americans at increased risk for GC include those with a family history or with cancer-predisposing syndromes, recent immigrants from high-incidence regions of the world, those with a history of Hp infection, and those with precancerous changes of the stomach.[29] It behooves both clinicians and policy makers to be cognizant of high-risk groups and to offer appropriate counseling for the role of preventative strategies such as GC screening.

IM is a critical precursor lesion to GC, and prevalence of IM in populations correlates with GC incidence. In the US, the prevalence of IM has been estimated to be between 5% and 10% of the general population.[52,53] High-risk subgroups including certain racial and ethnic minorities may have IM prevalence several-fold higher.[54,55] Within the US, there seems to be a close association between prevalence of IM with

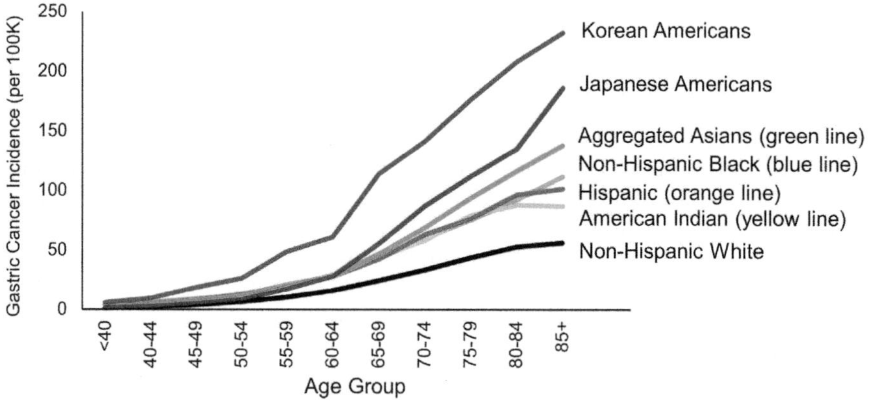

Fig. 4. Crude incidence of gastric cancer in United States (per 100,000; Y-axis) plotted by age group (X-axis). Asians, Blacks, Hispanics, and American Indian/Alaskan Natives face a several-fold increased risk compared with non-Hispanic Whites. (*Data from* the Surveillance, Epidemiology, and End Results (SEER) Program (www.seer.cancer.gov) Research Data (1973-2015), National Cancer Institute, DCCPS, Surveillance Research Program released in April 2018 based on the November 2017 submission.)

incidence of GC within racial subgroups (**Table 1**). These data suggest that all racial and ethnic groups are at risk for GC once IM has developed. Although gastritis and atrophy may reverse and normalize following Hp eradication, IM often persists.[56,57] Moreover, long-term clinical follow-up suggests that patients with IM remain at increased risk for GC even after eradication of Hp.[58,59]

The annual rate of progression onto GC from IM is estimated to be approximately 0.25%.[60] However, this aggregation of risk does not capture the variability of presentation in IM histologic severity or topographic distribution. In order to estimate histologic severity, scoring systems such as the operative link for gastritis assessment (OLGA)[61] for atrophic gastritis and the operative link for gastric IM (OLGIM) for IM have been developed (**Fig. 5**).[62] OLGA and OLGIM rely on both an assessment of the topographic extent of disease as well as the percentage of glandular involvement from each biopsy location using a visual-analogue scale.[63] The resultant stage score, ranging from 0 (no IM or no atrophy) to 4 (severe, extensive IM or atrophy), has been validated in several observational studies as risk-stratification tools for progression onto subsequent GC.[64–67] Use of the OLGA and OLGIM systems depends on consistent sampling of multiple locations of the stomach (including antrum, incisura, and corpus/body) in a systematic manner termed the "Sydney Protocol."[63] Another promising method of histologic risk stratification is through distinguishing complete IM from incomplete IM. Complete IM is characterized by well-defined goblet cells and a well-developed brush border, whereas in incomplete IM mucin droplets of varying sizes and shapes can be found and there is an absence of a brush border.[68] In specialized centers where mucin staining is available, complete IM will be found to display predominantly small intestinal phenotypic markers such as MUC2 and sucrase, whereas incomplete IM only selectively or incompletely expresses small intestinal markers but may express gastric phenotypic markers such as MUC5AC and large intestinal phenotypic markers such as Das-1.[69]

Current Recommendations

Recommendations for GC screening or precancerous lesion surveillance by US-based professional societies are depicted in **Table 2**. Currently, the American Society of Gastrointestinal Endoscopy (ASGE) has recommended endoscopic screening for GC in first-generation immigrants from high-risk regions (ie, Japan, China, Russia, and South America) older than 40 years, in particular if there is a family history of GC in a first-degree relative.[70] Regarding surveillance of patients with precancerous lesions, the ASGE recommends surveillance of patients with atrophic gastritis or IM when there is increased risk of GC due to ethnic/racial background, positive family history, or extensive anatomic distribution of disease.[14,70] By contrast, the American Gastroenterological Association (AGA) recommends against the *routine* use of

Table 1
Estimated prevalence of intestinal metaplasia and incidence of gastric cancer in racial/ethnic groups in the United States

Racial/Ethnic Group	Prevalence of IM (%)	Incidence of GC	References
Non-Hispanic Whites	7–9	6–8 per 100,000	4,21,52,54
Non-Hispanic Black	21	11 per 100,000	4,21,55
Hispanics	12–30	11 per 100,000	4,21,54,55
Chinese	26	15 per 100,000	51,54
Koreans	40	45 per 100,000	51,54

OLGA - Operative Link for Gastritis Assessment (Atrophic Gastritis)					
		Body			
		No Atrophy	Mild Atrophy	Moderate Atrophy	Marked Atrophy
Antrum (including incisura)	No Atrophy	Stage 0	Stage I	Stage II	Stage II
	Mild Atrophy	Stage I	Stage I	Stage II	Stage III
	Moderate Atrophy	Stage II	Stage II	Stage III	Stage IV
	Marked Atrophy	Stage III	Stage III	Stage IV	Stage IV

OLGIM - Operative Link for Gastric Intestinal Metaplasia					
		Body			
		No IM	Mild IM	Moderate IM	Marked IM
Antrum (including incisura)	No Intestinal Metaplasia (IM)	Stage 0	Stage I	Stage II	Stage II
	Mild IM	Stage I	Stage I	Stage II	Stage III
	Moderate IM	Stage II	Stage II	Stage III	Stage IV
	Marked IM	Stage III	Stage III	Stage IV	Stage IV

Fig. 5. Scoring of gastric precancerous lesions using the Operative Link systems. In these scoring systems, biopsies from the gastric antrum and body are individually scored for degree of atrophic gastritis and intestinal metaplasia using a visual-analogue scale (none, mild, moderate, marked). A summary stage for both atrophy and intestinal metaplasia is then assigned.

endoscopic surveillance in patients with IM but clarifies that this is a conditional recommendation based on very low-quality evidence.[71] The AGA guidelines further state that "Patients with IM at higher risk for GC who put a high value on potential but uncertain reduction in GC mortality, and who put a low value on potential risks of surveillance endoscopies, may reasonably elect for surveillance." The AGA guidelines identify patients with IM at higher risk for GC as those with incomplete IM, those with extensive IM, and those with a family history of GC. The AGA guidelines also identify patients at overall increased risk for GC including racial/ethnic minorities and immigrants from high-incidence regions. Notably neither the ASGE nor the AGA have made recommendation on the optimal interval for surveillance of IM if this strategy is pursued.

FUTURE SCREENING MODALITIES

Promising biomarkers currently under development or validation may revolutionize early GC detection and prevention. MicroRNAs (miRNAs) are small, noncoding molecules involved in biological processes including cell-cycle progression and apoptosis. Given their stability, presence in blood, and role in numerous pathways, miRNAs have been evaluated as potential biomarkers for GC. Five miRNAs have shown particular promise as screening tests for GC: miR-21[72–74] (inhibitor of tumor suppressor genes), miR-106a[75,76] (cell proliferation signal), miR-106b[77,78] (inhibitor of apoptosis), miR-223[73,79] (cell proliferation and invasion), and miR-421[80–82] (apoptosis resistance). Notably, these miRNAs have mostly been evaluated in cohorts from East Asia where the prevalence of Hp and incidence of GC is much higher. Additional prospective validation studies are required before translation of miRNAs to clinical practice.

Risk stratification of IM may also be improved through use of molecular markers. In a prospective cohort study of high-risk Singaporean Chinese patients, IM biopsy samples with shortened telomeres and chromosomal aberrations were found to be associated with subsequent progression to either dysplasia or frank carcinoma. By

Table 2
Guidelines issued by United States professional societies

Society	Year	Recommendation
Gastric Cancer Screening		
American Society of Gastrointestinal Endoscopy[70]	2015	Endoscopic screening for gastric cancer in first-generation immigrants from high-risk regions (eg, Japan, China, Russia, and South America) may be considered for those aged 40 y, particularly if there is a family history of gastric cancer in a first-degree relative
Surveillance of Intestinal Metaplasia (IM)		
American Society of Gastrointestinal Endoscopy[14,70]	2015	Endoscopic surveillance in patients with gastric atrophic gastritis or IM coupled with an increased risk of gastric cancer because of racial/ethnic background, extensive anatomic distribution, or family history
American Gastroenterological Association[71]	2019	Recommends against routine use of endoscopic surveillance in patients with IM. *Conditional recommendation, very low quality of evidence* Patients with IM at higher risk for gastric cancer who put a high value on potential but uncertain reduction in gastric cancer mortality, and who put a low value on potential risks of surveillance endoscopies, may reasonably elect for surveillance Patients with IM specifically at higher risk of gastric cancer include those with • Incomplete vs complete IM • Extensive vs limited IM • Family history of gastric cancer Patients at overall increased risk for gastric cancer include • Racial/ethnic minorities • Immigrants from high-incidence regions

Existing recommendations from United States–based professional societies regarding screening of gastric cancer or surveillance of precancerous lesions such as IM.

contrast, IM with normal-like epigenetic patterns were associated with stability or regression.[65] Although requiring validation, such a molecular signature for IM progression may serve as a valuable tool to allow for focused and highly personalized strategies of surveillance while also avoiding unnecessary endoscopies in low-risk subjects.

SUMMARY

GC remains a devastating disease for the 27,000 Americans diagnosed each year. Compared with East Asia, survival from GC in the US and Europe is lower, reflecting a later stage of diagnosis. In high-incidence nations of East Asia, national screening programs have been adopted. An emerging body of observational data suggests that endoscopic screening may prevent GC-specific mortality in targeted populations. There exist high-risk populations within the US who may benefit from targeted screening, including racial/ethnic groups (American Indians, Alaska Indians, Asians, Blacks, Hispanics), first-generation immigrants from high-incidence regions, and those with a family history of GC. Individuals diagnosed with IM, particularly extensive IM or histologically severe IM, may benefit from endoscopic surveillance. Emerging molecular technologies may help to identify high-risk individuals who should be screened, as well as stratify IM for risk of cancer progression.

CLINICS CARE POINTS

- Racial/ethnic minorities and first-generation immigrants are at increased risk for GC and may benefit from endoscopic cancer screening.
- Patients diagnosed with incomplete, extensive, or severe IM should be offered endoscopic surveillance.
- Use of narrow-band imaging and chromoendoscopy during endoscopy can improve the detection of GC.

DISCLOSURE

RJH is supported by the National Cancer Institute of the National Institutes of Health under Award Number K08CA252635. The content is solely the responsibility of the authors and does not necessarily represent the official views of the National Institutes of Health.

SUPPLEMENTARY DATA

Supplementary data related to this article can be found online at https://doi.org/10.1016/j.giec.2021.03.005.

REFERENCE

1. Collaborators GBDSC. The global, regional, and national burden of stomach cancer in 195 countries, 1990-2017: a systematic analysis for the Global Burden of Disease study 2017. Lancet Gastroenterol Hepatol 2020;5:42–54.
2. World Health Organization International Agency for Research on Cancer (IARC). Globocan 2012: estimated cancer incidence, mortality and prevalence worldwide in 2018. 2018. Available at: http://gco.iarc.fr/. Accessed January 23, 2019.

3. Cancer Facts and Figures 2019. American Cancer Society. Atlanta, GA. Available at: https://www.cancer.org/cancer/stomach-cancer/about/key-statistics.html. Accessed June 1, 2020.
4. SEER*Explorer: An interactive website for SEER cancer statistics [Internet]. Surveillance Research Program, National Cancer Institute. Available at: https://seer.cancer.gov/explorer/. Accessed December 30, 2019.
5. Colquhoun A, Arnold M, Ferlay J, et al. Global patterns of cardia and non-cardia gastric cancer incidence in 2012. Gut 2015;64:1881–8.
6. Hamashima C, Shibuya D, Yamazaki H, et al. The Japanese guidelines for gastric cancer screening. Jpn J Clin Oncol 2008;38:259–67.
7. Jun JK, Choi KS, Lee HY, et al. Effectiveness of the Korean National Cancer Screening Program in Reducing Gastric Cancer Mortality. Gastroenterology 2017;152:1319–1328 e7.
8. Nomura A, Stemmermann GN, Chyou PH, et al. Helicobacter pylori infection and gastric carcinoma among Japanese Americans in Hawaii. N Engl J Med 1991; 325:1132–6.
9. Parsonnet J, Friedman GD, Vandersteen DP, et al. Helicobacter pylori infection and the risk of gastric carcinoma. N Engl J Med 1991;325:1127–31.
10. Hooi JKY, Lai WY, Ng WK, et al. Global Prevalence of Helicobacter pylori Infection: Systematic Review and Meta-Analysis. Gastroenterology 2017; 153:420–9.
11. Eslick GD, Lim LL, Byles JE, et al. Association of Helicobacter pylori infection with gastric carcinoma: a meta-analysis. Am J Gastroenterol 1999;94:2373–9.
12. Peleteiro B, Bastos A, Ferro A, et al. Prevalence of Helicobacter pylori infection worldwide: a systematic review of studies with national coverage. Dig Dis Sci 2014;59:1698–709.
13. Correa P. Human gastric carcinogenesis: a multistep and multifactorial process–First American Cancer Society Award Lecture on Cancer Epidemiology and Prevention. Cancer Res 1992;52:6735–40.
14. Committee ASoP, Evans JA, Chandrasekhara V, et al. The role of endoscopy in the management of premalignant and malignant conditions of the stomach. Gastrointest Endosc 2015;82:1–8.
15. Kim SG, Jung HK, Lee HL, et al. Guidelines for the diagnosis and treatment of Helicobacter pylori infection in Korea, 2013 revised edition. J Gastroenterol Hepatol 2014;29:1371–86.
16. Leung WK, Sung JJ. Review article: intestinal metaplasia and gastric carcinogenesis. Aliment Pharmacol Ther 2002;16:1209–16.
17. Uemura N, Okamoto S, Yamamoto S, et al. Helicobacter pylori infection and the development of gastric cancer. N Engl J Med 2001;345:784–9.
18. Sipponen P, Kimura K. Intestinal metaplasia, atrophic gastritis and stomach cancer: trends over time. Eur J Gastroenterol Hepatol 1994;6(Suppl 1):S79–83.
19. Carter AJ, Delarosa B, Hur H. An analysis of discrepancies between United Kingdom cancer research funding and societal burden and a comparison to previous and United States values. Health Res Policy Syst 2015;13:62.
20. Maruthappu M, Head MG, Zhou CD, et al. Investments in cancer research awarded to UK institutions and the global burden of cancer 2000-2013: a systematic analysis. BMJ Open 2017;7:e013936.
21. Lui FH, Tuan B, Swenson SL, et al. Ethnic disparities in gastric cancer incidence and survival in the USA: an updated analysis of 1992-2009 SEER data. Dig Dis Sci 2014;59:3027–34.

22. Anderson LA, Tavilla A, Brenner H, et al. Survival for oesophageal, stomach and small intestine cancers in Europe 1999-2007: Results from EUROCARE-5. Eur J Cancer 2015;51:2144–57.
23. Minicozzi P, Walsh PM, Sanchez MJ, et al. Is low survival for cancer in Eastern Europe due principally to late stage at diagnosis? Eur J Cancer 2018;93:127–37.
24. Hamashima C, Choi IJ, Jung HY. The 2020 Stanford Gastric Cancer Summit. 2020. Available at: https://med.stanford.edu/care/gastric-cancer-summit-at-stanford/Gastric-Cancer-Summit-Videos.html. Stanford, CA. Accessed August 1, 2020.
25. Jung KW, Won YJ, Kong HJ, et al. Survival of korean adult cancer patients by stage at diagnosis, 2006-2010: national cancer registry study. Cancer Res Treat 2013;45:162–71.
26. Hamashima C. Update version of the Japanese Guidelines for Gastric Cancer Screening. Jpn J Clin Oncol 2018;48:673–83.
27. Hamashima C, Goto R. Potential capacity of endoscopic screening for gastric cancer in Japan. Cancer Sci 2017;108:101–7.
28. Kim Y, Jun JK, Choi KS, et al. Overview of the National Cancer screening programme and the cancer screening status in Korea. Asian Pac J Cancer Prev 2011;12:725–30.
29. Huang RJ, Koh H, Hwang JH, et al. A Summary of the 2020 Gastric Cancer Summit at Stanford University. Gastroenterology 2020;159(4):1221–6.
30. Dooley CP, Larson AW, Stace NH, et al. Double-contrast barium meal and upper gastrointestinal endoscopy. A comparative study. Ann Intern Med 1984;101: 538–45.
31. Longo WE, Zucker KA, Zdon MJ, et al. Detection of early gastric cancer in an aggressive endoscopy unit. Am Surg 1989;55:100–4.
32. Choi KS, Jun JK, Park EC, et al. Performance of different gastric cancer screening methods in Korea: a population-based study. PLoS One 2012;7: e50041.
33. Lee KJ, Inoue M, Otani T, et al. Gastric cancer screening and subsequent risk of gastric cancer: a large-scale population-based cohort study, with a 13-year follow-up in Japan. Int J Cancer 2006;118:2315–21.
34. Miyamoto A, Kuriyama S, Nishino Y, et al. Lower risk of death from gastric cancer among participants of gastric cancer screening in Japan: a population-based cohort study. Prev Med 2007;44:12–9.
35. Hamashima C, Okamoto M, Shabana M, et al. Sensitivity of endoscopic screening for gastric cancer by the incidence method. Int J Cancer 2013;133: 653–9.
36. Taghavi SA, Membari ME, Eshraghian A, et al. Comparison of chromoendoscopy and conventional endoscopy in the detection of premalignant gastric lesions. Can J Gastroenterol 2009;23:105–8.
37. Song KH, Hwang JA, Kim SM, et al. Acetic acid chromoendoscopy for determining the extent of gastric intestinal metaplasia. Gastrointest Endosc 2017;85: 349–56.
38. Dinis-Ribeiro M. Chromoendoscopy for early diagnosis of gastric cancer. Eur J Gastroenterol Hepatol 2006;18:831–8.
39. Chiu PW, Teoh AY, To KF, et al. Endoscopic submucosal dissection (ESD) compared with gastrectomy for treatment of early gastric neoplasia: a retrospective cohort study. Surg Endosc 2012;26:3584–91.

40. Cho JH, Cha SW, Kim HG, et al. Long-term outcomes of endoscopic submucosal dissection for early gastric cancer: a comparison study to surgery using propensity score-matched analysis. Surg Endosc 2016;30:3762–73.
41. Zhang X, Li M, Chen S, et al. Endoscopic screening in asian countries is associated with reduced gastric cancer mortality: a meta-analysis and systematic review. Gastroenterology 2018;155:347–354 e9.
42. Hamashima C, Saito S, Nakayama T, et al. The standardized development method of the Japanese guidelinesfor cancer screening. Jpn J Clin Oncol 2008;38:288–95.
43. ASoP Committee, Ben-Menachem T, Decker GA, et al. Adverse events of upper GI endoscopy. Gastrointest Endosc 2012;76:707–18.
44. Miki K. Gastric cancer screening by combined assay for serum anti-Helicobacter pylori IgG antibody and serum pepsinogen levels - "ABC method". Proc Jpn Acad Ser B Phys Biol Sci 2011;87:405–14.
45. Abnet CC, Zheng W, Ye W, et al. Plasma pepsinogens, antibodies against Helicobacter pylori, and risk of gastric cancer in the Shanghai Women's Health Study Cohort. Br J Cancer 2011;104:1511–6.
46. Tu H, Sun L, Dong X, et al. A serological biopsy using five stomach-specific circulating biomarkers for gastric cancer risk assessment: a multi-phase study. Am J Gastroenterol 2017;112:704–15.
47. Wang X, Lu B, Meng L, et al. The correlation between histological gastritis staging- 'OLGA/OLGIM' and serum pepsinogen test in assessment of gastric atrophy/intestinal metaplasia in China. Scand J Gastroenterol 2017;52:822–7.
48. Huang YK, Yu JC, Kang WM, et al. Significance of serum pepsinogens as a biomarker for gastric cancer and atrophic gastritis screening: a systematic review and meta-analysis. PLoS One 2015;10:e0142080.
49. Zagari RM, Rabitti S, Greenwood DC, et al. Systematic review with meta-analysis: diagnostic performance of the combination of pepsinogen, gastrin-17 and anti-Helicobacter pylori antibodies serum assays for the diagnosis of atrophic gastritis. Aliment Pharmacol Ther 2017;46:657–67.
50. Castro C, Dinis-Ribeiro M, Rodrigues ANG, et al. Western long-term accuracy of serum pepsinogen-based gastric cancer screening. Eur J Gastroenterol Hepatol 2018;30:274–7.
51. Huang RJ, Sharp N, Talamoa RO, et al. One size does not fit all: marked heterogeneity in incidence of and survival from gastric cancer among asian american subgroups. Cancer Epidemiol Biomarkers Prev 2020;29(5):903–9.
52. Sonnenberg A, Lash RH, Genta RM. A national study of Helicobactor pylori infection in gastric biopsy specimens. Gastroenterology 2010;139:1894–901.e2 [quiz: e12].
53. Sonnenberg A, Genta RM. Changes in the gastric mucosa with aging. Clin Gastroenterol Hepatol 2015;13:2276–81.
54. Choi CE, Sonnenberg A, Turner K, et al. High prevalence of gastric preneoplastic lesions in east asians and hispanics in the USA. Dig Dis Sci 2015;60:2070–6.
55. Huang RJ, Ende AR, Singla A, et al. Prevalence, risk factors, and surveillance patterns for gastric intestinal metaplasia among patients undergoing upper endoscopy with biopsy. Gastrointest Endosc 2020;91:70–77 e1.
56. Hwang YJ, Kim N, Lee HS, et al. Reversibility of atrophic gastritis and intestinal metaplasia after Helicobacter pylori eradication - a prospective study for up to 10 years. Aliment Pharmacol Ther 2018;47:380–90.

57. Chiang TH, Maeda M, Yamada H, et al. Risk stratification for gastric cancer after Helicobacter pylori eradication: A population-based study on Matsu Islands. J Gastroenterol Hepatol 2020;36(3):671–9.
58. Ito M, Takata S, Tatsugami M, et al. Clinical prevention of gastric cancer by Helicobacter pylori eradication therapy: a systematic review. J Gastroenterol 2009; 44:365–71.
59. Take S, Mizuno M, Ishiki K, et al. Risk of gastric cancer in the second decade of follow-up after Helicobacter pylori eradication. J Gastroenterol 2019;55(3):281–8.
60. Song H, Ekheden IG, Zheng Z, et al. Incidence of gastric cancer among patients with gastric precancerous lesions: observational cohort study in a low risk Western population. BMJ 2015;351:h3867.
61. Rugge M, Meggio A, Pennelli G, et al. Gastritis staging in clinical practice: the OLGA staging system. Gut 2007;56:631–6.
62. Capelle LG, de Vries AC, Haringsma J, et al. The staging of gastritis with the OLGA system by using intestinal metaplasia as an accurate alternative for atrophic gastritis. Gastrointest Endosc 2010;71:1150–8.
63. Dixon MF, Genta RM, Yardley JH, et al. Classification and grading of gastritis. The updated Sydney System. International Workshop on the Histopathology of Gastritis, Houston 1994. Am J Surg Pathol 1996;20:1161–81.
64. den Hollander WJ, Holster IL, den Hoed CM, et al. Surveillance of premalignant gastric lesions: a multicentre prospective cohort study from low incidence regions. Gut 2018;68(4):585–93.
65. Huang KK, Ramnarayanan K, Zhu F, et al. Genomic and epigenomic profiling of high-risk intestinal metaplasia reveals molecular determinants of progression to gastric cancer. Cancer Cell 2018;33:137–150 e5.
66. Rugge M, Genta RM, Fassan M, et al. OLGA gastritis staging for the prediction of gastric cancer risk: a long-term follow-up study of 7436 patients. Am J Gastroenterol 2018;113(11):1621–8.
67. Yue H, Shan L, Bin L. The significance of OLGA and OLGIM staging systems in the risk assessment of gastric cancer: a systematic review and meta-analysis. Gastric Cancer 2018;21:579–87.
68. Correa P, Piazuelo MB, Wilson KT. Pathology of gastric intestinal metaplasia: clinical implications. Am J Gastroenterol 2010;105:493–8.
69. Huang RJ, Choi AY, Truong CD, et al. Diagnosis and Management of Gastric Intestinal Metaplasia: Current Status and Future Directions. Gut Liver 2019;13: 596–603.
70. ASGE Standards of Practice Committee, Wang A, Shaukat A, et al. Race and ethnicity considerations in GI endoscopy. Gastrointest Endosc 2015;82:593–9.
71. Gupta S, Li D, El Serag HB, et al. AGA clinical practice guidelines on management of gastric intestinal metaplasia. Gastroenterology 2019;158(3):693–702.
72. Zheng Y, Cui L, Sun W, et al. MicroRNA-21 is a new marker of circulating tumor cells in gastric cancer patients. Cancer Biomark 2011;10:71–7.
73. Li BS, Zhao YL, Guo G, et al. Plasma microRNAs, miR-223, miR-21 and miR-218, as novel potential biomarkers for gastric cancer detection. PLoS One 2012;7: e41629.
74. Wang B, Zhang Q. The expression and clinical significance of circulating microRNA-21 in serum of five solid tumors. J Cancer Res Clin Oncol 2012;138: 1659–66.
75. Zhou H, Guo JM, Lou YR, et al. Detection of circulating tumor cells in peripheral blood from patients with gastric cancer using microRNA as a marker. J Mol Med (Berl) 2010;88:709–17.

76. Yuan R, Wang G, Xu Z, et al. Up-regulated Circulating miR-106a by DNA Methylation Promised a Potential Diagnostic and Prognostic Marker for Gastric Cancer. Anticancer Agents Med Chem 2016;16:1093–100.
77. Tsujiura M, Ichikawa D, Komatsu S, et al. Circulating microRNAs in plasma of patients with gastric cancers. Br J Cancer 2010;102:1174–9.
78. Cai H, Yuan Y, Hao YF, et al. Plasma microRNAs serve as novel potential biomarkers for early detection of gastric cancer. Med Oncol 2013;30:452.
79. Wang H, Wang L, Wu Z, et al. Three dysregulated microRNAs in serum as novel biomarkers for gastric cancer screening. Med Oncol 2014;31:298.
80. Zhou H, Xiao B, Zhou F, et al. MiR-421 is a functional marker of circulating tumor cells in gastric cancer patients. Biomarkers 2012;17:104–10.
81. Wu J, Li G, Yao Y, et al. MicroRNA-421 is a new potential diagnosis biomarker with higher sensitivity and specificity than carcinoembryonic antigen and cancer antigen 125 in gastric cancer. Biomarkers 2015;20:58–63.
82. Zhao G, Xu L, Hui L, et al. Level of circulated microRNA-421 in gastric carcinoma and related mechanisms. Int J Clin Exp Pathol 2015;8:14252–6.

Chemoprevention Against Gastric Cancer

Shailja C. Shah, MD, MPH[a,b,*], Richard M. Peek Jr, MD[a]

KEYWORDS

- Gastric neoplasm • Helicobacter pylori • Aspirin
- Nonsteroidal anti-inflammatory drugs • Chemoprevention

KEY POINTS

- *Helicobacter pylori* eradication remains the mainstay form of chemoprevention against noncardia gastric adenocarcinoma.
- However, the observations that the incidence of non-*H. pylori* associated gastric cancer is rising, and gastric cancer still develops in people after *H. pylori* eradication highlights the importance of investigations defining other effective chemopreventive agents.
- To date, many agents including aspirin, non-steroidal anti-inflammatory drugs, metformin, statins, and alpha-difluoromethylornithine have been investigated in their role as chemopreventive agents in gastric cancer.
- Future randomized controlled clinical trials particularly for high-risk populations, such as people with gastric preneoplastic mucosal changes are needed in order to provide guidance on how to position the use of these agents for gastric cancer prevention.

BACKGROUND

Gastric cancer is the fifth most common cancer and third leading cause of cancer-related mortality globally, accounting for approximately 1 million new cases annually and more than 780,000 cancer-related deaths.[1] Prevention and early detection are two foundational pillars for addressing the substantial burden of gastric cancer. Early detection provides the opportunity for potentially curative resection if gastric cancer is diagnosed before submucosal invasion. However, except in the few countries where

Grant support: S.C. Shah is funded by a 2019 American Gastroenterological Association Research Scholar Award and Veterans Affairs Career Development Award under award number ICX002027A-01. R.M. Peek is funded by the NIH/NCI through the following awards: R01 DK58587, R01 CA 77955, P01 116087. The content is solely the responsibility of the listed authors and does not necessarily represent the official views of the funding agencies listed.
Writing assistance: None.
[a] Division of Gastroenterology, Hepatology and Nutrition, Department of Medicine, Vanderbilt University Medical Center, 1030C MRB IV, 2215 Garland Avenue, Nashville, TN 37232-0252, USA;
[b] Veterans Affairs Tennessee Valley Health System, Nashville Campus, Nashville, TN, USA
* Corresponding author.
E-mail address: shailja.c.shah@vumc.org

Gastrointest Endoscopy Clin N Am 31 (2021) 519–542
https://doi.org/10.1016/j.giec.2021.03.006
1052-5157/21/Published by Elsevier Inc.

endoscopic screening for gastric cancer occurs, gastric cancer is most often diagnosed in the advanced stages, which is when symptoms present and prompt a diagnostic evaluation. Unfortunately, there are no curative options for advanced stage disease and the 5-year survival rates are dismal at best. The vast majority of countries, including the United States, do not screen for gastric cancer. Focused efforts on gastric prevention, therefore, are key and represent the mainstay in these countries. Attention to primary, secondary, and tertiary gastric cancer prevention, even in those countries where gastric cancer screening does occur, decreases the downstream health and economic burden associated with a gastric cancer diagnosis.

Cancer risk determinants can be divided into modifiable (eg, diet, smoking) and nonmodifiable (eg, genetics, age) factors. Accordingly, interventions aimed at cancer risk attenuation and prevention are focused on altering modifiable factors; for example, via smoking cessation and nutritional education programs. Chemoprevention is a critical adjunct, because these interventions alone are rarely sufficient. Chemoprevention in the form of *Helicobacter pylori* eradication already forms the foundation for gastric cancer prevention. However, the benefit is significantly attenuated once more advanced gastric mucosal changes have occurred, because the risk of gastric cancer persists despite *H pylori* eradication. As described elsewhere in this article, *H pylori* eradication therapy decreases but does not eliminate the risk of metachronous cancer (tertiary prevention), thus suggesting that there is a field effect that persists even in the absence of ongoing *H pylori* infection. Further complicating the picture is that there is an increase in observed non–*H pylori* associated noncardia gastric adenocarcinoma in some populations, particularly as the prevalence of *H pylori* decreases.[2] For these reasons, chemopreventive agents aside from *H pylori* eradication alone should likewise be considered tenets to any successful gastric cancer control program.

In this article, we will discuss chemopreventive agents for intestinal-type noncardia gastric cancer, with a predominant focus on *H pylori* eradication therapy and nonsteroidal anti-inflammatory drugs (NSAIDs), including aspirin, because these agents have the strongest and largest body of supporting data. Other putative chemopreventive agents are discussed within the context of both clinical and experimental data.

Mechanisms

Having an in-depth understanding of the pathogenesis of intestinal-type noncardia gastric adenocarcinoma (NCGA), along with modifying factors, is foundational to chemoprevention research and the discovery of effective chemopreventive agents. NCGA develops as a stepwise progression from chronic nonatrophic gastritis to atrophic gastritis, intestinal metaplasia, and dysplasia, before the final malignant transformation in a very small proportion of individuals.[3,4] The most common trigger for this so-called Correa cascade is chronic infection with *H pylori*. Three nested case-control studies, all published in 1991, demonstrated that people with *H pylori* infection had a significant 3-fold to 6-fold higher likelihood of developing gastric cancer compared with individuals without *H pylori* infection.[5–7] Accordingly, the World Health Organization and International Agency for Research on Cancer classified *H pylori* as a definite biological carcinogen. A meta-analysis published by the Helicobacter and Cancer Collaborative Group in 2001 with 10 additional years of data confirmed these findings.[8] Even though only a small percentage of individuals infected with *H pylori* (<1%–3%) will have malignant complications, this number still represents a massive burden of preventable disease because *H pylori* is estimated to infect more than one-half the global population; indeed, approximately 90% of NCGA are attributable to *H pylori* infection.[9–11] Other environmental triggers for the inflammation–

preneoplasia–neoplasia sequence, including chronic bile reflux, high dietary consumption of salt and nitrites, the non–*H pylori* microbiome and metabolic byproducts, and autoimmunity, can act independently or potentiate the pathologic effects of *H pylori*.[12]

The complex interactions between these triggers, along with underlying host genetic factors and microbial factors, including *H pylori* strain–specific factors, together lead to a field effect of gastric mucosal changes; however, the exact molecular and genetic underpinnings remain unclear. Depending on ongoing insults, progression may or may not occur. DNA damage, as the downstream consequence of ongoing inflammation and subsequent oxidative stress, is a fundamental process in gastric carcinogenesis, even in the absence of *H pylori.* One study in a Mongolian gerbil experimental model demonstrated that administering a diet containing a potent antioxidant derived from canola oil (4-vinyl-2,6-dimethoxyphenol) resulted in a substantially lower incidence of gastric adenocarcinoma, even though the *H pylori* bacterial density was not changed.[13] Similar findings were replicated in transgenic mice, where administration of 4-vinyl-2,6-dimethoxyphenol was associated with significantly lower levels of cyclo-oxygenase (COX)-2, IL-1B, and IL-12B expression and significantly lower likelihood of spontaneous gastric tumor development.[14] Collectively, these data confirm that inflammation severity, not just *H pylori* infection alone, is likely the more important factor in NCGA pathogenesis and underscores the importance of chemopreventive strategies apart from simply *H pylori* eradication alone.

H pylori Eradication Treatment as Chemoprevention Against Gastric Cancer

H pylori typically persists for the lifetime of the host unless eradicated with antibiotics and high-dose acid suppression for a set duration. Before the formal discovery of *H pylori* by J. Robin Warren and Barry Marshall in the late 1970s,[15] the environmental trigger for the Correa cascade was unknown and was thought most likely to be dietary. Several subsequent studies unequivocally confirmed that chronic *H pylori* infection led to chronic gastritis with or without continued progression along the carcinogenic cascade.[6–8,16]

Since that time, several observational and interventional studies evaluating the effect of *H pylori* eradication versus no eradication on gastric cancer incidence have been published, albeit with mixed results, because some studies have yielded null findings. The mixed results likely reflect differences in study population, design, length of follow-up, presence of preneoplastic lesions at the time of *H pylori* eradication, the exposure measure (eg, *H pylori* eradication treatment but without subsequent confirmation testing as the exposure group vs *H pylori* eradication treatment and confirmed successful eradication as the exposure group), outcome measures (eg, some studies analyzed changes in atrophic gastritis or gastric intestinal metaplasia as surrogate markers, and not gastric cancer incidence per se), and the reference population (eg, general population as the reference group vs individuals with *H pylori* infection but who received placebo/no treatment, or unsuccessful treatment as the reference group), among others. Prospective large population-based studies are no longer likely to be performed, especially in countries with low to intermediate gastric cancer incidence, owing to cost and logistical barriers, not to mention ethical considerations.[17] The long sojourn time between *H pylori* infection and gastric cancer occurrence and the overall rarity of gastric cancer on a population level are leading barriers for such studies. For chemoprevention trials, follow-up should ideally extend past 10 years. Thus, even in a high-risk population, the estimated sample size to detect a 50% decrease over 10 years between an *H pylori* eradicated versus noneradicated group would be more than 17,000 per group.[18] Ethical considerations provide another formidable barrier because, even though only a minority of individuals with *H pylori* will develop malignant complications, we are not able to definitively predict who will or will not progress; this line of reasoning forms the rationale for the recommendation of most major medical societies to universally eradicate *H pylori* when diagnosed. Thus, withholding eradication treatment or providing a placebo treatment for a known carcinogen would be unethical.[17] Notably, in countries where *H pylori* eradication therapy is still not universally recommended, such as in South Korea, randomized controlled trials (RCTs) of *H pylori* eradication versus no eradication have continued to be conducted; these studies have provided risk reduction estimates in distinct high-risk populations, including those with family history of gastric cancer[19] or prior history of gastric cancer[20,21] (discussed elsewhere in this article), although the ethics of these studies has been questioned. The same group that published these referenced studies is currently conducting an RCT of *H pylori* eradication therapy versus placebo to investigate the effect of *H pylori* eradication on gastric cancer incidence in the general population (HELPER study, NCT02112214); the anticipated completion date for this 10-year follow-up study is 2029.

Multiple retrospective cohort studies have been published, the majority in Asian-Pacific countries, analyzing the association between *H pylori* eradication treatment and primary prevention of gastric cancer.[22] Important differences across studies are those already listed elsewhere in this article, with the major differences including variability with respect to *H pylori* eradication regimens (most used clarithromycin-based regimens), rigor with respect to *H pylori* diagnosis determination, whether or not *H pylori* eradication confirmation testing was performed (and modality), reference groups, study time period, and duration and completeness of follow-up, as well as the baseline demographics of the cohort itself (eg, several studies had a greater than 70% male predominance, with variability in the mean age at study entry).[22] Moreover, most of these studies were not designed to separately analyze outcomes according to the presence or absence of symptoms or the presence or absence of gastric pathology, such as gastric or duodenal ulcers or already existing gastric (pre)neoplasia; or, this factor was analyzed in a limited fashion. Notwithstanding, a meta-analysis of cohort studies published before May 2015 demonstrated that *H pylori* eradication treatment was associated with a pooled 48% lower risk (incidence rate ratio, 0.52; 95% confidence interval [CI], 0.41–0.64) of incident gastric cancer, which was not significantly different compared with the pooled estimate for RCTs (incidence rate ratio, 0.60; 95% CI, 0.44–0.81) (P = .34 by meta-regression).[22] There was a trend toward greater benefit with a longer duration of follow-up after eradication (P = .06), but this difference was not statistically significant; the mean follow-up for the included studies ranged from 24 to 121 months. This meta-analysis also supported prior studies suggesting that the benefit of *H pylori* eradication for primary prevention is greater in populations with a higher gastric cancer incidence compared with a lower incidence. It should be emphasized, however, that this meta-analysis included only 2 studies conducted outside of the Asian-Pacific region, and one was conducted in Colombia,[23] a country with a high gastric cancer incidence; thus, only 1 study was from a country with a low to intermediate incidence of gastric cancer (Finland).[24] Of note, the Finnish study, which was conducted from 1986 to 1998, used a decrease in *H pylori* serum antibody titers as a surrogate for *H pylori* eradication, which may have led to misclassification.

Since the publication of that meta-analysis, 2 retrospective cohort studies from Western populations (Sweden, the United States) were published, both with different study designs.[25,26] The population-based retrospective cohort study from Sweden (2005–2012) compared the incidence of NCGA in patients who received *H pylori* eradication treatment to the general Swedish population as the reference group.[26] The majority of individuals were 18 to 59 years old, and the mean follow-up time for this study was only 3.7 years (maximum, 7.5 years; minimum not specified, but presumably 1 year). Details regarding the *H pylori* positivity rate in the general population comparator group, as well as the presence of symptoms or gastric pathology, and whether or not individuals had received *H pylori* treatment before study entry were not available or provided in the study. The exposure group included patients with gastric pathology based on *International Classification of Disease* codes, including gastric ulcers, duodenal ulcers, and atrophic gastritis. Moreover, eradication confirmation testing was not universally performed after *H pylori* treatment and thus *H pylori* eradication cannot be confirmed in the primary exposure group; acknowledging this limitation, the authors did conduct a separate analysis among individuals who received more than 1 prescription of *H pylori* treatment during follow-up. Notwithstanding, after correction of an error in the statistical analysis,[27] the authors reported that, among 95,176 Swedish individuals who received *H pylori* eradication therapy, 0.1% (n = 69) developed NCGA over 351,018 person-years of follow-up time. The age- and sex-standardized risk of gastric cancer in the *H pylori* treated group compared with the general population decreased with increasing time since eradication therapy, such that the risk was 4.2-fold higher (95% CI, 3.04–5.66) and 3.1-fold higher (95% CI, 1.88–4.76) after 1 to 3 years and 3 to 5 years of follow-up, respectively. After 5 to 7.5 years of follow-up, however, the rate in the *H pylori* treated group was not significantly different compared with the general population (standardized incidence ratio, 2.06; 95% CI, 0.75–4.48); however, this finding was based on only 6 cases of NCGA.[27] There was a higher risk of NCGA among those with persistent *H pylori* infection, as indicated by at least 2 courses of eradication treatment during follow-up (standardized incidence ratio, 10.5; 95% CI, 3.82–22.8), compared with individuals who received only 1 course of *H pylori* treatment during follow-up (standardized incidence ratio, 2.38; 95% CI, 1.80–3.10).

One recently published retrospective cohort study conducted in United States veterans included a limited secondary analysis investigating the impact of *H pylori* eradication treatment among those with confirmed *H pylori* who also had subsequent *H pylori* testing to evaluate the success of treatment.[26] It was not stated whether patients were symptomatic or had known gastric (pre)neoplasia. Notably, only 2.2% of the starting cohort (n = 8020 of 371,813) had sufficient data available to be included in this secondary analysis. Based on this restricted sample of patients who had confirmatory testing, which is subject to bias, the authors did demonstrate that successful *H pylori* eradication was associated with a 76% lower likelihood (standardized hazard ratio, 0.24; 95% CI, 0.15–0.41) of distal gastric cancer compared with unsuccessful *H pylori* eradication. The follow-up time specifically for this subanalysis was not provided. Other methodological limitations need to be considered when interpreting the findings of this study[28]; for example, approximately 70% (n = 258,362 of 371,813) of the cohort were deemed to have *H pylori* exposure based solely on prescriptions for anti–*H pylori* therapy without confirmatory laboratory testing identified in the medical record.

Multiple RCTs have also been published that compare *H pylori* eradication versus no eradication and the subsequent incidence of gastric cancer, and thus complement the observational evidence provided from cohort studies. Unfortunately, there is a similar dearth of evidence from low or intermediate risk populations from Western countries. Recently, the Cochrane Gut Group updated their systematic review and meta-analysis, which was published in 2015, that compared the incidence of gastric cancer in asymptomatic individuals from the general population randomized to *H*

Table 1
RCTs evaluating the association between *H pylori* eradication and gastric cancer

First Author, Publication year	Country/Region	Study Population	Intervention	Follow-up	Outcome Measures
Choi et al,[19] 2020	Korea, single center	Participants with a family history of gastric cancer, n = 1826 randomized (n = 1587 evaluated for *H pylori* eradication)	1. Lansoprazole 30 mg, Amoxicillin 1g, Clarithromycin 500 mg BID × 7 d 2. Placebo × 7 d *H pylori* eradication = 70.1%	Median duration of follow-up was 9.2 y (IQR, 6.2–10.6) and 10.2 y (IQR, 8.9–11.6) for incident gastric cancer and overall survival, respectively	1. Incident gastric cancer 2. Overall survival 3. Incident gastric adenoma
Correa et al[23] 2000 Correa et al,[106] 2001	Colombia, 2 communities in Narino Province	Participants with confirmed histologic diagnoses of gastric preneoplasia, n = 976 randomized (n = 852 in intention to treat; n = 631 complete case analyses); age 29–69, mean 51.1 y; 46.1% male	1. Bismuth 262 mg, amoxicillin 500 mg, metronidazole 375 mg TID × 14 d • With or without dietary supplements 2. Placebo • With or without dietary supplements *H pylori* eradication rate = 58.0%	Cited analysis, 6 y. *Note: multiple points of follow-up have been published to date, with the most recent a 16-y analysis.*[107]	1. Progression of preneoplastic lesions (based on histologic score, and global assessment). • Gastric cancer outcome published separately[108] 2. Relative risk of progression, no change, regression of histologic lesions
Leung et al,[34] 2004	China, 11 villages in Yantai County, Shandong Province	Participants with vs without dyspepsia, who underwent upper endoscopy with biopsy. n = 587 randomized (34% with gastric preneoplasia at baseline); age 35–75 y, mean, 52.0 y; 47.8% male *Note: 33.7% with preneoplasia at baseline*	1. Omeprazole 20 mg, amoxicillin 1g, clarithromycin 500 mg BID × 7 d 2. Placebo × 7 d *H pylori* eradication rate = 55.6%	Cited analysis, 5 y *Note: 10-y follow-up also published.*[108]	1. Histologic outcomes at 2 and 5 y (subsequently, 8 and 10 y)

Saito et al 2005 (abstract only; full study not published as of Feb. 2020)	Japan, 145 centers	Participants were healthy volunteers with *H pylori* infection. n = 629 randomized; age 20–59 y, mean not reported	1. Lansoprazole 30 mg, amoxicillin 1.5 g, clarithromycin 400 mg once daily × 7 d 2. No eradication *H pylori* eradication rate = 74.4%	Follow-up stated as "≥4 y"	1. Histologic regression or progression of atrophy by at least 1 grade (*Note: did not report on gastric cancer incidence, although this was a priori planned outcome*)
Wong 2004[32]	China, 7 villages in Changle Country, Fujian Province	Participants undergoing screening endoscopy (age 35–65 y, mean 42.2 y). n = 2423 evaluated, and n = 1628 with *H pylori* infection but without endoscopic lesions (eg, peptic ulcer) were randomized *Note: 37.7% with premalignant lesions at baseline (gastric atrophy, intestinal metaplasia, gastric cancer)*	1. Omeprazole 20 mg, amoxicillin/clavulanic acid 750 mg, metronidazole 400 mg BID × 14 d 2. Placebo × 14 d *H pylori* eradication rate = 83.7%	Follow-up time, 7.5 y	1. Incidence of gastric cancer 2. Incidence in those with vs without premalignant lesions
Wong et al,[30] 2012	China, 12 villages Linqu County, Shandong Province	Participants with *H pylori* infection and advanced gastric lesions (severe chronic atrophy, intestinal metaplasia, dysplasia); age 35–64 y, mean 53 y n = 1024 randomized, 2 × 2 factorial design *ALL participants had*	1. Omeprazole 20 mg, amoxicillin 1g, clarithromycin 500 mg BID × 7 d a. PLUS placebo BID, OR b. PLUS celecoxib 2. Placebo 3. Celecoxib + placebo *H pylori* eradication rate = 63.5%	Follow-up time, 5 y	1. Gastric cancer 2. Regression or progression of gastric premalignant lesions

(*continued on next page*)

Table 1
(continued)

First Author, Publication year	Country/Region	Study Population	Intervention	Follow-up	Outcome Measures
		premalignant lesions at baseline			
You et al,[33] 2006	China, 13 villages Linqu County, Shandong Province	Participants were selected randomly and underwent upper-endoscopy, n = 2258 participants randomized; age 35–64 y, mean 46.8 y 2 × 2 × 2 factorial design *Note:* H pylori *confirmed via serologic testing* *64% had preneoplastic lesions at baseline*	1. Omeprazole 20 mg, Amoxicillin 1g BID × 14 d a. with or without vitamin or garlic supplementation 2. Placebo ± vitamin or garlic supplementation • "Vitamins" = vitamin C, E, selenium • Garlic = garlic oil and Kyolic aged garlic extract	Follow-up time, 14.7 y *Note: multiple points of follow-up have been published to date, with the most recent a 22-y analysis.*[82]	1. Prevalence of dysplasia or gastric cancer 2. Prevalence of other precancerous lesions (severe chronic atrophic gastritis, intestinal metaplasia) 3. Average 'severity' score

Abbreviation: BID, 2 times per day; IQR, interquartile range; TID, 3 times per day.
Data from Refs.[19,23,29,30,32–34,82,106–108]

pylori eradication therapy versus no therapy. Their comprehensive literature search through February 2, 2020, identified 7 distinct baseline RCTs (ie, no overlapping study populations) that met the full inclusion criteria. Six of these RCTs were performed in Asian countries, and the seventh was performed in Colombia.[19,23,29–34] No RCTs analyzing *H pylori* eradication versus no eradication on gastric cancer incidence have been conducted in countries with populations at low or intermediate risk for NCGA. **Table 1** provides descriptions of these base RCTs, which resulted in a number of subsequent publications that are organized in the full Cochrane Review.[29] Based on meta-analysis of 8323 individuals in these 7 RCTs (modified intention to treat), compared with placebo or no treatment, *H pylori* eradication treatment was associated with a significant 46% lower risk (relative risk [RR], 0.46; 95% CI, 0.40–0.72) of incident gastric cancer on 4 to 22 years of follow-up time; the number needed to treat to have 1 person benefit was 72 (95% CI, 55–118). There was no significant heterogeneity observed across the studies. The quality of evidence was downgraded from high to moderate for this primary analysis based on a few important considerations. First, although 4 studies were deemed low risk of bias, 2 were deemed high risk and 1 was at unclear risk. Second, the *H pylori* eradication regimens used in these 7 studies varied; indeed, many of these studies started enrolling before 1994, which is when proton-pump inhibitors became more widely available. Last, some studies used a factorial design, with some arms including *H pylori* eradication therapy and vitamin supplementation, for example; as such, it was sometimes not possible to isolate fully whether the observed relative risk reduction in gastric cancer was wholly attributable to *H pylori* eradication. Based on meta-analysis of the 4 RCTs (n = 6301) that reported on gastric cancer-related mortality, randomization to *H pylori* eradication therapy versus no therapy/placebo was associated with a significant 49% lower risk of gastric-cancer related mortality (RR, 0.61; 95% CI, 0.40–0.92) on follow-up ranging from 7 to 22 years, with a number needed to treat to benefit of 137 (95% CI, 89–667).

Concomitant gastric preneoplasia

As described elsewhere in this article, one of the leading mechanisms underlying the chemopreventive effect of *H pylori* eradication treatment is that successful eradication of *H pylori* substantially decreases and ideally eliminates persistent inflammation. Indeed, the majority of individuals with *H pylori* nonatrophic gastritis and nonsevere atrophic gastritis will have normalization of these mucosal changes after successful *H pylori* eradication. The return of normal gastric mucosa also restores gastric acid production and facilitates the restoration of the normal gastric microbiota,[35] which likely also contributes to the beneficial effect of *H pylori* eradication in these early, reversible mucosal stages. However, if there are severe mucosal changes present, including severe gastric atrophy with or without gastric intestinal metaplasia, studies suggest that the benefit of *H pylori* eradication treatment, even with confirmed eradication of *H pylori* organisms, is attenuated and potentially even null. The presence of gastric intestinal metaplasia has been considered the first irreversible stage in the Correa cascade and the earliest point of no return, although a handful of cohort studies have challenged this notion of irreversibility.[36] Our understanding of the chemopreventive effects of *H pylori* eradication once preneoplastic gastric mucosal changes have developed is limited at best and largely reflects the difficulty in conducting robust clinical studies to investigate this question with rigor. As such, most studies have included mixed populations with or without gastric preneoplastic changes—under which nonmetaplastic and metaplastic gastric atrophy both qualify.

A few studies have provided some insight, however. The authors of the updated Cochrane meta-analysis of RCTs cited elsewhere in this article conducted a subgroup analysis of 3425 individuals who had gastric preneoplasia at baseline and demonstrated that there was no difference in gastric cancer incidence between those randomized to *H pylori* eradication treatment versus placebo or no treatment; 2.4% of participants randomized to treatment (42 of 1734 participants) compared with 3.4% of participants randomized to placebo or no treatment (57 of 1691 participants) developed gastric cancer on follow-up.[29] It should be noted, however, that the authors included dysplasia (grade not specified) as a preneoplastic mucosal change. A recent comprehensive systematic review with meta-analysis that was focused specifically on the natural history and outcomes of gastric intestinal metaplasia reported that, among individuals with confirmed gastric intestinal metaplasia and no higher grade pathology, *H pylori* eradication treatment versus placebo was associated with a 17% higher risk of progression (RR, 1.17; 95% CI, 1.01–1.36) to more advanced histology (moderate certainty in evidence), although the authors noted that the estimate was largely driven by data from 1 trial, the Shandong Interventional Trial.[33,36] This same trial though had conflicting results in another analysis, because *H pylori* eradication treatment in individuals with confirmed gastric intestinal metaplasia was also associated with regression to improved histology.[33,36,37] For the outcome of gastric cancer incidence specifically, *H pylori* eradication treatment versus placebo was associated with a significantly decreased risk in patients with or without gastric intestinal metaplasia (RR, 0.68; 95% CI, 0.48–0.96) on follow-up ranging from 4 to 16 years; however, when limited to only individuals with gastric intestinal metaplasia, there was similarly no substantial benefit on follow-up ranging from 5 to 12 years (RR, 0.76; 95% CI, 0.36–1.61).[17] Importantly, the data informing these meta-analyses were drawn primarily from 3 main RCTs, 2 from China and 1 from Colombia. The findings were somewhat driven by 1 large RCT from the Fujian Province, China with 7.5 years of follow-up; in this study, compared with placebo, the eradication of *H pylori* was associated with a decreased risk of gastric cancer only in individuals without precancerous lesions (atrophy, intestinal metaplasia, or dysplasia) at the outset, but there was no difference between the treatment and placebo groups when the analysis included individuals with precancerous lesions, including dysplasia.

Despite the conflicting evidence, *H pylori* eradication as chemoprevention for gastric cancer among individuals with gastric intestinal metaplasia (and other premalignant mucosal pathology) is still recommended by most international guidelines.[38–41] Because these individuals remain at risk of gastric cancer despite *H pylori* eradication, most international medical societies also suggest ongoing endoscopic surveillance for early detection of neoplasia, although the recommendations remain mixed in the absence of high-quality evidence derived from RCTs. Importantly, this finding underscores the need for more studies to better define mechanisms driving neoplastic progression in the absence of ongoing *H pylori* infection, such as the role of the non–*H pylori* microbiome and metabolites. Indeed, a better understanding of these mechanisms will help to inform the identification of adjunctive chemopreventive agents to ideally reverse these mucosal abnormalities and restore normal gastric mucosa, or at least halt further progression.

H pylori eradication for gastric cancer prevention in specific populations

Family history of gastric cancer. *H pylori* and family history of gastric cancer are the 2 strongest risk factors for gastric cancer. Approximately 10% of gastric cancers demonstrate familial aggregation. Having a family history of gastric cancer in a first-degree relative compared with no family history is associated with an approximately 3-fold higher risk of gastric cancer, although this risk varies from 2-fold up to 10-fold higher in case-control studies, depending on the ethnic group and country of origin.[42] In addition to sharing genetics, family members share environmental exposures, behaviors, and cultural practices, as well as dietary habits and preferences. Furthermore, family members can share the same strains of *H pylori* as well as develop similar host immune responses to chronic *H pylori* infection; they may also have a greater susceptibility to infection.[43–47] To this end, studies have demonstrated that individuals who have a family history of gastric cancer more often have *H pylori* infection and more often demonstrate precancerous gastric mucosal changes that are more severe compared with individuals without a family history. Although there are guideline recommendations for endoscopic screening in individuals with a family history of gastric cancer in a first-degree family member, there is a notable dearth of studies analyzing strategies for chemoprevention in this high-risk population. One recent double-blind, placebo-controlled RCT from South Korea, in which 1838 first-degree relatives of individuals with gastric cancer were randomized to *H pylori* treatment versus placebo, demonstrated that *H pylori* eradication treatment was associated with a 55% decreased risk of incident gastric cancer (hazard ratio [HR], 0.45; 95% CI, 0.21–0.94) during a median follow-up of 9.2 years, based on the modified intention-to-treat analysis (n = 1676).[19] Gastric cancer occurred with significantly lower frequency in those with successful *H pylori* eradication compared with those with persistent infection (0.8% vs 2.9%; HR, 0.27; 95% CI, 0.10–0.70).[19] There is a relative consensus globally for recommending a test and treat strategy for *H pylori* as a chemopreventive measure among individuals with a positive family history of gastric cancer,[41,48] but recommendations are mixed in some Western countries, namely the United States,[49,50] owing to lack of high-quality evidence supporting this practice.

Metachronous gastric cancer (tertiary prevention). To date, there have been at least 3 RCTs of *H pylori* eradication versus no eradication for reducing the risk of metachronous gastric cancer, with 2 studies[20,51] reporting a decreased risk of subsequent gastric cancer and a third study[52] demonstrating no statistically significant difference in the incidence of metachronous gastric cancer in those who were randomized to *H pylori* treatment versus no treatment ($P = .15$). Several observational studies have also been performed, with overall mixed results, either demonstrating a benefit or a null association, which likely reflects sample size considerations and significant differences in study design. Notably, no studies outside of Asia have investigated the effect of *H pylori* eradication for tertiary chemoprevention. A meta-analysis of 10 studies, including both RCTs and cohort studies that were published before May 2015, demonstrated that, compared with the reference group, *H pylori* eradication was associated with 54% lower risk of metachronous gastric cancer (RR, 0.46; 95% CI, 0.35–0.60).[22] The duration of follow-up for these studies ranged from a minimum of 24 months to a maximum of 58 months. A third RCT published in 2018 (and, thus, not included in the previously referenced meta-analysis) with median follow-up of 5.9 years, reported that, compared with placebo, *H pylori* eradication therapy was associated with a significant 50% decrease in the risk of metachronous gastric cancer (HR, 0.50; 95% CI, 0.26–0.94) based on a modified intention-to-treat analysis; moreover, among individuals who had baseline atrophy of the corpus lesser curvature, those who received *H pylori* eradication treatment more often had improvement in atrophy grade at 3 years compared with individuals who received placebo (48.4% vs 15.0%; $P<.001$).[20]

These data, coupled with the observation that the vast majority of individuals with NCGA have background preneoplastic mucosal changes at diagnosis, provide further evidence for the field effect that occurs within the context of chronic *H pylori* exposure. Moreover, multiple studies in the past decade have confirmed that ongoing *H pylori* infection may lead to genome instability and aberrant gene expression as a result of *H pylori*–mediated epigenetic changes and dysregulated DNA repair, among other potentially carcinogenic events.[53] Taken together, these data do lend support to the strategy of treatment of *H pylori* in the presence of gastric premalignant mucosal changes. However, the extrapolation of these data outside of the populations included in these studies is problematic, given the variability in and interaction between host genetic risk and *H pylori* strain specific virulence that might characterize other diverse populations. Thus, although *H pylori* eradication therapy for tertiary prevention of gastric cancer seems reasonable, studies are needed across diverse populations, especially low to intermediate risk populations from Western countries.

Collectively, these data suggest there is insufficient evidence to support broad population-based testing and treatment of *H pylori* as a screening strategy in populations with a low incidence of gastric cancer, but this might be reasonable for higher risk populations, including those residing within countries that are overall low risk based on population aggregation.[48,54] Several questions remain when considering how to best translate the current evidence into clinical practice, particularly among high-risk populations residing in otherwise low-risk geographic regions; for example, determining the optimal age for *H pylori* screening and treatment because gastric premalignant changes are more frequent in older individuals who have greater cumulative *H pylori* exposure, as well as determining how to balance the desire for chemoprevention with the increasing rates of *H pylori* eradication failure and antibiotic resistance.

Aspirin and Nonsteroidal Anti-inflammatory Drugs as Chemoprevention Against Gastric Cancer

Aspirin and nonaspirin NSAIDs have both been investigated extensively for their role in cancer prevention, with their protective effect appearing most relevant for adenocarcinomas.[55] The daily intake of aspirin or nonaspirin NSAIDs has been associated with risk reductions of up to 63% in colorectal cancer and up to nearly 40% for breast, lung, and prostate adenocarcinomas. The exact molecular basis of this chemopreventive effect is not fully elucidated and likely varies depending on the cancer location, cancer phenotype, and individual characteristics, such as host genetic composition and environmental contributors. That said, several biologically plausible hypotheses have been proposed, the majority of which are COX dependent, although COX-independent pathways also seem to be relevant. NSAIDs, including aspirin, inhibit COX-1 and COX-2 production. The inhibition of COX-2 seems to be most relevant in chemoprevention against malignancies of the gastrointestinal tract, namely, colorectal and (noncardia) gastric cancers. Several studies have consistently demonstrated that COX-2 levels are significantly higher in gastrointestinal malignancies; indeed, higher COX-2 expression is observed in gastric cancer tissue compared with tissue samples obtained from normal gastric mucosa in the same individual. This finding suggests a role for increased prostaglandin biosynthesis and COX-2 overexpression in carcinogenesis, as well as lymphovascular invasion and metastasis.[55] COX-2 is involved in several other pathways that, when dysregulated, are also implicated in carcinogenesis; these pathways include promotion of angiogenesis and cell proliferation, as well as inhibition of apoptosis. NSAIDs including aspirin, presumably through blockade of COX-2, have antitumor growth effects, including the inhibition of angiogenesis and the upregulation of mediators leading to apoptosis (eg, activation of caspase-3).[56–58] Aspirin and nonaspirin NSAIDs might also exert chemopreventive benefit through COX-independent pathways, including activation of nuclear factor-κB, activated protein 1, Wnt-ß-catenin, and extracellular signal-regulated kinase, among others.[59–62] Some of these pathways exert important roles in *H pylori*–induced gastric carcinogenesis, adding a further layer of complexity.

Numerous cohort and case control studies, along with several meta-analyses, analyzing the association between aspirin and nonaspirin NSAIDs and risk of gastric cancer, have been published to date. The results are generally consistent and demonstrate an inverse association between regular NSAID use and the risk of noncardia gastric cancer. Notably, the protective association for noncardia gastric cancer does seem to be driven more so by aspirin, with the data for nonaspirin NSAID use generally demonstrating a lesser risk attenuation or a null association. Again, these mixed findings may relate more to study design considerations such as rigor of the statistical analysis with respect to confounder adjustment and exposure misclassification, particularly because NSAIDs can be obtained over the counter in most countries. Many studies that analyzed nonaspirin NSAIDs did not adjust for aspirin use, which is important because some studies have demonstrated as high as 56% overlap between nonaspirin NSAID users and aspirin users.[63] At least 2 studies have analyzed the association according to histology of noncardia gastric cancer, both with congruent findings that the risk reduction was stronger for intestinal-type, compared with diffuse-type histology, which tends to have a greater genetic predisposition as opposed to the former, where environmental factors are key drivers.[63,64]

Most studies report a risk reduction for noncardia gastric cancer among regular aspirin users of approximately 20% to 50%, although these values vary depending on the definition of regular use (typically at least once weekly), the duration of use, the rigor of the analysis, the completeness of the data, and other population characteristics, including geography and *H pylori* status. One of the most recently published meta-analyses, which analyzed 33 studies from Asia, Europe, and North America and included nearly 2 million individuals, demonstrated that the use of aspirin at least monthly was associated with a 16% to 26% significantly lower risk of noncardia gastric cancer.[65] Based on a meta-analysis of 3 studies, aspirin use compared with nonuse was also associated with a significantly lower risk of gastric cancer-related mortality. Another recent meta-analysis of both any NSAID use, aspirin only, and nonaspirin NSAID use reported significant 30% (RR, 0.70; 95% CI, 0.59–0.84), 36% (RR, 0.64; 95% CI, 0.53–0.78), and 26% (RR, 0.74; 95% CI, 0.60–0.93) respective reductions in the risk of noncardia gastric cancer; whereas, none were associated with cardia gastric cancer.[66] Subgroup analyses demonstrated consistent findings irrespective of study design (cohort vs case control).

Individual studies conducted in populations with a higher gastric cancer risk, including those conducted in Asia and among individuals with *H pylori* exposure, have generally demonstrated greater risk decreases with regular aspirin use versus nonuse. One large territory-wide study from Hong Kong, which included 63,605 individuals with *H pylori* infection who were successfully eradicated between 2003 and 2012, demonstrated that regular aspirin use (at least once weekly) compared with no use or infrequent use was associated with a significantly reduced risk of gastric cancer (HR, 0.30; 95% CI, 0.15–0.61) on follow-up out to a median of 7.6 years (interquartile range, 5.1–10.3 years). A greater decrease in risk was observed with increasing aspirin frequency, dose, and duration of use (all P trends <.001).[62] The risk reduction associated with aspirin doses of less than 100 mg was 62% (HR, 0.38; 95% CI, 0.18–0.79) versus 85% in users of aspirin 100 mg or higher (HR, 0.15; 95% CI, 0.03–0.65), although the CI was wider in the latter group owing to smaller sample size (n = 4607 [8%] vs 1725 [3%]). The mechanisms underlying the greater magnitude of risk reduction observed in this cohort of *H pylori* eradicated individuals compared with cohorts with mixed *H pylori* infected and uninfected individuals are not well defined. NSAID use has been demonstrated to decrease *H pylori* proliferation and enhance the antimicrobial effect of anti–*H pylori* treatment, as well as attenuate potential *H pylori*–induced carcinogenic pathways; indeed, *H pylori* infection is associated with increased prostaglandin synthesis and COX-2 expression, which might be blocked by NSAID consumption.[67–71] The chemopreventive benefit of NSAID use, especially aspirin, after *H pylori* has been eliminated, however, has been incompletely investigated. It is likely that many participants in the referenced study from Hong Kong[62] already had underlying gastric premalignant mucosal changes; whether regular NSAID use decreases the likelihood of malignant transformation, which is known to occur even after successful *H pylori* eradication,[36] is undetermined. Notably, 1 RCT of rofecoxib 25 mg/d versus placebo in individuals with histologically confirmed intestinal metaplasia and successful *H pylori* eradication reported no significant difference in the frequency of intestinal metaplasia regression or in the severity of intestinal metaplasia after 2 years of follow-up.[72] It is possible that NSAIDs, including aspirin, are more relevant with respect to the prevention of actual malignant transformation, as opposed to earlier phases of progression. This remains an important area of investigation because there are limited options for gastric cancer risk attenuation in this high-risk population, save perhaps interval endoscopic surveillance, which is costly and has limitations.

Although these data are overall promising, particularly for aspirin, evidence from RCTs is needed to guide positioning of NSAIDs as chemopreventive agents against gastric cancer. The most pressing knowledge gaps that need to be bridged include defining the high-risk populations who might benefit most from NSAID chemoprevention and in whom there is minimal harm; the minimum effective dose, frequency, and duration of use needed for benefit; and the ideal drug (eg, aspirin vs selective COX-2 inhibitors, such as celecoxib, which have fewer adverse gastrointestinal effects compared with nonselective agents), which should also consider individual comorbidities (eg, cardiovascular risk, bleeding risk). To date, no RCTs have been conducted analyzing NSAID use and gastric cancer incidence or mortality as the primary outcome. One related RCT was conducted using the Women's Health Study cohort. In this study, nearly 40,000 women age 45 years or older who were generally healthy were randomly assigned to every other day aspirin 100 mg or placebo and were followed for the outcome of an invasive cancer diagnosis at any site. Over an average follow-up of 10 years, there was no significant association between aspirin use and the risk of invasive gastric cancer.[73] However, this study was likely underpowered for gastric cancer because only 20 cases occurred (cardia vs noncardia not specified); the population is also a low-risk population for gastric cancer, because the Women's Health Study recruited female health professionals and the overall demographic included less than 10% non-White races/ethnicities.[74] A secondary analysis of individual level data from 8 eligible RCTs where study participants were randomized to daily aspirin versus no aspirin and originally followed for the primary outcome of cardiovascular events, demonstrated the potential benefit of regular use of aspirin for chemoprevention and decreasing the risk of cancer-related mortality. Among 23,535 participants randomized to aspirin use, there was a lesser all-cancer mortality, including gastrointestinal cancers specifically (HR, 0.46; 95% CI, 0.27–0.77), after 5 years of follow-up. For cancers overall, the benefit was greater with longer duration of aspirin use, but aspirin doses in excess of 75 mg did not impact the risk estimates. For gastric adenocarcinoma specifically (cardia vs noncardia not specified), there was a lower risk of death only after 10 to 20 years of follow-up (HR, 042; 95% CI, 0.23–0.79). Competing risk of death is certainly a consideration in this study; the cancer incidence was not reported.

α-Difluoromethylornithine as Chemoprevention Against Gastric Cancer in Patients with Gastric Preneoplasia

Polyamines have been implicated in gastric carcinogenesis. These effectors, which are generated by ornithine deoxycarboxylase, have been associated with disruption of DNA repair mechanisms and inducing DNA damage, as well as altering the host immune response in gastric tissue. The expression of ornithine deoxycarboxylase in the gastric mucosa is part of the host innate immune response to *H pylori* infection.[75,76] Treatment with α-difluoromethylornithine (DFMO), which is an inhibitor of ornithine deoxycarboxylase, has been demonstrated to directly reduce *H pylori* virulence and attenuate risk of gastric dysplasia and carcinoma in Mongolian gerbils via a decrease in polyamine concentration in gastric tissue and abrogating polyamine-driven oxidative stress.[76] At least in experimental studies, DFMO also enhances DNA repair and decreases apoptosis-resistant cells with DNA damage; in this way, DFMO directly impacts genome stability in *H pylori*–infected gastric mucosa.[75–78] As such, DFMO has been proposed as a chemopreventive agent specifically in *H pylori*–associated gastric carcinogenesis and human trials are ongoing. Studies have demonstrated a chemopreventive effect of DFMO (in combination with sulindac) with respect to colorectal adenoma recurrence, which is hypothesized to be via a similar mechanism of polyamine inhibition.[79–81]

Other Chemopreventive Agents Against Gastric Cancer

Several other medications and dietary interventions have been investigated for their chemopreventive effects against gastric cancer, mostly with mixed findings and without high-quality data. Studies of nutritional intakes and cancer risk are inevitably difficult to conduct in a rigorous manner owing to the large sample sizes and long follow-up time that are needed, not to mention the challenges with respect to residual confounding, accurate exposure assessment, and determining the level of sustained dietary modification that is needed for an effect. This said, dietary interventions are attractive as chemoprevention, owing to the fact that they are generally safe, cost effective, and feasible. As such, certain dietary interventions might have an adjunctive role in addition to other lifestyle modifications that are known to decrease noncardia gastric cancer (as well as the risk of other cancer types). Dietary interventions include limiting the consumption of salted foods, high nitrite foods, processed foods, and red meats, and increasing the consumption of fresh vegetables and fruits, particularly citrus fruits and those high in beta-carotene, vitamin C, and antioxidants, and possibly garlic and allium vegetables. Garlic and its derivatives have antioxidant, antimicrobial, and immunomodulatory properties, among other benefits.[82] Studies have demonstrated that garlic is associated with a decreased risk of metachronous colorectal adenomas, and possibly also gastric cancer.[82–84] Calcium and magnesium might also have benefit in decreases noncardia gastric cancer risk.[85] Curcumin has been investigated in mechanistic studies, but clinical data are limited. Clinical and experimental data suggest a possible benefit of green tea and ginseng consumption.[86–90] Selenium, which is an essential trace element that is consumed in the diet, has also been investigated as a chemopreventive agent in gastric cancer given its antioxidant properties, in addition to anti-inflammatory, proapoptotic, and antiangiogenic properties.[91]

One RCT from Linqu County, Shandong Province of China randomly assigned 2258 *H pylori* seropositive individuals to *H pylori* treatment, vitamin supplementation, garlic supplementation, or placebo (2 × 2 × 2 factorial design) and 1107 *H pylori* seronegative individuals to vitamin supplementation, garlic supplementation, or placebo (2 × 2 factorial design). The vitamin supplementation intervention included the administration of vitamin C, vitamin E, and selenium for 7.3 years (1995–2003), whereas the garlic supplementation intervention included administration of garlic extract and oil over this same time period. Notably, *H pylori* treatment was amoxicillin 1 g and omeprazole 20 mg 2 times per day for 2 weeks and it is not stated whether or not nonserologic testing and confirmation of eradication was performed. The authors did report excellent compliance among participants. Based on 22 years of follow-up, *H pylori* treatment (odds ratio [OR], 0.48; 95% CI, 0.32–0.71), and vitamin supplementation (OR, 0.64; 95% CI, 0.46–0.91), but not garlic supplementation (OR, 0.81; 95% CI, 0.57–1.13) were associated with reduced incidence of gastric cancer. All 3 interventions, compared with placebo, were associated with a significantly decreased gastric cancer–related mortality; however, the effects of vitamin supplementation on gastric cancer incidence and garlic supplementation on mortality generally occurred later, and only after 14.7 years of follow-up. Separate analyses were not conducted for noncardia versus cardia, but the authors noted that the majority of gastric cancers were noncardia.[82] Other RCTs of dietary interventions with or without concomitant *H pylori* eradication treatment have been conducted in other high-risk populations.[23] The coadministration of vitamins and antioxidants with *H pylori* eradication therapy does seem to have a greater chemopreventive effect compared with eradication treatment alone.[29] The factorial design of some of these trials, however, make it difficult to isolate the effect, if even present, of any singular exposure. Also complicating this field are the baseline risk of gastric cancer in the study population and the modifying effects of other environmental, cultural, and nongenetic factors, including nutritional deficiencies, as well as genetic factors; these factors limit generalizability. These findings do warrant exploration in other high-risk populations for the primary reasons stated elsewhere in this article—dietary modifications are generally safe, low-cost, and sustainable interventions that can be implemented on a larger scale, and might have other off-target benefits related to risk reduction of other disease pathology.

Metformin and statins have also been investigated clinically for their chemopreventive effects for gastric cancer based on supportive data from experimental studies. Metformin decreases gastric cancer cell viability, invasion, and migration via downregulation of COX expression, as well as through downregulation of hypoxia inducible factor 1α, pyruvate kinase M2, phosphatidylinositol 3-kinase/protein kinase b, and poly (ADP-ribose) polymerase expression.[92–95] By inhibiting phosphatidylinositol 3-kinase/protein kinase b and poly (ADP-ribose) polymerase pathways specifically, metformin also induces cell cycle arrest and apoptosis in gastric cancer cells. There are numerous observational studies, the majority of which are limited to individuals with type 2 diabetes (indication bias), which analyze the association between metformin and gastric cancer incidence. Collectively, the conclusions are mixed, with some studies, including large population-based studies, demonstrating null findings, whereas others demonstrate a protective effect.[96–101] These inconsistent data relate to significant differences in study design with respect to the study population, the rigor of the statistical analysis, including confounder adjustment and assessment of the exposure, such as new user versus prevalent user designs, as well as variable accounting of immortal time bias,[102] and preclude strong conclusions. Many studies did not adjust for relevant medications including aspirin, NSAIDs, statins, and insulin, or other relevant confounders such as *H pylori* exposure, smoking, and body mass index. One recent meta-analysis that included eligible cohort studies published through October 2019 demonstrated that using 8 cohort studies with approximately 1.2 million type 2 diabetics, metformin use was associated with 21% decrease in gastric cancer risk (HR, 0.79; 95% CI, 0.62–1.00); separate estimates were not provided for noncardia versus cardia gastric cancer.[96] Meta-analyses of the studies that analyzed sulfonylurea derivatives and noninsulin antidiabetic agents demonstrated a null association with gastric cancer incidence. Geographic differences seem to be relevant, because the magnitude of the protective association was amplified when meta-analysis was limited to the 3 studies from Asian populations only (HR, 0.54; 95% CI, 0.38–0.78), but the benefit was significantly attenuated when limited to the 5 studies from Western populations (HR, 0.99; 95% CI, 0.99–0.99). One recent cohort analysis conducted among diabetic patients from Hong Kong who were successfully eradicated for *H pylori* demonstrated that metformin use was associated with a significantly lower risk of gastric cancer compared with nonusers, and there was a trend toward an increased benefit with increasing duration and dose of metformin.[99] The authors also conducted a propensity score adjustment, as well as repeated their analysis using time varying covariates and lag time analysis with similar findings.[102,103]

There is also biological plausibility underlying a hypothesized chemopreventive effect of statins for gastric cancer, but high-quality and consistent clinical data are lacking.[104,105] Well-conducted RCTs among specific high-risk populations are needed to adjudicate the findings presented herein regarding aspirin, NSAIDs, metformin, and statin use, among other putative chemopreventive agents to establish their effectiveness, or lack thereof, in noncardia gastric cancer. Despite otherwise promising data at least for aspirin and metformin, these cannot yet be recommended outside of their primary indications.

SUMMARY

There is ample evidence of the benefit of *H pylori* eradication in primary chemoprevention against intestinal-type noncardia gastric cancer when eradication occurs before the development of advanced preneoplastic mucosal changes. There might still be benefit thereafter, but the data are overall mixed and the benefit seems to be attenuated at best. Experimental as well as clinical data support other agents as primary chemoprevention, all with biological plausibility and the majority already used clinically for benign conditions. Although the largest body of evidence is available for NSAIDs, particularly aspirin, there are still no RCTs analyzing primary prevention of gastric cancer as the outcome. Dietary modifications as chemoprevention in gastric cancer also show promise and are particularly attractive given their favorable safety profile. Unfortunately, despite the substantial burden of gastric cancer globally, little progress has been made to rigorously analyze chemopreventive agents. To move the needle forward, the research agenda should ideally be focused on primary prevention trials, as well as on investigations aiming to personalize the selection of chemoprevention agents in high risk individuals. Several major knowledge gaps persist, including defining the role of agents, such as aspirin or metformin, as chemoprevention after *H pylori* eradication in individuals who have developed gastric preneoplasia, as well as identifying the age at which these interventions are most beneficial in specific populations. Another challenge remains in identifying effective chemoprevention for non-*H pylori*–associated gastric cancer. Focused investigation is needed in the face of an expanding aging population and the projected increase in gastric cancer-related deaths so that we can appropriately position gastric cancer chemopreventive agents in the armamentarium of gastric cancer control programs.

CLINICS CARE POINTS

- Several randomized controlled trials have confirmed that chemoprevention through *H. pylori* eradication is associated with a reduced risk of noncardia gastric adenocarcinoma; however, the chemopreventive benefit is significantly

attenuated in patients who have already developed gastric premalignant mucosal changes.
- Additional studies are especially needed to define underlying mechanisms of neoplastic progression following *H. pylori* eradication and in patients without *H. pylori* to help target discovery of chemoprevention agents.
- Several case-control and cohort studies support an association between aspirin and potentially non-aspirin non-steroidal anti-inflammatory drugs and noncardia gastric cancer.
- This review describes the current literature surrounding several posited chemopreventive agents for gastric cancer, and provides a critical appraisal of the current evidence.

DISCLOSURES/CONFLICT OF INTEREST STATEMENT

The authors have no potential conflicts (financial, professional, nor personal) that are relevant to this article.

REFERENCES

1. Bray F, Ferlay J, Soerjomataram I, et al. Global cancer statistics 2018: GLOBOCAN estimates of incidence and mortality worldwide for 36 cancers in 185 countries. CA Cancer J Clin 2018;68:394–424.
2. Anderson WF, Rabkin CS, Turner N, et al. The Changing Face of Noncardia Gastric Cancer Incidence Among US Non-Hispanic Whites. J Natl Cancer Inst 2018;110:608–15.
3. Correa P, Piazuelo MB, Wilson KT. Pathology of gastric intestinal metaplasia: clinical implications. Am J Gastroenterol 2010;105:493–8.
4. Correa P, Piazuelo MB. Helicobacter pylori infection and gastric adenocarcinoma. US Gastroenterol Hepatol Rev 2011;7:59–64.
5. Nomura A, Stemmermann GN, Chyou PH, et al. Helicobacter pylori infection and gastric carcinoma among Japanese Americans in Hawaii. N Engl J Med 1991; 325:1132–6.
6. Parsonnet J, Friedman GD, Vandersteen DP, et al. Helicobacter pylori infection and the risk of gastric carcinoma. N Engl J Med 1991;325:1127–31.
7. Forman D, Newell DG, Fullerton F, et al. Association between infection with Helicobacter pylori and risk of gastric cancer: evidence from a prospective investigation. BMJ 1991;302:1302–5.
8. Helicobacter and Cancer Collaborative Group. Gastric cancer and Helicobacter pylori: a combined analysis of 12 case control studies nested within prospective cohorts. Gut 2001;49:347–53.
9. McColl KEL. Clinical practice. Helicobacter pylori infection. N Engl J Med 2010; 362:1597–604.
10. Hooi JKY, Lai WY, Ng WK, et al. Global Prevalence of Helicobacter pylori Infection: systematic Review and Meta-Analysis. Gastroenterology 2017;153:420–9.
11. Plummer M, Franceschi S, Vignat J, et al. Global burden of gastric cancer attributable to Helicobacter pylori. Int J Cancer 2015;136:487–90.
12. Nozaki K, Shimizu N, Inada K, et al. Synergistic promoting effects of Helicobacter pylori infection and high-salt diet on gastric carcinogenesis in Mongolian gerbils. Jpn J Cancer Res 2002;93:1083–9.
13. Cao X, Tsukamoto T, Seki T, et al. 4-Vinyl-2,6-dimethoxyphenol (canolol) suppresses oxidative stress and gastric carcinogenesis in Helicobacter pylori-infected carcinogen-treated Mongolian gerbils. Int J Cancer 2008;122:1445–54.

14. Cao D, Jiang J, Tsukamoto T, et al. Canolol inhibits gastric tumors initiation and progression through COX-2/PGE2 pathway in K19-C2mE transgenic mice. PLoS One 2015;10:e0120938.
15. Warren JR, Marshall B. Unidentified curved bacilli on gastric epithelium in active chronic gastritis. Lancet 1983;1:1273–5.
16. Kuipers EJ, Uyterlinde AM, Peña AS, et al. Long-term sequelae of Helicobacter pylori gastritis. Lancet 1995;345:1525–8.
17. Graham DY, Asaka M. RE: Effects of helicobacter pylori treatment on gastric cancer incidence and mortality in subgroups. J Natl Cancer Inst 2014;106. https://doi.org/10.1093/jnci/dju352.
18. Graham DY, Shiotani A. The time to eradicate gastric cancer is now. Gut 2005; 54:735–8.
19. Choi IJ, Kim CG, Lee JY, et al. Family history of gastric cancer and helicobacter pylori treatment. N Engl J Med 2020;382:427–36.
20. Choi IJ, Kook M-C, Kim Y-I, et al. Helicobacter pylori therapy for the prevention of metachronous gastric cancer. N Engl J Med 2018;378:1085–95.
21. Cho SJ, Choi IJ, Kook MC, et al. Randomised clinical trial: the effects of Helicobacter pylori eradication on glandular atrophy and intestinal metaplasia after subtotal gastrectomy for gastric cancer. Aliment Pharmacol Ther 2013;38: 477–89.
22. Lee Y-C, Chiang T-H, Chou C-K, et al. Association between helicobacter pylori eradication and gastric cancer incidence: a systematic review and meta-analysis. Gastroenterology 2016;150:1113–24.e5.
23. Correa P, Fontham ET, Bravo JC, et al. Chemoprevention of gastric dysplasia: randomized trial of antioxidant supplements and anti-helicobacter pylori therapy. J Natl Cancer Inst 2000;92:1881–8.
24. Kosunen TU, Pukkala E, Sarna S, et al. Gastric cancers in Finnish patients after cure of Helicobacter pylori infection: a cohort study. Int J Cancer 2011;128: 433–9.
25. Doorakkers E, Lagergren J, Engstrand L, et al. Helicobacter pylori eradication treatment and the risk of gastric adenocarcinoma in a Western population. Gut 2018;67:2092–6.
26. Kumar S, Metz DC, Ellenberg S, et al. Risk factors and incidence of gastric cancer after detection of helicobacter pylori infection: a large cohort study. Gastroenterology 2020;158:527–36.e7.
27. Doorakkers E, Lagergren J, Engstrand L, et al. Reply to: Helicobacter pylori eradication treatment and the risk of gastric adenocarcinoma in a western population. Gut 2020;69:1149–50.
28. Shah SC. Practice update: risk factors and incidence of gastric cancer after detection of helicobacter pylori infection. J Scan Pract Update 2019. Available at: https://www.practiceupdate.com/content/risk-factors-and-incidence-of-gastric-cancer-after-detection-of-helicobacter-pylori-infection/91600/65/9/1. Accessed November 6, 2020.
29. Ford AC, Yuan Y, Forman D, et al. Helicobacter pylori eradication for the prevention of gastric neoplasia. Cochrane Database Syst Rev 2020;7:CD005583.
30. Wong BCY, Zhang L, Ma J, et al. Effects of selective COX-2 inhibitor and Helicobacter pylori eradication on precancerous gastric lesions. Gut 2012;61: 812–8.
31. Saito D, Boku N, Fujioka T, et al. Impact of H-pylori eradication on gastric cancer prevention: endoscopic results of the Japanese intervention trial (JITHP-study). A Randomized multi-center trial. Gastroenterology 2005.

32. Wong BC-Y, Lam SK, Wong WM, et al. Helicobacter pylori eradication to prevent gastric cancer in a high-risk region of China: a randomized controlled trial. JAMA 2004;291:187–94.
33. You W, Brown LM, Zhang L, et al. Randomized double-blind factorial trial of three treatments to reduce the prevalence of precancerous gastric lesions. J Natl Cancer Inst 2006;98:974–83.
34. Leung WK, Lin SR, Ching JYL, et al. Factors predicting progression of gastric intestinal metaplasia: results of a randomised trial on Helicobacter pylori eradication. Gut 2004;53:1244–9.
35. Noto JM, Peek RM. The gastric microbiome, its interaction with Helicobacter pylori, and its potential role in the progression to stomach cancer. PLoS Pathog 2017;13:e1006573.
36. Gawron AJ, Shah SC, Altayar O, et al. AGA technical review on gastric intestinal metaplasia-natural history and clinical outcomes. Gastroenterology 2020;158: 705–31.e5.
37. Li W-Q, Ma J-L, Zhang L, et al. Effects of Helicobacter pylori treatment on gastric cancer incidence and mortality in subgroups. J Natl Cancer Inst 2014; 106. https://doi.org/10.1093/jnci/dju116.
38. Gupta S, Li D, El Serag HB, et al. AGA clinical practice guidelines on management of gastric intestinal metaplasia. Gastroenterology 2020;158:693–702.
39. Pimentel-Nunes P, Libânio D, Marcos-Pinto R, et al. Management of epithelial precancerous conditions and lesions in the stomach (MAPS II): European Society of Gastrointestinal Endoscopy (ESGE), European Helicobacter and Microbiota Study Group (EHMSG), European Society of Pathology (ESP), and Sociedade Portuguesa de Endoscopia Digestiva (SPED) guideline update 2019. Endoscopy 2019;51:365–88.
40. Banks M, Graham D, Jansen M, et al. British Society of Gastroenterology guidelines on the diagnosis and management of patients at risk of gastric adenocarcinoma. Gut 2019;68:1545–75.
41. Sugano K, Tack J, Kuipers EJ, et al. Kyoto global consensus report on Helicobacter pylori gastritis. Gut 2015;64:1353–67.
42. Yaghoobi M, Bijarchi R, Narod SA. Family history and the risk of gastric cancer. Br J Cancer 2010;102:237–42.
43. Shin CM, Kim N, Yang HJ, et al. Stomach cancer risk in gastric cancer relatives: interaction between Helicobacter pylori infection and family history of gastric cancer for the risk of stomach cancer. J Clin Gastroenterol 2010;44:e34–9.
44. Chang Y-W, Han Y-S, Lee D-K, et al. Role of Helicobacter pylori infection among offspring or siblings of gastric cancer patients. Int J Cancer 2002;101:469–74.
45. Nam JH, Choi IJ, Cho S-J, et al. Helicobacter pylori infection and histological changes in siblings of young gastric cancer patients. J Gastroenterol Hepatol 2011;26:1157–63.
46. Brenner H, Bode G, Boeing H. Helicobacter pylori infection among offspring of patients with stomach cancer. Gastroenterology 2000;118:31–5.
47. El-Omar EM, Oien K, Murray LS, et al. Increased prevalence of precancerous changes in relatives of gastric cancer patients: critical role of H. pylori. Gastroenterology 2000;118:22–30.
48. Malfertheiner P, Megraud F, O'Morain CA, et al. Management of Helicobacter pylori infection-the Maastricht V/Florence Consensus Report. Gut 2017;66:6–30.
49. El-Serag HB, Kao JY, Kanwal F, et al. Houston consensus conference on testing for Helicobacter pylori Infection in the United States. Clin Gastroenterol Hepatol 2018;16:992–1002.e6.

50. Chey WD, Leontiadis GI, Howden CW, et al. ACG clinical guideline: treatment of Helicobacter pylori infection. Am J Gastroenterol 2017;112:212–39.
51. Fukase K, Kato M, Kikuchi S, et al. Effect of eradication of Helicobacter pylori on incidence of metachronous gastric carcinoma after endoscopic resection of early gastric cancer: an open-label, randomised controlled trial. Lancet 2008; 372:392–7.
52. Choi J, Kim SG, Yoon H, et al. Eradication of Helicobacter pylori after endoscopic resection of gastric tumors does not reduce incidence of metachronous gastric carcinoma. Clin Gastroenterol Hepatol 2014;12:793–800.e1.
53. Hanada K, Graham DY. Helicobacter pylori and the molecular pathogenesis of intestinal-type gastric carcinoma. Expert Rev Anticancer Ther 2014;14:947–54.
54. Fock KM, Katelaris P, Sugano K, et al. Second Asia-Pacific Consensus Guidelines for Helicobacter pylori infection. J Gastroenterol Hepatol 2009;24: 1587–600.
55. Harris RE, Beebe-Donk J, Doss H, et al. Aspirin, ibuprofen, and other non-steroidal anti-inflammatory drugs in cancer prevention: a critical review of non-selective COX-2 blockade (review). Oncol Rep 2005;13:559–83.
56. Wang WH, Huang JQ, Zheng GF, et al. Non-steroidal anti-inflammatory drug use and the risk of gastric cancer: a systematic review and meta-analysis. J Natl Cancer Inst 2003;95:1784–91.
57. Wong BC, Zhu GH, Lam SK. Aspirin induced apoptosis in gastric cancer cells. Biomed Pharmacother 1999;53:315–8.
58. Jiang X-H, Lam S-K, Lin MCM, et al. Novel target for induction of apoptosis by cyclo-oxygenase-2 inhibitor SC-236 through a protein kinase C-beta(1)-dependent pathway. Oncogene 2002;21:6113–22.
59. Wu C-Y, Wu M-S, Kuo KN, et al. Effective reduction of gastric cancer risk with regular use of nonsteroidal anti-inflammatory drugs in Helicobacter pylori-infected patients. J Clin Oncol 2010;28:2952–7.
60. Yamamoto Y, Yin MJ, Lin KM, et al. Sulindac inhibits activation of the NF-kappaB pathway. J Biol Chem 1999;274:27307–14.
61. Cuzick J, Otto F, Baron JA, et al. Aspirin and non-steroidal anti-inflammatory drugs for cancer prevention: an international consensus statement. Lancet Oncol 2009;10:501–7.
62. Cheung KS, Chan EW, Wong AYS, et al. Aspirin and risk of gastric cancer after helicobacter pylori eradication: a territory-wide study. J Natl Cancer Inst 2018; 110:743–9.
63. Epplein M, Nomura AMY, Wilkens LR, et al. Nonsteroidal antiinflammatory drugs and risk of gastric adenocarcinoma: the multiethnic cohort study. Am J Epidemiol 2009;170:507–14.
64. Akre K, Ekström AM, Signorello LB, et al. Aspirin and risk for gastric cancer: a population-based case-control study in Sweden. Br J Cancer 2001;84:965–8.
65. Niikura R, Hirata Y, Hayakawa Y, et al. Effect of aspirin use on gastric cancer incidence and survival: a systematic review and meta-analysis. JGH Open 2020;4:117–25.
66. Huang X-Z, Chen Y, Wu J, et al. Aspirin and non-steroidal anti-inflammatory drugs use reduce gastric cancer risk: a dose-response meta-analysis. Oncotarget 2017;8:4781–95.
67. Hudson N, Balsitis M, Filipowicz F, et al. Effect of Helicobacter pylori colonisation on gastric mucosal eicosanoid synthesis in patients taking non-steroidal anti-inflammatory drugs. Gut 1993;34:748–51.

68. Takahashi M, Katayama Y, Takada H, et al. The effect of NSAIDs and a COX-2 specific inhibitor on Helicobacter pylori-induced PGE2 and HGF in human gastric fibroblasts. Aliment Pharmacol Ther 2000;14(Suppl 1):44–9.
69. Wang WH, Wong WM, Dailidiene D, et al. Aspirin inhibits the growth of Helicobacter pylori and enhances its susceptibility to antimicrobial agents. Gut 2003; 52:490–5.
70. Chang SH, Chung JG, Huang LJ, et al. Ibuprofen affects arylamine N-acetyltransferase activity in Helicobacter pylori from peptic ulcer patients. J Appl Toxicol 1998;18:179–85.
71. Lee C-W, Rickman B, Rogers AB, et al. Combination of sulindac and antimicrobial eradication of Helicobacter pylori prevents progression of gastric cancer in hypergastrinemic INS-GAS mice. Cancer Res 2009;69:8166–74.
72. Leung WK, Ng EKW, Chan FKL, et al. Effects of long-term rofecoxib on gastric intestinal metaplasia: results of a randomized controlled trial. Clin Cancer Res 2006;12:4766–72.
73. Cook NR, Lee I-M, Gaziano JM, et al. Low-Dose Aspirin in the Primary Prevention of Cancer. JAMA 2005;294:47.
74. Available at: whs.bwh.harvard.edu/images/WHS website-Overview of study.pdf. Accessed November 3, 2020.
75. Hardbower DM, Asim M, Luis PB, et al. Ornithine decarboxylase regulates M1 macrophage activation and mucosal inflammation via histone modifications. Proc Natl Acad Sci U S A 2017;114:E751–60.
76. Chaturvedi R, de Sablet T, Asim M, et al. Increased Helicobacter pylori-associated gastric cancer risk in the Andean region of Colombia is mediated by spermine oxidase. Oncogene 2015;34:3429–40.
77. Sierra JC, Suarez G, Piazuelo MB, et al. α-Difluoromethylornithine reduces gastric carcinogenesis by causing mutations in Helicobacter pylori cagY. Proc Natl Acad Sci U S A 2019;116:5077–85.
78. Barry DP, Asim M, Leiman DA, et al. Difluoromethylornithine is a novel inhibitor of Helicobacter pylori growth, CagA translocation, and interleukin-8 induction. PLoS One 2011;6:e17510.
79. Zell JA, Lin BS, Madson N, et al. Role of obesity in a randomized placebo-controlled trial of difluoromethylornithine (DFMO) + sulindac for the prevention of sporadic colorectal adenomas. Cancer Causes Control 2012;23:1739–44.
80. Thompson PA, Wertheim BC, Zell JA, et al. Levels of rectal mucosal polyamines and prostaglandin E2 predict ability of DFMO and sulindac to prevent colorectal adenoma. Gastroenterology 2010;139:797–805, 805.e1.
81. Raj KP, Zell JA, Rock CL, et al. Role of dietary polyamines in a phase III clinical trial of difluoromethylornithine (DFMO) and sulindac for prevention of sporadic colorectal adenomas. Br J Cancer 2013;108:512–8.
82. Li W-Q, Zhang J-Y, Ma J-L, et al. Effects of Helicobacter pylori treatment and vitamin and garlic supplementation on gastric cancer incidence and mortality: follow-up of a randomized intervention trial. BMJ 2019;366:l5016.
83. Tanaka S, Haruma K, Kunihiro M, et al. Effects of aged garlic extract (AGE) on colorectal adenomas: a double-blinded study. Hiroshima J Med Sci 2004;53: 39–45.
84. Li H, Li H, Wang Y, et al. An intervention study to prevent gastric cancer by micro-selenium and large dose of allitridum. Chin Med J 2004;117:1155–60.
85. Shah SC, Dai Q, Zhu X, et al. Associations between calcium and magnesium intake and the risk of incident gastric cancer: a prospective cohort analysis of the National Institutes of Health-American Association of Retired Persons

(NIH-AARP) Diet and Health Study. Int J Cancer 2019. https://doi.org/10.1002/ijc.32659.
86. Tsukamoto T, Nakagawa M, Kiriyama Y, et al. Prevention of gastric cancer: eradication of helicobacter pylori and beyond. Int J Mol Sci 2017;18. https://doi.org/10.3390/ijms18081699.
87. Yang C, Du W, Yang D. Inhibition of green tea polyphenol EGCG((-)-epigallocatechin-3-gallate) on the proliferation of gastric cancer cells by suppressing canonical wnt/β-catenin signalling pathway. Int J Food Sci Nutr 2016;67:818–27.
88. Shibata K, Moriyama M, Fukushima T, et al. Green tea consumption and chronic atrophic gastritis: a cross-sectional study in a green tea production village. J Epidemiol 2000;10:310–6.
89. Inoue M, Tajima K, Hirose K, et al. Tea and coffee consumption and the risk of digestive tract cancers: data from a comparative case-referent study in Japan. Cancer Causes Control 1998;9:209–16.
90. Kamangar F, Gao Y-T, Shu X-O, et al. Ginseng intake and gastric cancer risk in the Shanghai Women's Health Study cohort. Cancer Epidemiol Biomarkers Prev 2007;16:629–30.
91. Steevens J, van den Brandt PA, Goldbohm RA, et al. Selenium status and the risk of esophageal and gastric cancer subtypes: the Netherlands cohort study. Gastroenterology 2010;138:1704–13.
92. Chen G, Feng W, Zhang S, et al. Metformin inhibits gastric cancer via the inhibition of HIF1α/PKM2 signaling. Am J Cancer Res 2015;5:1423–34.
93. Kato K, Gong J, Iwama H, et al. The antidiabetic drug metformin inhibits gastric cancer cell proliferation in vitro and in vivo. Mol Cancer Ther 2012;11:549–60.
94. Courtois S, Durán RV, Giraud J, et al. Metformin targets gastric cancer stem cells. Eur J Cancer 2017;84:193–201.
95. Yu G, Fang W, Xia T, et al. Metformin potentiates rapamycin and cisplatin in gastric cancer in mice. Oncotarget 2015;6:12748–62.
96. Shuai Y, Li C, Zhou X. The effect of metformin on gastric cancer in patients with type 2 diabetes: a systematic review and meta-analysis. Clin Transl Oncol 2020;22:1580–90.
97. Zhang J, Wen L, Zhou Q, et al. Preventative and therapeutic effects of metformin in gastric cancer: a new contribution of an old friend. Cancer Manag Res 2020;12:8545–54.
98. Zhou X-L, Xue W-H, Ding X-F, et al. Association between metformin and the risk of gastric cancer in patients with type 2 diabetes mellitus: a meta-analysis of cohort studies. Oncotarget 2017;8:55622–31.
99. Cheung KS, Chan EW, Wong AYS, et al. Metformin use and gastric cancer risk in diabetic patients after helicobacter pylori eradication. J Natl Cancer Inst 2019;111:484–9.
100. Murff HJ, Roumie CL, Greevy RA, et al. Metformin use and incidence cancer risk: evidence for a selective protective effect against liver cancer. Cancer Causes Control 2018;29:823–32.
101. Zheng J, Xie S-H, Santoni G, et al. Metformin use and risk of gastric adenocarcinoma in a Swedish population-based cohort study. Br J Cancer 2019;121:877–82.
102. Khosrow-Khavar F, Kurteva S, Douros A. RE: metformin use and gastric cancer risk in diabetic patients after helicobacter pylori eradication. J Natl Cancer Inst 2019;111:1107–8.
103. Cheung KS, Leung WK. Response to Khosrow-Khavar, Kurteva, and Douros. J Natl Cancer Inst 2019;111:1109.

104. Kuoppala J, Lamminpää A, Pukkala E. Statins and cancer: a systematic review and meta-analysis. Eur J Cancer 2008;44:2122–32.
105. Browning DRL, Martin RM. Statins and risk of cancer: a systematic review and metaanalysis. Int J Cancer 2007;120:833–43.
106. Correa P, Fontham ETH, Bravo JC, et al. RESPONSE: Re: chemoprevention of gastric dysplasia: randomized trial of antioxidant supplements and anti-Helicobacter pylori therapy. JNCI J Natl Cancer Inst 2001;93:559–60.
107. Mera RM, Bravo LE, Camargo MC, et al. Dynamics of Helicobacter pylori infection as a determinant of progression of gastric precancerous lesions: 16-year follow-up of an eradication trial. Gut 2018;67:1239–46.
108. Zhou L, Lin S, Ding S, et al. Relationship of Helicobacter pylori eradication with gastric cancer and gastric mucosal histological changes: a 10-year follow-up study. Chin Med J 2014;127:1454–8.

Endoscopic Advances for Gastric Neoplasia Detection

Andrew Canakis, DO[a], Raymond Kim, MD[b,*]

KEYWORDS

- Gastric neoplasia • Image enhancement endoscopy • Narrow band imaging
- Blue laser imaging • i-scan • Flexible spectral imaging color enhancement
- Probe-based confocal laser • Endocytoscopy

KEY POINTS

- Advances in endoscopic gastric neoplasia detection provides clinicians with the opportunity to decrease mortality rates through early detection of subtle lesions and targeted biopsies.
- The validated classification system used with narrow band imaging is able to predict and correlate endoscopic gastric findings with histopathologic diagnoses.
- Further multicenter studies with supporting clinical evidence, standardized definitions, and adequate training are needed before these newer modalities are routinely used in practice.
- Decision model analyses are needed to determine if these modalities can improve detection rates while reducing costs and unnecessary biopsies.

INTRODUCTION

Gastric cancer (GC) is the third most common cause of cancer-related death worldwide and represents a major health burden because of its high incidence and mortality rates,[1] with more than 700,000 related deaths annually.[2] The multistep progression toward GC includes well-defined stages from chronic active gastritis, chronic atrophic gastritis, gastric intestinal metaplasia (GIM), dysplasia, and ultimately invasive carcinoma.[3] Endoscopic screening and surveillance strategies are now proving critical in

Conflict of Interest Statement: A. Canakis has no potential conflicts (financial, professional, or personal) that are relevant to the content presented in this article. R. Kim is a consultant to Medtronic.

[a] Department of Medicine, Boston University School of Medicine, Boston Medical Center, 72 East Concord Street, Evans 124, Boston, MA 02118, USA; [b] Division of Gastroenterology & Hepatology, University of Maryland Medical Center, University of Maryland School of Medicine, 22 South Greene Street, Baltimore, MD 21201, USA
* Corresponding author.
E-mail address: rkim@som.umaryland.edu
Twitter: @AndrewCanakis (A.C.)

Gastrointest Endoscopy Clin N Am 31 (2021) 543–561
https://doi.org/10.1016/j.giec.2021.03.007
1052-5157/21/Published by Elsevier Inc.

reducing mortality and costs, especially because when patients are symptomatic they are usually diagnosed at an advance stage with a dismal 5-year survival rate.[4,5] However, in Japan, the implementation of a national GC screening program has improved the 5-year survival rate to more than 60%,[6] and in Korea a 47% reduction of GC mortality was reported by endoscopic screening. It has been shown that the main driver of cost is diagnosing gastric neoplasia in a curable stage and preventing advanced-staged disease and mortality.[7] Fortunately, the prolonged time interval over several years before final malignant transformation, coupled with identifiable preneoplastic stages on histopathology provides a massive opportunity for early detection of gastric neoplasia via endoscopic screening.[4] As such, GC is being increasingly recognized as a preventable and curable cancer, especially in light of expanding availability and experience with effective, endoscopic therapeutic options, such as endoscopic submucosal dissection (ESD).[4,8]

In this context, advances in endoscopic gastric neoplasia detection have rapidly evolved, and now provides clinicians with the opportunity to decrease mortality rates through early detection of subtle lesions. Although white light endoscopy (WLE) is currently the primary method for detecting lesions, its macroscopic, diagnostic limitations and poor histopathologic correlation have led to the development of newer technologies that improve mucosal and microvascular visualization.[9] In this article, we explore image-enhancement endoscopy (IEE) methods, such as chromoendoscopy (CE), narrow band imaging (NBI), blue light imaging, i-scan technology, flexible spectral imaging color enhancement (FICE), and a few more (**Table 1**).

DISCUSSION

Conventional Chromoendoscopy

CE uses dye-based staining techniques to aid in the visualization and detection of mucosal irregularities during endoscopy to improve the yield of targeted biopsies.[10] CE can either be applied through staining directed at a suspicious lesion or blindly by voluminously spraying and screening the entire area of interest.[11] There are three types of stains used (absorptive, contrast, and reactive stains) with different transient properties that can enhance the mucosal topography and delineate anatomic borders. (1) Absorptive stains (ie, methylene blue, acetic acid, crystal violet, and Lugol) have differential absorptive properties based on cell type, and in the case of methylene blue, the dye is absorbed by intestinal epithelial cells, and not the epithelia of squamous or gastric mucosa.[10,11] (2) Contrast, or nonabsorptive stains (ie, indigo carmine), do not react with the cells; instead the dye accentuates the topography, mucosal surface, and border of a lesion by accumulating in the grooves and crevices of a mucosal lesion.[10,12] (3) Reactive stains, such as Congo red and phenol red, change color during a chemical reaction when it comes into contact with acidic and alkaline environments on the surface, respectively. Congo red can detect ectopic sites of excessive acid production, whereas phenol red can detect *Helicobacter pylori* infection within the stomach.[11,12]

The CE equipment is widely available, easy to use, inexpensive, and safe. However, this technique can often lengthen procedure times, add to staff burden, and requires extensive experience to interpret staining patterns.[13,14] Yet, its application in the clinical setting has shown promise in detecting early GC (EGC).[15] A meta-analysis of 10 studies, including 699 patients with 902 lesions, found that compared with standard WLE, CE exhibited higher detection rates for EGC and premalignant lesions.[16] It is important to highlight that only two of the studies in this analysis used methylene blue, whereas the majority examined indigo carmine, the most commonly used stain.

Table 1
Summary of advances in endoscopic techniques

Techniques	Company	Manufacture Technology	How It Works
Conventional chromoendoscopy	—	Absorptive stains (methylene blue, acetic acid, crystal violet, Lugol); contrast stains (indigo carmine); reactive stains (Congo red, phenol red)	During an endoscopy, the topical application of specialized biodegradable stains or dyes are deployed to the area of interest to improve the enhancement of tissue characterization
Autofluorescence imaging	Olympus	Evis Exera II/III processors, Video System Center (CV-260SL)	A trimodal video processor enables real-time detection of natural tissue fluorescence that combines autofluorescence signals with green light to create false color images via a special rotary filter
Narrow band imaging	Olympus	Evis Exera II/III processors, Video System Center (CV-260SL, CV-290)	Real-time images are captured with a special optical filter (narrow bands of 415 nm and 540 nm) that illuminates mucosal surfaces at specific wavelengths to create greater contrast images between vascular and mucosal structures
Flexible spectral imaging color enhancement	Fujifilm	EPX-4400 system, VP-4400HD and VP-4450HD processors, XL-4400 and XL-4450 light source	Video processor imaging, reconstruction technology that generates reconfigured pixilated images of a single wavelength to create enhanced color images of vascular and surface tissue
Blue laser imaging	Fujifilm	VP-4450HD processor, XL-4450 HD light source, L590 series endoscopes	Computerized processing system that uses a combination of white (450 nm) and blue light (410 nm) laser sources to create mucosal surface pattern images

(*continued on next page*)

Table 1
(*continued*)

Techniques	Company	Manufacture Technology	How It Works
Probe-based confocal laser endomicroscopy	Pentax	Probe: Cellvizio 100 Series System with Confocal Miniprobes; GastroFlex UHD Miniprobe Endoscope: Pentax ISC-1000 system with EC3870CIK scope	Low-power, laser tissue illumination that creates high-magnification, high-resolution images with tissue fluorescence using exogenous contrast agents
i-scan digital contrast	Pentax	EPK-i5000 and EPK-i7000 HD processor, Series I and 90K gastroscopies	Software-based, digital post-processing imaging system that provides combinations of surface, contrast, and/or tone enhancement
Endocytoscopy	Olympus	Probe-based system (XEC-300, XEC-120) with CLV-180 light source and CV-180 video processor Integrated endoscope system (XGIF-Q260EC1,XCF-Q260EC1) with a CLV-260SL light source and CV-260SL video processor	Fixed-focus, high-power objective lens allows for real-time visualization of cellular structures
Near-infrared Raman spectroscopy	Multiple companies	Four major components: (1) laser systems (eg, Nd:YAG and diode laser), (2) collection optics, (3) Raman spectrophotometers, and (4) detectors (deep-depletion charge-couple or charge-injection devices)	An optical vibrational technique that uses near infrared light to detect the scattering of monochromatic light (and photon absorption) to characterize biomolecular tissue changes

A few studies have suggested that when methylene blue is absorbed by colonocytes[17] and esophageal[18] cells there is a risk of oxidative DNA damage when exposed to white light, which is not seen with indigo carmine.

Still, methylene blue has shown promise in detecting premalignant gastric lesions.[19] In a study of 136 patients by Dinis-Ribeiro and colleagues,[20] methylene blue was shown to have a diagnostic accuracy of 84% and 83% when detecting GIM and dysplasia, for which the study proposed a classification system based on these findings. A few years later Areia and colleagues[21] externally validated and reproduced these findings in a multicenter study of 42 subjects with premalignant lesions. Another prospective study of 33 patients, with prior biopsies showing GIM, demonstrated the advantage of CE over conventional endoscopy with 40 and 16 positive biopsies of premalignant lesions detected, respectively.[22]

Although there are limited studies examining methylene blue for gastric neoplasia detection, indigo carmine is widely used, and in combination with acetic acid, numerous studies have shown its ability to accurately detect dysplasia and EGC.[23–27] Taking advantage of the contrast changes when acetic acid is used, one study was able to differentiate grades of neoplasia based on the dynamic changes in the whitening with time.[28] In response to this, a subsequent group attempted to classify neoplastic changes into five categories,[29] and later showed acetic acid's superiority over conventional endoscopy in characterizing staining patterns with EGC changes.[23] In an effort to enhance this effect, indigo carmine was added to an acetic acid mixture and when compared with conventional endoscopy it showed better results in defining lateral borders of GC (67% vs 84%).[27] Before ESD, one prospective of 108 EGC lesions found that the accuracy of delineating EGC margins in WLE, acetic acid, and acetic acid plus indigo carmine was 50%, 76%, and 91%, respectively.[30] In this context, current clinical evidence supports the use of this modality when CE is used.

Autofluorescence Endoscopy

Autofluorescence endoscopy (AFI) uses the fluorescent properties of gastric tissue to create real-time endoscopic images that generates blue and green light from tissue illumination.[31] By taking advantage of fluorophores (eg, collagen, flavins, and porphyrins) and their ability to emit fluorescent light at certain wavelengths, AFI can capture normal, metaplastic, and dysplastic changes accordingly.[32,33] In autofluorescence, shorter wavelength light interacts with the fluorophores, which then emit light at longer wavelengths in the submucosal layer.[33]

The utility of AFI in detecting gastric neoplasia is unclear because of conflicting evidence in the literature, and it is not typically used in routine practice.[34–38] A prospective study of 51 patients with 91 gastric lesions compared WLE with AFI in detecting gastric neoplasia, and found AFI was less sensitive (64% vs 74%) and specific (49% vs 83%).[34] Furthermore, of the 39 biopsy-proven neoplastic lesions, 22 were detected by WLE and AFI, whereas only seven were seen by WLE and five by AFI alone. The same group conducted another study of 62 patients with 47 biopsy-proven neoplastic lesions using trimodal imaging endoscopy, which added NBI and AFI to WLE, and found that they were able to increase detection rates by 13%, although AFI alone still displayed lower detection rates compared with WLE.[35] Although these two studies by Kato and colleagues34,35 did not show promising results for EGC, So and colleagues[38] conducted a randomized prospective study comparing trimodal imaging endoscopy with WLE in 64 patients and found that there were improved detection rates for GIM when using trimodal imaging endoscopy (68% vs 34%). To explore the role of AFI in surveillance following ESD, Imaeda and colleagues[37] investigated

242 surveillance endoscopies and found that WLE missed five EGC lesions, which were all detected by AFI.

In the context of conflicting data, AFI is unlikely to be a stand-alone modality because of its high false-positive rate and inconsistent autofluorescence pattern for EGC.[31,36] Additionally, the low-resolution image quality, nonspecific indirect detection of dysplasia, and inability to examine deeper tissue further hinders its use.[32]

Narrow Band Imaging

NBI has emerged as an accurate and reliable technique in identifying EGC by optically filtering white light. Since its introduction in 2005 it has become the most widely used IEE technology. The system is activated by a button on the endoscope, which powers a filter located between the xenon lamp and red-green-blue rotatory filter.[10,11] This enables narrow band blue (415 nm) and green (540 nm) light to generate false color images on the endoscopy monitor for which 100-fold magnification is possible.[10] Because hemoglobin is a chromophore, blue and green light are absorbed and then reflected at different depths resulting in enhanced visualization of the superficial capillary network (green light) and deeper subsurface vasculature (blue light).[10,11,39]

NBI has been well validated as a tool that correlates endoscopic gastric findings with histopathologic diagnoses when used with magnifying endoscopy.[39] As such, magnifying endoscopy with NBI (ME-NBI) can characterize EGC tissue based on microvascular patterns and surface microstructures, for which Yao and colleagues[40] introduced a widely used classification system that can enhance diagnostic accuracy. This systematic classification system is defined by the presence or absence of a demarcation line (DL), between the lesion and surrounding noncancerous mucosa, and an irregular microvascular pattern within the lesion itself.[40] Using these two findings, the group was able to prospectively differentiate benign and cancerous lesions with a sensitivity, specificity, and accuracy of 93%, 99%, and 99%, respectively.[40] A simple diagnostic algorithm has been introduced for the endoscopist to follow when encountering suspicious lesions.[41]

Furthermore, ME-NBI has been able to predict and correlate the vascular histologic findings of intralobular and corkscrew pattern with differentiated and undifferentiated carcinoma, respectively.[42,43] ME-NBI has also shown promise when looking at smaller gastric lesions, and one study of 362 patients with depressed lesions less than 10 mm found that variations in microvessel shape had a diagnostic accuracy of 92%.[44] When compared with CE, ME-NBI demonstrated a higher sensitivity (78% vs 44%), specificity (82% vs 93%), and diagnostic accuracy (88% vs 70%) in identifying lesions less than or equal to 5 mm.[45] As **Table 2** illustrates, ME-NBI has been properly investigated in EGC as a reliable modality to detect microvascular and mucosal patterns.

Magnified White Light Versus Narrow Band Imaging

There have been a multitude of studies comparing NBI with WLE. A randomized controlled trial showed that ME-NBI was more accurate in diagnosing cancer in small depressed lesions.[46] When comparing the 40 GCs (20 in each group), the accuracy (90% vs 65%) and specificity (94% vs 68%) were statistically significant and greater in the ME-NBI cohort; when using the modalities together the accuracy and specificity improved to 97%. Another prospective randomized trial of 353 patients with EGC, showed that WLE alone had marginal accuracy (65%), specificity (68%), and sensitivity (40%) findings.[47] However, when applying ME-NBI after WLE, the accuracy, specificity, and sensitivity markedly improved to 97%, 97%, and 95%, respectively. Another group also illustrated the superiority ME-NBI over WLE when using a triad-

Table 2
Summary of studies looking at NBI and early gastric cancer detection

Author, Year	Country	Study Design	Number of Gastric Lesions (Type)	M-NBI Sensitivity (C-WLI), %	M-NBI Specificity (C-WLI), %	M-NBI Accuracy (C-WLI), %
Kanesaka et al,[44] 2015	Japan	Post hoc analysis, multicenter prospective	343 (40 cancer, 303 benign)	[a]25; 55; 13; 70	[a]90; 24; 99; 95	[a]83, 28, 89, 92
Fujiwara et al,[45] 2015	Japan	Single center, retrospective	103 (32 cancer, 71 noncancerous)	78	92.9	88.3
Yao et al,[94] 2014	Japan	Multicenter, prospective	371 (20 cancer, 351 noncancerous)	85.7	99.4	98.1
Yamada et al,[47] 2014	Japan	Post hoc analysis, multicenter, prospective, RCT	M-NBI group: 177 (20 cancer, 155 noncancerous)	95 (40)	97 (68)	97 (65)
Ezoe et al,[46] 2011	Japan	Multicenter, prospective, RCT	M-NBI group: 177 (20 cancer, 157 noncancerous)	60 (40)	94.3 (67.9)	90.4 (64.8)
Kato et al,[48] 2010	Japan	Single center, prospective, comparative	201 (14 cancer, 187 noncancerous)	92.9 (42.9)	94.7 (61)	—
Yao et al,[95] 2007	Japan	Single center, prospective, blinded	158 (14 cancer, 144 gastritis)	92.9	99.3	98.7

Abbreviations: C-WLI, conventional white-light imaging; M-NBI, magnifying narrow band imaging; RCT, randomized controlled trial.
[a] Microvascular findings based were characterized by dilation, tortuosity, difference in caliber, and variation in shape (% listed in that order).

based diagnosis of disappearance of fine mucosal structure, microvascular dilation, and heterogeneity in detecting superficial GC.[48]

Many of these promising studies suggest that ME-NBI is an accurate tool that may enable clinicians to avoid unnecessary biopsies while improving targeted biopsies and serving as a potential method to make an optical diagnosis. One comparative meta-analysis of 14 studies with more than 2000 patients, found that the pooled sensitivity, specificity, and area under curve for EGC when using ME-NBI was 86%, 96%, and 96%, respectively.[49] These findings were influenced by the type and size of the lesion, where depressed lesions less than 10 mm in diameter exhibited lower sensitivities. Yet, the specificity for these small depressed lesions remained high and still outperformed WLE. Another meta-analysis of 2153 gastric lesions echoed these findings and found that ME-NBI was superior to WLE in terms of sensitivity (83% vs 48%), specificity (96% vs 67%), and area under curve (96% vs 62%).[50] Once again these were promising results; however, this was a prospective randomized multicenter study of 579 patients that found no statistical difference in the GC detection rates between the ME-NBI (7/286) and WLE (3/293).[51]

Narrow Band Imaging's Role in Endoscopic Submucosal Dissection

ESD now offers clinicians with the chance to obtain complete curative resection in cases of EGG. The defining features of successful ESD are the ability to determine the horizonal margins and depth of the lesion, a finding that is enhanced by the application of ME-NBI. One of the first comparative studies between indigo carmine CE and ME-NBI, showed the higher diagnostic accuracy of ME-NBI (97% vs 78%) in delineating EGC tumor margins.[52] As **Table 3** shows, similar findings have been reported in other comparative studies favoring the utility of ME-NBI in determining the horizonal extent of EGC lesions. However, it is important to highlight that one randomized controlled study by Nagahama and colleagues[53] reported similar margin delineation rates between ME-NBI and indigo carmine CE (88% vs 86%). Despite this finding most studies to date have favored the use of ME-NBI.

Briefly, in terms of defining the invasion depth for EGC, the main diagnostic approach is conventional endoscopy and endoscopic ultrasound; however, some studies have shown that roughly 20% of patients undergoing such evaluations may not be eligible for ESD because of the diagnostic limitations.[39] ME-NBI has been shown to improve the diagnostic yield of differentiated EGC based on the presence or absence of microvascular structures and patterns.[54,55] It is interesting to mention that a recent artificial intelligence (AI) study compared WLE, NBI, and CE using indigo carmine and found that each method was highly accurate in predicting invasion depth but there was no significant difference in accuracy between each system.[56] Another study compared an AI computer-aided system using ME-NBI with 11 experts in diagnosis EGC and found that the AI system was equivalent to and better than several experts.[57] At this point in time further studies are needed to clarify the role of NBI and AI in serving as supplementary tools when approaching ESD.

Limitations of Narrow Band Imaging

Although there are promising advantages of this technology, there are a few limitations of NBI to highlight. First, the significant experience needed to effectively use this system is time consuming, and accurately identifying horizontal margins before ESD can also to procedure times and endoscopy costs.[39] Second, in the stomach darker imaging of distant lesions is limited when examining a broader area.[58] Last, its reliability in delineating undifferentiated cancers is limited, and should be limited to differentiated type GC until further data results.[39,55] At this point in time, most of the data are

Table 3
Comparative studies of NBI using endoscopic submucosal dissection in EGC lesions

Author, Year	Study Design (Country)	Comparative Modality	Total Number of EGC Lesions (# in M-NBI Group)	Accuracy (%)
Nagahama et al,[53] 2018	Multicenter, RCT (Japan)	Indigo carmine CE	343 (175)	M-NBI: 88 CE: 85.7
Asada-Hirayama et al,[96] 2016	Single center, prospective (Japan)	Indigo carmine CE	109 (58)	M-NBI: 89.4 CE: 75.9
Nagahama et al,[97] 2011	Single center, case series (Japan)	Indigo carmine CE	350 (62)	M-NBI: 72.6 CE: 81.1
Kiyotoki et al,[52] 2010	Single center, RCT (Japan)	Indigo carmine CE	83 (38)	M-NBI: 97.4 CE: 77.8

Abbreviations: CE, chromoendoscopy; EGC, early gastric cancer; M-NBI, magnifying narrow band imaging.

primarily from high-prevalence regions; however, its generalization to low-prevalence regions has to be approached with caution.

Flexible Spectral Imaging Color Enhancement and Bright Image Enhanced Endoscopy Using Blue Laser Imaging

Flexible spectral imaging color enhancement

FICE was introduced in 2005 as an IEE system that mathematically processes endoscopic images at dedicated wavelengths without the need for an optical filter.[58] Using a computed spectral estimation technique, endoscopists can view reconfigured high-resolution contrast images without magnification or compromising on brightness. As such, this optical band imaging system can differentiate malignant and normal mucosa based on surface pattern enhancement influenced by neoplastic laminar blood flow and structural distortion.[58]

There are only a few studies looking at the reliability of FICE as a screening tool in detecting EGC. The first study to demonstrate the clinical utility of FICE was conducted in Japan in which Osawa and colleagues[59] prospectively identified 96% (26/27 cases) of depressed-type EGC. Shortly afterward, the same group conducted a prospective study, where they examined 81 lesions with elevated-type EGC, and were able to easily identify DLs using FICE without magnification in the background of whitish atrophic mucosa.[60] These findings were validated in a retrospective study by Mouri and colleagues,[61] who found that setting the wavelength at 530 nm enhanced EGC visualization in close to 50% of cases studied. Although these results are promising, one meta-analysis showed that there are still insufficient data and differing pattern definitions for neoplasia to aggregate the results for FICE.[62] Furthermore, comparative studies against other modalities are still needed and require further investigation.

Bright image enhanced endoscopy using blue laser imaging

Blue laser imaging (BLI) evolved as an adaptive technologic method that combines narrow band laser light and white light to produce enhanced color images of deep mucosal microvasculature and superficial microtubule patterns.[58] Serving as a computer-based CE system, BLI enables distant high-resolution vascular contrast detection during a screening endoscopy.[63] As such, boundaries of malignant lesions are identified and magnified. The added advantage of distant light dark imaging and the ability to examine mucosal microstructures makes BLI more appealing when comparing it with NBI.[63] The characteristics between BLI and FICE are seen in **Table 4**.

As a newer technology there are only a handful of GC studies to date.[63–66] Kaneko and colleagues[64] measured and compared observable distances of GC between BLI and NBI, for which they demonstrated the ability of BLI to identify 14 GC lesions at a further distance (27 mm vs 16 mm). At distance of 40 mm, only one lesion was detected by NBI, whereas six were observed using BLI. In a prospective study analyzing 127 gastric lesions (32 cancerous and 95 noncancerous), a group in Japan showed that the accuracy (92% vs 72%), sensitivity (94% vs 47%), and specificity (92% vs 80%) of BLI was notable higher when compared with WLE.[65] Similar findings were also reported in another comparative study of EGC lesions.[63] Recently, a randomized controlled study of 122 gastric lesions with clear DL seen on BLI were compared with and without biopsy confirmation, and the researchers showed that biopsy confirmation may not be needed when DL are identified by BLI.[66] Further comparative studies are needed to define the role of BLI in clinical practice and its potential to increase the efficacy of ESD.

Probe-Based Confocal Laser Endomicroscopy

Probe-based confocal laser endomicroscopy (pCLE) is a new endoscopic technique that enables real-time high-resolution microscopic imaging.[67] This imaging modality uses confocal probes that are passed along the accessory channel whereby laser light is focused at a certain tissue depth, reflected, and then refocused through a pinhole via the same lens. This specific method of tissue illumination creates images at the cellular and microvascular level, which offers clinicians the ability to make an optical biopsy in real time.[68] This technology is exciting because it has the potential to decrease biopsy-related costs and adverse events, while at the same time offering

Table 4
Descriptions and comparisons between flexible spectral imaging color enhancement and blue laser imaging

	Flexible Spectral Imaging Color Enhancement	Blue Laser Imaging
Color information	Blue-green-red	Blue-green
Light source	Xenon laser	Laser
Processor	Fujinon VP-4450HD, VP-4400HD	Fujinon VP-4450 HD
Wavelengths/ images	Divides white light into 3 wavelengths to create color-enhanced image	Two different laser wavelengths; laser light (410 nm) and white light (450 nm) combine to produce images
Viewing characteristics	Bright images ± magnification	Bright images with a contrast mode and bright mode

the potential to make informed real-time treatment decisions.[69] To advance the application of pCLE, the Miami Classification was introduced in 2009 as a way to implement a standardized classification system for its diagnostic use.[69] The routine use of this method is hindered by its well-documented learning curve for image interpretation that depends on experience and adequate training.[70]

Although pCLE is a promising technique there are only a few studies examining GC. To compare pCLE with WLE, Park and colleagues[71] demonstrated the superiority of pCLE in undifferentiated-type GCs. Another study of 20 resected or biopsied lesions found that pCLE made an accurate diagnosis in 19/20 cases.[68] Favorable results were also seen in two meta-analysis, which reported sensitivities and specificities ranging from 85% to 91% and 99%, respectively.[67,72] Lastly, a recent prospective, pathologist-blinded study compared pCLE with standard biopsies in 74 lesions (21 gastric and 53 esophageal) and reported comparable results.[73] Although these limited studies show the potential for pCLE, larger randomized studies are needed to solidify its clinical reliability for GC detection.

I-Scan

Introduced in 2007, i-scan is a new technology that uses the reflective proprieties of mucosal surfaces to create real-time, multichannel images using special processing technology.[9] There are three modes for this method (ie, surface enhancement, contrast enhancement, and tone enhancement) that mathematically process white light images by the press of a button on the endoscope, enabling endoscopists to simultaneously view two or more modes at the same time.[74] These special functions allow for enhanced screening detection of early gastric lesions. Briefly, surface enhancement and contrast enhancement provide light-dark contrast and add blue color in dark areas, respectively.[74] As such, these algorithms use pixel luminance information to provide enhancement of depressed areas and surface architecture.[9,74] The last method, tone enhancement, is able to process individual components of red-green-blue light frequencies to create a detailed reconfigured color image that enhances detailed mucosal structures.[9,74]

Although this technology is exciting, there are currently limited data to support its routine use for diagnosing gastric neoplasia. Li and colleagues[75] conducted one of the first prospective studies using i-scan where they examined 43 patients with small (<1 cm) superficial gastric lesions. In comparing all three modes, surface enhancement and tone enhancement displayed a slightly higher diagnostic yield than contrast enhancement. Overall, when comparing i-scan readings with the gold standard of histology, its value was limited in neoplasia detection. The study reported a specificity of 77% and a positive predictive value of 50%.[75] Similar findings were demonstrated in another study that compared i-scan with WLE in 10 patients with gastric neoplasia, in which the accuracy of WLE (92%) and i-scan (91%) were comparable.[76] Consequently, more experience and head-to-head studies are needed with i-scan technology.

Endocytoscopy

Initially developed in 2003, endocytoscopy (ECS) has evolved as an in vivo magnification technology that provides ultrahigh microscopic imaging with a ×520 magnification power.[77] Through contact light microscopy, ECS enables visualization at the individual cellular level where a high-powered lens projects a magnified image using intraprocedural staining.[78] As such, GC is identified, and there has been favorable interobserver agreement between pathologists and endoscopists.[77] However, there are limited data on GC detection, especially because image quality is hindered by poor dye staining from gastric secretions.[79] One of the first studies examined 28 gastric lesions and reported a sensitivity of 56% and specificity of 89%.[80] A larger study of 100 lesions reported favorable results (regardless of expertise) for which the sensitivity, specificity, and accuracy were 78%, 93%, and 87%, respectively.[81] Another group showed that the "enlarged nuclear sign" could aid in EGC diagnosis with similar interobserver sensitivities (83%–87%), specificities (85%–95%), and accuracies (84%–91%).[78] The high accuracy of ECS has shown promise, but larger blinded studies are still needed to determine if it can provide additional advantage to conventional endoscopy and NBI.[78,79]

The intersection of ECS and AI with machine learning has also been explored, with promising results.[82,83] In one study by Hirasawa and colleagues,[82] endoscopic images of 67 GC lesions were detected with an overall sensitivity of 92%, and 99% when looking at lesions with diameters more than 6 mm. The lesions missed by the AI system were all superficially depressed. Another study by Zhu and colleagues[83] found that this deep learning application outperformed their endoscopists, with higher accuracy and specificity rates, when detecting the invasion depth of GC. These studies provide a glimpse of what these future technologies can provide, whereby improved diagnostic methods and efficient workflow can reduce costs and better identify patients for ESD.[77]

Near-Infrared Raman Spectroscopy

Raman spectroscopy measures the inelastic scattering of monochromatic light with a 1.8-mm endoscopic probe that process molecular vibrations when it comes into direct contact with tissue.[84] As such, molecular features of cellular components and biochemical tissues (ie, proteins, lipids, glycoproteins, and DNA) are analyzed and identified.[84] In combination with a near-infrared laser, this modality can penetrate deeper levels of tissues via photon absorption with less interference to provide endoscopists with detailed molecular fingerprints that can differentiate neoplastic changes.[85]

There have been numerous studies exploring the diagnostic ability of near-infrared Raman spectroscopy (NIR) to identify GC changes.[86–93] In an early study of 76 gastric samples (21 histologically proven dysplasia), Teh and colleagues[91] found that specific spectral ranges of dysplasia were seen from 1200 to 1500 cm^{-1} and 1600 to 1800 cm^{-1} with a peak at 1450 cm^{-1}. Using these spectral patterns in a diagnostic algorithm based on principal component analysis and linear discriminant analysis, they reported a sensitivity and specificity of 95% and 91%, respectively.[91] A subsequent study by the same group reported similar findings when detecting GC and noted that Raman peaks at 875 cm^{-1} and 1745 cm^{-1} were the most significant intensities to differentiate normal and GC tissues.[93] In a larger study of 1277 in vivo Raman spectra acquired from 83 patients, Bergholt and colleagues[86] further confirmed the ability of NIR to detect intestinal-type adenocarcinoma with sensitivity of 85% and specificity of 96%. Additionally, this method has also been able to differentiate benign versus malignant gastric ulcers.[87]

These studies show that Raman spectroscopy is a quick, noninvasive way to make an accurate and early diagnosis of gastric neoplasia. What is even more exciting is that NIR has also been able to discriminate between differentiated and undifferentiated GC at early and advance stages with accuracies ranging from 93% to 98%.[90] Yet, there are currently no studies comparing Raman spectroscopy with other endoscopic detection techniques. The advancements of NIR have propelled this technology to the forefront of GC diagnostic studies, although there are a few limitations to highlight. Because this method detects molecular structures, there are instances where two similar molecules (eg, arachidonic and eicosapentaenoic acid) may be indistinguishable.[88] There are also times where it is sensitive to process interference from pressure changes or during heating when the sample can be damaged.[88] However, these limitations have not hindered the rapid advances of NIR where a noninvasive, reagent free tissue diagnosis is feasible and accurate.

SUMMARY

With advancement of techniques for endoscopic detection of gastric neoplasia clinicians are now provided with the opportunity to decrease mortality rates through the early detection of subtle lesions and subsequent targeted biopsies. In this article we reviewed various IEE methods including CE, AFI, NBI, ME-NBI, FICE, BLI, pCLE, i-scan, ECS, and NIR and their available scientific data. Despite the recent evolution of these technologies, most of these image-enhancing modalities still lack randomized controlled studies to prove their benefit in detecting EGC compared with conventional WLE. Because of the relative lack of comparative data, no specific GI organization recommends IEE for gastric malignancy screening at this time, nor do there exist algorithms to select the appropriate IEE method.

There is, however, stronger evidence supported by multiple randomized controlled studies that some of these newer technologies including ME-NBI and BLI with their superior mucosal and microvascular visualization enhance therapeutic endoscopic treatment outcomes by better delineating tumor margins.

It is hoped that the continued evolution of techniques and availability of data from large-scale comparative studies will alleviate these limitations.

CLINICS CARE POINTS

- When screening for an early gastric cancer, WLE is the currently recommended standard.
- CE with indigo carmine or methylene blue is used for the detection of early gastric cancer.
- AFI is unlikely to be a stand-alone modality because of its high false-positive rate.
- Nonmagnified NBI has a potential to improve early gastric cancer detection but it has limitations with its dark field view.
- When endoscopic resection of the early gastric cancer is performed with ESD, IEE including CE, NBI, ME-NBI, and BLI can be used for a better delineation of the tumor margins.

DISCLOSURE

There are no relevant disclosures.

REFERENCES

1. Torre LA, Bray F, Siegel RL, et al. Global cancer statistics, 2012. CA Cancer J Clin 2015;65(2):87–108.
2. Cancer of the Stomach - Cancer Stat Facts. SEER. Available at: https://seer.cancer.gov/statfacts/html/stomach.html. Accessed September 7, 2020.
3. Correa P. Human gastric carcinogenesis: a multistep and multifactorial process: first American Cancer Society Award Lecture on Cancer Epidemiology and Prevention. Cancer Res 1992;52(24):6735–40.

4. Canakis A, Pani E, Saumoy M, et al. Decision model analyses of upper endoscopy for gastric cancer screening and preneoplasia surveillance: a systematic review. Ther Adv Gastroenterol 2020;13. 1756284820941662.
5. Sitarz R, Skierucha M, Mielko J, et al. Gastric cancer: epidemiology, prevention, classification, and treatment. Cancer Manag Res 2018;10:239–48.
6. CANCER STATISTICS IN JAPAN '16【Cancer information Service, National Cancer Center Japan】. Available at: https://ganjoho.jp/en/professional/statistics/brochure/2016_en.html. Accessed September 12, 2020.
7. Saumoy M, Schneider Y, Shen N, et al. Cost effectiveness of gastric cancer screening according to race and ethnicity. Gastroenterology 2018;155(3):648–60.
8. Akintoye E, Obaitan I, Muthusamy A, et al. Endoscopic submucosal dissection of gastric tumors: a systematic review and meta-analysis. World J Gastrointest Endosc 2016;8(15):517–32.
9. Li H, Hou X, Lin R, et al. Advanced endoscopic methods in gastrointestinal diseases: a systematic review. Quant Imaging Med Surg 2019;9(5):905–20.
10. Kaltenbach T, Sano Y, Friedland S, et al, American Gastroenterological Association. American Gastroenterological Association (AGA) Institute technology assessment on image-enhanced endoscopy. Gastroenterology 2008;134(1):327–40.
11. Hussain I, Ang TL. Evidence based review of the impact of image enhanced endoscopy in the diagnosis of gastric disorders. World J Gastrointest Endosc 2016;8(20):741–55.
12. Kheir AO, Soetikno R, Kaltenbach T. Chromoendoscopy. In: Konda VJA, Waxman I, editors. Endoscopic imaging techniques and tools. Springer International Publishing; 2016. p. 29–48.
13. Huang RJ, Choi AY, Truong CD, et al. Diagnosis and management of gastric intestinal metaplasia: current status and future directions. Gut Liver 2019;13(6):596–603.
14. Trivedi PJ, Braden B. Indications, stains and techniques in chromoendoscopy. QJM Int J Med 2013;106(2):117–31.
15. Ohnita K, Isomoto H, Shikuwa S, et al. Magnifying chromoendoscopic findings of early gastric cancer and gastric adenoma. Dig Dis Sci 2011;56(9):2715–22.
16. Zhao Z, Yin Z, Wang S, et al. Meta-analysis: the diagnostic efficacy of chromoendoscopy for early gastric cancer and premalignant gastric lesions. J Gastroenterol Hepatol 2016;31(9):1539–45.
17. Davies J, Burke D, Olliver JR, et al. Methylene blue but not indigo carmine causes DNA damage to colonocytes in vitro and in vivo at concentrations used in clinical chromoendoscopy. Gut 2007;56(1):155–6.
18. Olliver JR, Wild CP, Sahay P, et al. Chromoendoscopy with methylene blue and associated DNA damage in Barrett's oesophagus. Lancet 2003;362(9381):373–4.
19. Morales TG, Bhattacharyya A, Camargo E, et al. Methylene blue staining for intestinal metaplasia of the gastric cardia with follow-up for dysplasia. Gastrointest Endosc 1998;48(1):26–31.
20. Dinis-Ribeiro M, da Costa-Pereira A, Lopes C, et al. Magnification chromoendoscopy for the diagnosis of gastric intestinal metaplasia and dysplasia. Gastrointest Endosc 2003;57(4):498–504.
21. Areia M, Amaro P, Dinis-Ribeiro M, et al. External validation of a classification for methylene blue magnification chromoendoscopy in premalignant gastric lesions. Gastrointest Endosc 2008;67(7):1011–8.

22. Taghavi SA, Membari ME, Eshraghian A, et al. Comparison of chromoendoscopy and conventional endoscopy in the detection of premalignant gastric lesions. Can J Gastroenterol 2009;23(2):105–8.
23. Tanaka K, Toyoda H, Kadowaki S, et al. Surface pattern classification by enhanced-magnification endoscopy for identifying early gastric cancers. Gastrointest Endosc 2008;67(3):430–7.
24. Kono Y, Takenaka R, Kawahara Y, et al. Chromoendoscopy of gastric adenoma using an acetic acid indigo carmine mixture. World J Gastroenterol 2014; 20(17):5092–7.
25. Numata N, Oka S, Tanaka S, et al. Useful condition of chromoendoscopy with indigo carmine and acetic acid for identifying a demarcation line prior to endoscopic submucosal dissection for early gastric cancer. BMC Gastroenterol 2016;16. https://doi.org/10.1186/s12876-016-0483-7.
26. Song KH, Hwang JA, Kim SM, et al. Acetic acid chromoendoscopy for determining the extent of gastric intestinal metaplasia. Gastrointest Endosc 2017; 85(2):349–56.
27. Lee BE, Kim GH, Park DY, et al. Acetic acid-indigo carmine chromoendoscopy for delineating early gastric cancers: its usefulness according to histological type. BMC Gastroenterol 2010;10:97.
28. Yagi K, Aruga Y, Nakamura A, et al. The study of dynamic chemical magnifying endoscopy in gastric neoplasia. Gastrointest Endosc 2005;62(6):963–9.
29. Tanaka K, Toyoda H, Kadowaki S, et al. Features of early gastric cancer and gastric adenoma by enhanced-magnification endoscopy. J Gastroenterol 2006; 41(4):332–8.
30. Kawahara Y, Takenaka R, Okada H, et al. Novel chromoendoscopic method using an acetic acid–indigo carmine mixture for diagnostic accuracy in delineating the margin of early gastric cancers. Dig Endosc 2009;21(1):14–9.
31. Song L-MWK, Banerjee S, Desilets D, et al. Autofluorescence imaging. Gastrointest Endosc 2011;73(4):647–50.
32. Falk GW. Autofluorescence endoscopy. Gastrointest Endosc Clin N Am 2009; 19(2):209–20.
33. Ragunath K. Autofluorescence endoscopy: not much gain after all? Endoscopy 2007;39(11):1021–2.
34. Kato M, Kaise M, Yonezawa J, et al. Autofluorescence endoscopy versus conventional white light endoscopy for the detection of superficial gastric neoplasia: a prospective comparative study. Endoscopy 2007;39(11):937–41.
35. Kato M, Kaise M, Yonezawa J, et al. Trimodal imaging endoscopy may improve diagnostic accuracy of early gastric neoplasia: a feasibility study. Gastrointest Endosc 2009;70(5):899–906.
36. Kato M, Uedo N, Ishihara R, et al. Analysis of the color patterns of early gastric cancer using an autofluorescence imaging video endoscopy system. Gastric Cancer 2009;12(4):219–24.
37. Imaeda H, Hosoe N, Kashiwagi K, et al. Surveillance using trimodal imaging endoscopy after endoscopic submucosal dissection for superficial gastric neoplasia. World J Gastroenterol 2014;20(43):16311–7.
38. So J, Rajnakova A, Chan Y-H, et al. Endoscopic tri-modal imaging improves detection of gastric intestinal metaplasia among a high-risk patient population in Singapore. Dig Dis Sci 2013;58(12):3566–75.
39. Kim J-W. Usefulness of narrow-band imaging in endoscopic submucosal dissection of the stomach. Clin Endosc 2018;51(6):527–33.

40. Yao K, Oishi T, Matsui T, et al. Novel magnified endoscopic findings of microvascular architecture in intramucosal gastric cancer. Gastrointest Endosc 2002; 56(2):279–84.
41. Muto M, Yao K, Kaise M, et al. Magnifying endoscopy simple diagnostic algorithm for early gastric cancer (MESDA-G). Dig Endosc 2016;28(4):379–93.
42. Nakayoshi T, Tajiri H, Matsuda K, et al. Magnifying endoscopy combined with narrow band imaging system for early gastric cancer: correlation of vascular pattern with histopathology (including video). Endoscopy 2004;36(12):1080–4.
43. Ok K-S, Kim GH, Park DY, et al. Magnifying endoscopy with narrow band imaging of early gastric cancer: correlation with histopathology and mucin phenotype. Gut Liver 2016;10(4):532–41.
44. Kanesaka T, Uedo N, Yao K, et al. A significant feature of microvessels in magnifying narrow-band imaging for diagnosis of early gastric cancer. Endosc Int Open 2015;3(6):E590–6.
45. Fujiwara S, Yao K, Nagahama T, et al. Can we accurately diagnose minute gastric cancers ($\leq$5 mm)? Chromoendoscopy (CE) vs magnifying endoscopy with narrow band imaging (M-NBI). Gastric Cancer 2015;18(3):590–6.
46. Ezoe Y, Muto M, Uedo N, et al. Magnifying narrowband imaging is more accurate than conventional white-light imaging in diagnosis of gastric mucosal cancer. Gastroenterology 2011;141(6):2017–25.e3.
47. Yamada S, Doyama H, Yao K, et al. An efficient diagnostic strategy for small, depressed early gastric cancer with magnifying narrow-band imaging: a post-hoc analysis of a prospective randomized controlled trial. Gastrointest Endosc 2014;79(1):55–63.
48. Kato M, Kaise M, Yonezawa J, et al. Magnifying endoscopy with narrow-band imaging achieves superior accuracy in the differential diagnosis of superficial gastric lesions identified with white-light endoscopy: a prospective study. Gastrointest Endosc 2010;72(3):523–9.
49. Hu Y-Y, Lian Q-W, Lin Z-H, et al. Diagnostic performance of magnifying narrow-band imaging for early gastric cancer: a meta-analysis. World J Gastroenterol 2015;21(25):7884–94.
50. Zhang Q, Wang F, Chen Z-Y, et al. Comparison of the diagnostic efficacy of white light endoscopy and magnifying endoscopy with narrow band imaging for early gastric cancer: a meta-analysis. Gastric Cancer 2016;19(2):543–52.
51. Ang TL, Pittayanon R, Lau JYW, et al. A multicenter randomized comparison between high-definition white light endoscopy and narrow band imaging for detection of gastric lesions. Eur J Gastroenterol Amp Hepatol 2015;27(12):1473–8.
52. Kiyotoki S, Nishikawa J, Satake M, et al. Usefulness of magnifying endoscopy with narrow-band imaging for determining gastric tumor margin. J Gastroenterol Hepatol 2010;25(10):1636–41.
53. Nagahama T, Yao K, Uedo N, et al. Delineation of the extent of early gastric cancer by magnifying narrow-band imaging and chromoendoscopy: a multicenter randomized controlled trial. Endoscopy 2018;50(6):566–76.
54. Yagi K, Nakamura A, Sekine A, et al. Magnifying endoscopy with narrow band imaging for early differentiated gastric adenocarcinoma. Dig Endosc 2008;20(3): 115–22.
55. Kikuchi D, Iizuka T, Hoteya S, et al. Usefulness of magnifying endoscopy with narrow-band imaging for determining tumor invasion depth in early gastric cancer. Gastroenterol Res Pract 2013;2013. https://doi.org/10.1155/2013/217695.
56. Nagao S, Tsuji Y, Sakaguchi Y, et al. Highly accurate artificial intelligence systems to predict the invasion depth of gastric cancer: efficacy of conventional white-

light imaging, nonmagnifying narrow-band imaging, and indigo-carmine dye contrast imaging. Gastrointest Endosc 2020;92(4):866–73.e1.
57. Horiuchi Y, Hirasawa T, Ishizuka N, et al. Performance of a computer-aided diagnosis system in diagnosing early gastric cancer using magnifying endoscopy videos with narrow-band imaging (with videos). Gastrointest Endosc 2020. https://doi.org/10.1016/j.gie.2020.04.079.
58. Osawa H, Yamamoto H. Present and future status of flexible spectral imaging color enhancement and blue laser imaging technology. Dig Endosc 2014;26(S1): 105–15.
59. Osawa H, Yoshizawa M, Yamamoto H, et al. Optimal band imaging system can facilitate detection of changes in depressed-type early gastric cancer. Gastrointest Endosc 2008;67(2):226–34.
60. Yoshizawa M, Osawa H, Yamamoto H, et al. Diagnosis of elevated-type early gastric cancers by the optimal band imaging system. Gastrointest Endosc 2009;69(1):19–28.
61. Mouri R, Yoshida S, Tanaka S, et al. Evaluation and validation of computed virtual chromoendoscopy in early gastric cancer. Gastrointest Endosc 2009;69(6): 1052–8.
62. Kikuste I, Marques-Pereira R, Monteiro-Soares M, et al. Systematic review of the diagnosis of gastric premalignant conditions and neoplasia with high-resolution endoscopic technologies. Scand J Gastroenterol 2013;48(10):1108–17.
63. Zhenming Y, Lei S. Diagnostic value of blue laser imaging combined with magnifying endoscopy for precancerous and early gastric cancer lesions. Turk J Gastroenterol 2019;30(6):549–56.
64. Kaneko K, Oono Y, Yano T, et al. Effect of novel bright image enhanced endoscopy using blue laser imaging (BLI). Endosc Int Open 2014;2(4):E212–9.
65. Dohi O, Yagi N, Majima A, et al. Diagnostic ability of magnifying endoscopy with blue laser imaging for early gastric cancer: a prospective study. Gastric Cancer 2017;20(2):297–303.
66. Nakano T, Dohi O, Naito Y, et al. Efficacy and feasibility of magnifying blue laser imaging without biopsy confirmation for the diagnosis of the demarcation of gastric tumors: a randomized controlled study. Dig Dis 2020. https://doi.org/10.1159/000510559.
67. Fugazza A, Gaiani F, Carra MC, et al. Confocal laser endomicroscopy in gastrointestinal and pancreatobiliary diseases: a systematic review and meta-analysis. Biomed Res Int 2016;2016:4638683.
68. Safatle-Ribeiro AV, Ryoka Baba E, Corsato Scomparin R, et al. Probe-based confocal endomicroscopy is accurate for differentiating gastric lesions in patients in a Western center. Chin J Cancer Res 2018;30(5):546–52.
69. Wallace M, Lauwers GY, Chen Y, et al. Miami classification for probe-based confocal laser endomicroscopy. Endoscopy 2011;43(10):882–91.
70. Lim LG, Yeoh KG, Salto-Tellez M, et al. Experienced versus inexperienced confocal endoscopists in the diagnosis of gastric adenocarcinoma and intestinal metaplasia on confocal images. Gastrointest Endosc 2011;73(6):1141–7.
71. Park CH, Kim H, Jo JH, et al. Role of probe-based confocal laser endomicroscopy-targeted biopsy in the molecular and histopathological study of gastric cancer. J Gastroenterol Hepatol 2019;34(1):84–91.
72. Zhang H-P, Yang S, Chen W-H, et al. The diagnostic value of confocal laser endomicroscopy for gastric cancer and precancerous lesions among Asian population: a system review and meta-analysis. Scand J Gastroenterol 2017;52(4): 382–8.

73. Kollar M, Krajciova J, Prefertusova L, et al. Probe-based confocal laser endomicroscopy versus biopsies in the diagnostics of oesophageal and gastric lesions: a prospective, pathologist-blinded study. United Eur Gastroenterol J 2020;8(4):436–43.
74. Kodashima S, Fujishiro M. Novel image-enhanced endoscopy with i-scan technology. World J Gastroenterol 2010;16(9):1043–9.
75. Li C-Q, Li Y, Zuo X-L, et al. Magnified and enhanced computed virtual chromoendoscopy in gastric neoplasia: a feasibility study. World J Gastroenterol 2013;19(26):4221–7.
76. Nishimura J, Nishikawa J, Nakamura M, et al. Efficacy of i-scan imaging for the detection and diagnosis of early gastric carcinomas. Gastroenterol Res Pract 2014;2014. https://doi.org/10.1155/2014/819395.
77. Teh J-L, Shabbir A, Yuen S, et al. Recent advances in diagnostic upper endoscopy. World J Gastroenterol 2020;26(4):433–47.
78. Abad MRA, Inoue H, Ikeda H, et al. Utilizing fourth-generation endocytoscopy and the 'enlarged nuclear sign' for in vivo diagnosis of early gastric cancer. Endosc Int Open 2019;7(8):E1002–7.
79. Kaise M, Ohkura Y, Iizuka T, et al. Endocytoscopy is a promising modality with high diagnostic accuracy for gastric cancer. Endoscopy 2015;47(1):19–25.
80. Eberl T, Jechart G, Probst A, et al. Can an endocytoscope system (ECS) predict histology in neoplastic lesions? Endoscopy 2007;39(6):497–501.
81. Kaise M, Kimura R, Nomura K, et al. Accuracy and concordance of endocytoscopic atypia for the diagnosis of gastric cancer. Endoscopy 2014;46(10):827–32.
82. Hirasawa T, Aoyama K, Tanimoto T, et al. Application of artificial intelligence using a convolutional neural network for detecting gastric cancer in endoscopic images. Gastric Cancer 2018;21(4):653–60.
83. Zhu Y, Wang Q-C, Xu M-D, et al. Application of convolutional neural network in the diagnosis of the invasion depth of gastric cancer based on conventional endoscopy. Gastrointest Endosc 2019;89(4):806–15.e1.
84. Kim HH. Endoscopic Raman spectroscopy for molecular fingerprinting of gastric cancer: principle to implementation. Biomed Res Int 2015;2015. https://doi.org/10.1155/2015/670121.
85. Luo S, Chen C, Mao H, et al. Discrimination of premalignant lesions and cancer tissues from normal gastric tissues using Raman spectroscopy. J Biomed Opt 2013;18(6):067004.
86. Bergholt MS, Zheng W, Ho KY, et al. Fiber-optic Raman spectroscopy probes gastric carcinogenesis in vivo at endoscopy. J Biophotonics 2013;6(1):49–59.
87. Bergholt MS, Zheng W, Lin K, et al. Raman endoscopy for in vivo differentiation between benign and malignant ulcers in the stomach. Analyst 2010;135(12):3162–8.
88. Duraipandian S, Sylvest Bergholt M, Zheng W, et al. Real-time Raman spectroscopy for in vivo, online gastric cancer diagnosis during clinical endoscopic examination. J Biomed Opt 2012;17(8):081418.
89. Huang Z, Teh SK, Zheng W, et al. In vivo detection of epithelial neoplasia in the stomach using image-guided Raman endoscopy. Biosens Bioelectron 2010;26(2):383–9.
90. Kawabata T, Kikuchi H, Okazaki S, et al. Near-infrared multichannel Raman spectroscopy with a 1064 nm excitation wavelength for ex vivo diagnosis of gastric cancer. J Surg Res 2011;169(2):e137–43.

91. Teh SK, Zheng W, Ho KY, et al. Diagnostic potential of near-infrared Raman spectroscopy in the stomach: differentiating dysplasia from normal tissue. Br J Cancer 2008;98(2):457–65.
92. Teh SK, Zheng W, Ho KY, et al. Near-infrared Raman spectroscopy for early diagnosis and typing of adenocarcinoma in the stomach. Br J Surg 2010;97(4):550–7.
93. Teh SK, Zheng W, Ho KY, et al. Diagnosis of gastric cancer using near-infrared Raman spectroscopy and classification and regression tree techniques. J Biomed Opt 2008;13(3):034013.
94. Yao K, Doyama H, Gotoda T, et al. Diagnostic performance and limitations of magnifying narrow-band imaging in screening endoscopy of early gastric cancer: a prospective multicenter feasibility study. Gastric Cancer 2014;17(4): 669–79.
95. Yao K, Iwashita A, Tanabe H, et al. Novel zoom endoscopy technique for diagnosis of small flat gastric cancer: a prospective, blind study. Clin Gastroenterol Hepatol 2007;5(7):869–78.
96. Asada-Hirayama I, Kodashima S, Sakaguchi Y, et al. Magnifying endoscopy with narrow-band imaging is more accurate for determination of horizontal extent of early gastric cancers than chromoendoscopy. Endosc Int Open 2016;4(6): E690–8.
97. Nagahama T, Yao K, Maki S, et al. Usefulness of magnifying endoscopy with narrow-band imaging for determining the horizontal extent of early gastric cancer when there is an unclear margin by chromoendoscopy (with video). Gastrointest Endosc 2011;74(6):1259–67.

Endoscopic Resection of Gastric Cancer

Ga Hee Kim, MD, PhD, Hwoon-Yong Jung, MD, PhD, AGAF*

KEYWORDS

- Early gastric cancer (EGC) • Endoscopic submucosal dissection (ESD)
- Endoscopic mucosal resection (EMR) • Stomach

KEY POINTS

- Endoscopic resection is an established first-line treatment modality for selected early gastric cancers.
- Compared with endoscopic mucosal resection, endoscopic submucosal dissection is generally associated with higher rates of en bloc, complete, and curative resections and lower rates of local recurrence.
- Long-term outcomes in terms of recurrence and death of tumors that fulfill both the absolute and the expanded criteria are excellent. Endoscopic resection might be considered a primary treatment modality, replacing radical gastrectomy.

Video content accompanies this article at http://www.giendo.theclinics.com.

INTRODUCTION

Endoscopic resection (ER) is recognized as a minimally invasive treatment strategy for premalignant gastrointestinal lesions, superficial esophageal cancer (SEC), early gastric cancer (EGC), and early colon cancer with low morbidity and mortality.[1] EGC is a well-established indication for ER for patients in East Asian and Western countries.[2,3] Recently, advancements in endoscopic techniques, including magnifying endoscopy and image-enhanced endoscopy, have enabled the diagnosis of superficial neoplasia.[4] With improvements in the early detection of EGC and advances in techniques used, ER has become widely performed. Several studies have reported favorable clinical outcomes of ER that are comparable to those of surgical resection (SR), with greater safety and sufficient oncologic outcomes.[5–10] ER for EGC was superior to SR and showed several advantages in terms of improving the patient's quality of life. Therefore, ER became a standard treatment for tumors meeting the specific criteria characteristic of very low risk of lymph node metastasis (LNM).[11]

Department of Gastroenterology, University of Ulsan College of Medicine, Asan Medical Center, Asan Digestive Disease Research Institute, 88, Olympic-ro 43-gil, Songpa-gu, Seoul
* Corresponding author.
E-mail address: hwoonymd@gmail.com

Gastrointest Endoscopy Clin N Am 31 (2021) 563–579
https://doi.org/10.1016/j.giec.2021.03.008 giendo.theclinics.com
1052-5157/21/

In this review article, the authors aim to discuss the techniques, indications, long-term follow-up results, clinical management, and adverse events of ER as treatment for gastric cancer.

Indications for Endoscopic Resection

Previous guidelines used for determining the indications for ER as treatment for EGC were established primarily based on the presumed risk of LNM observed in surgical specimens.[12] In addition, the traditional criteria for ER of EGC were established according to the technical limitation of traditional endoscopic mucosal resection (EMR) for removing gastric lesions larger than 2 cm in diameter en bloc.[13] The absolute indications for ER were as follows: (1) papillary or tubular (differentiated) adenocarcinoma, (2) ≤2 cm in diameter, (3) no ulceration within the tumor, and (4) no lymphatic-vascular involvement.[14–16]

Clinical observations have noted that the empirical indications for EMR are too strict and lead to unnecessary surgery.[17] Therefore, the expanded criteria for ER have been proposed, especially in cases whereby a large en bloc resection could be accomplished using endoscopic submucosal dissection (ESD).[18,19] With the accumulation of experience and technical advances, the indications for ER have widened and criteria have expanded, proposed for tumors with minimal risk of LNM. Previous studies investigated the long-term outcomes of ER in EGC meeting the expanded indication criteria, and the results were comparable with those in patients meeting the absolute indication criteria. The expanded indication included 4 discrete criteria: (1) intramucosal differentiated tumor without ulcers, size greater than 2 cm; (2) intramucosal differentiated tumor with ulcers, size ≤3 cm; (3) intramucosal undifferentiated tumor without ulcers, size ≤2 cm; and (4) submucosal invasion less than 500 μm (sm1), differentiated tumor, size ≤3 cm.[14–16]

According to a recent multicenter study conducted in Japan (JCOG0607) that included patients with differentiated mucosal cancer measuring greater than 2 cm in diameter without ulcers and those with differentiated mucosal cancer measuring ≤3 cm with ulcers, the 5-year overall survival (OS) in the enrolled patients was 97.0% (95% confidence interval [CI], 95.0% to 98.2%).[20] Based on the updated 2018 Japanese Gastric Cancer Association (JGCA) guidelines, the absolute indications for ESD were as follows: (1) a differentiated-type adenocarcinoma without ulcerative findings, in which the depth of invasion is clinically diagnosed as T1a and the diameter is greater than 2 cm, and (2) a differentiated-type adenocarcinoma with ulcerative findings, in which the depth of invasion is clinically diagnosed as T1a and the diameter is ≤3 cm.[11] In addition, the expanded indication now considers an undifferentiated-type adenocarcinoma without ulcerative findings, in which the depth of invasion is clinically diagnosed as T1a and the diameter is ≤2 cm. As such, the use of ESD for tumors that fulfilled these expanded criteria subcategories should be considered along with the risk of performing SR, given the increased risk of LNM. The number of patients undergoing ESD for EGC has continuously increased as a result of the criteria expansion.

Principles of Endoscopic Resection

Endoscopic mucosal resection

The first EMR technique was introduced in 1984 in Japan,[21] and various techniques have been developed since. The EMR with a cap-fitted panendoscope method was developed in 1992 for the resection of SEC and is directly applicable to the resection of EGC.[22] The technique uses a transparent plastic cap mounted to the tip of a standard endoscope. A snare is prelooped inside the groove of the inner aspect of the distal part of the cap, thus allowing the operator to cut lesions that are suctioned into the cap. Using this technique, intramucosal cancers of 2 cm or less in diameter can be safely removed. The EMR technique using ligation, which was subsequently extended to EMR using multiband ligation, uses band ligation to create a "pseudopolyp" by suctioning the lesion into the banding cap and deploying a band underneath it.[23] There is a wide variety of EMR methods used in the clinical setting, but the basic steps in performing this procedure are as follows (**Fig. 1**): (1) delineation of the lateral margin with or without chromoendoscopy, (2) placement of markings using a brief burst of electrocautery or argon plasma coagulation, (3) submucosal injection to lift the lesion, and (4) resection of the lesion. Before the development of ESD, EMR with circumferential precutting (EMR-P) was the most effective method for cutting larger lesions in 1 piece.[24] EMR-P for intramucosal cancers less than 2 cm may be considered an alternative to ESD (Video 1).[25] However, larger-sized lesions (>2 cm) cannot be completely resected by EMR at once, and piecemeal resection can potentially increase the risk of local recurrence and cause inadequate histologic staging.[26,27]

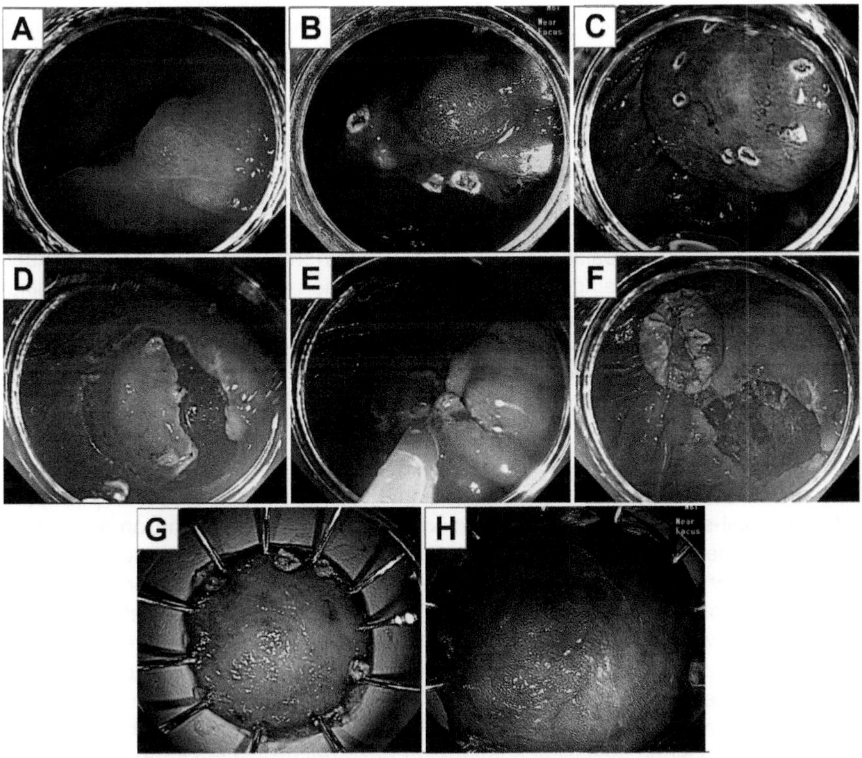

Fig. 1. EMR-P. (*A*) Adenoma of about10 mm in size with high-grade dysplasia on the lesser curvature side of the antrum. (*B*) Narrow band imaging (NBI) finding of adenoma and circumferential marking. (*C*) After saline injection, an elevated lesion shows hyperemic discoloration at the center. (*D*) Circumferential precutting using snare tip. (*E*) Cutting of submucosal tissue using a snare. (*F*) Tissue containing adenoma resected with by the EMR procedure after hemostasis. (*G*) Retrieved specimen. (*H*) NBI finding of resected specimen. The final diagnosis of this 53-year-old patient was 2a type EGC with a 7 × 6-mm sized well-differentiated adenocarcinoma, which invaded into lamina propria.

Endoscopic submucosal dissection

The ESD technique has been widely used to remove tumors greater than 2 cm in diameter with acceptable complication rates and higher en bloc and complete resection rates than conventional EMR. Using this technique, the submucosal layer is dissected with through-the-scope endoscopic knives. ESD was first published in 1999 and can be used for resection of large lesions en bloc and allows precise pathologic staging.[28] Complete en bloc resection regardless of tumor size, location, and presence of fibrosis is now possible.

The procedure is performed in the following order: identification of the lesion, marking around the lesion, submucosal injection, mucosal incision, submucosal dissection, and tissue retrieval (**Fig. 2**). Before performing ESD, endoscopic examination, including white-light imaging, narrow-band imaging, and chromoendoscopy, was performed to determine the exact margin of the tumor. Mucosal markings were made mainly by forced coagulation effect 3 to 5 mm outside apart from the border of the lesion (Video 2). After placing several dots around the lesion, normal saline mixed with epinephrine and methylene blue was injected into the submucosal layer. The solution was repeatedly injected into the target mucosa until the layer was sufficiently lifted and the tumor area appeared brown. This change is attributed to the thickness of the tumor. A small incision was made using a needle knife followed by a circumferential precutting outside the marking. Submucosal dissection was performed from the oral side, as the tumor was located in the distal location. If the tumor is located in the proximal or middle stomach, dissection begins at the anal side. Various knives, including insulation-tipped (IT), IT-2, hook, flex, triangle tip, flush and dual knives, were used to dissect the submucosal layer parallel to the muscular layer until the lesion was completely removed. The dissection is usually performed from the posterior wall side to the dependent position. It is preferable to dissect the submucosal layer located in a dependent position. Hemostasis was performed by applying hemostatic forceps or hemoclips or using argon plasma coagulation to prevent delayed bleeding. All nonbleeding visible vessels were coagulated after the completion of ER. The resected tissue was stretched and fixed with a pin to ensure that all marked areas have been removed before the resection. The tissues were then fixed in 10% formalin solution and sent to the pathologists.

Endoscopic mucosal resection versus endoscopic submucosal dissection

The classical EMR method is easy to perform, has less complications, and is applicable for small-sized lesions, although 1 treatment effect depending on the size of the lesion has been reported. Moreover, the en bloc resection and complete resection rates are greatly reduced. When the classical EMR method was used for lesions less than 1 cm in size, the rate of complete resection was approximately 60% and remained high, whereas the rate of complete resection of lesions greater than 2 cm in size was low (20%–30%). Complete resection of lesions greater than 3 cm is difficult to achieve.[29] The success rate of conventional EMR was influenced by tumor size and shape and decreased in patients with lesions of size greater than 2 cm, of depressed type, and located along the lesser curvature or posterior wall of the body.[27] In a meta-analysis of 18 observational studies including 6723 lesions, patients who underwent ESD had an increased incidence of en bloc resection (odds ratio [OR]: 9.00; 95% CI: 6.66 to 12.17; $P<.001$), complete resection (OR: 8.43; 95% CI: 5.04–14.09; $P<.001$), and curative resection (OR: 2.92; 95% CI: 1.85–4.61; $P<.001$) compared with those who underwent EMR. Furthermore, ESD was associated with a lower risk of local recurrence (OR: 0.18; 95% CI: 0.09–0.34; $P<.001$).[30] There was no significant difference between ESD and EMR for the risk of bleeding (OR: 1.26; 95% CI:

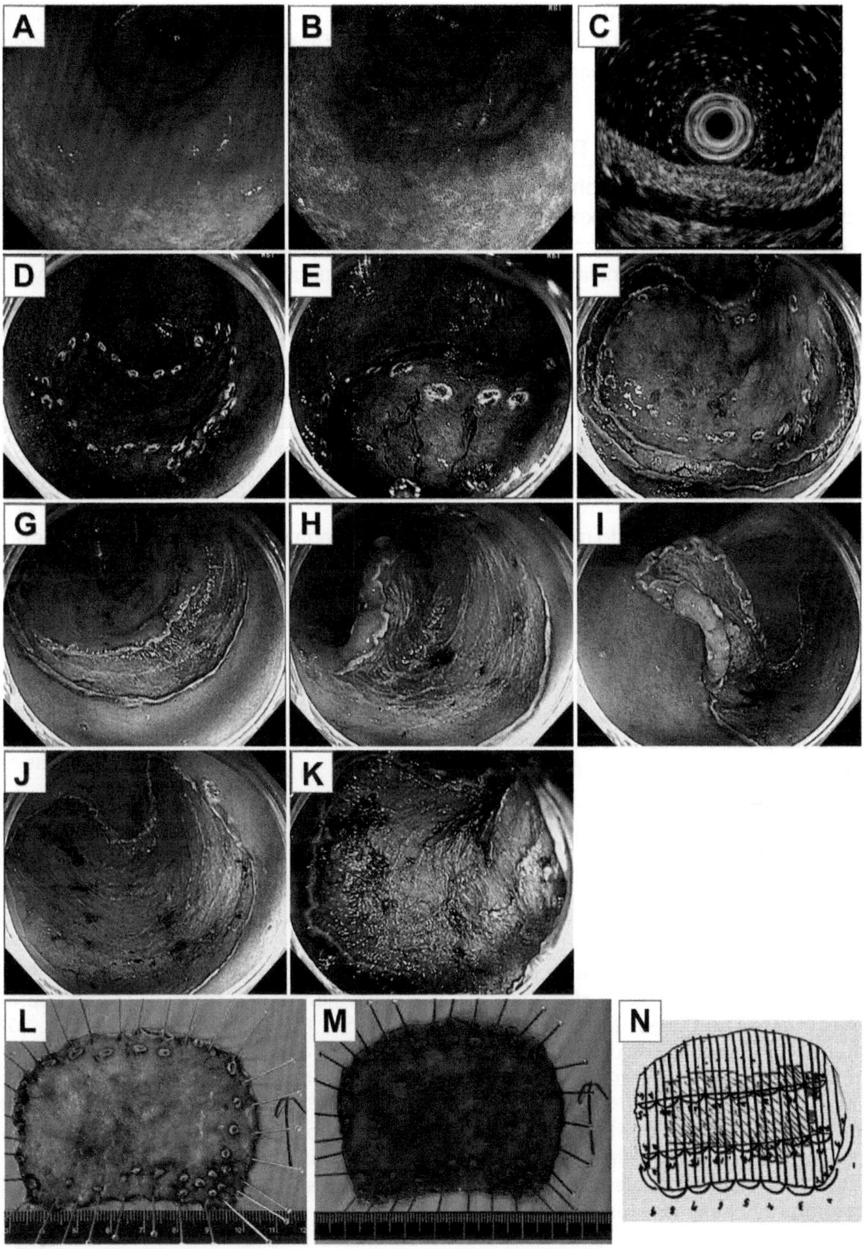

Fig. 2. ESD. (*A*) Hyperemic flat elevated and depressed lesion of about 5 × 3 cm in size on the greater curvature side of the antrum. (*B*) The tumor area is distinguishable under NBI mode because the neoplasm has many vascular structures and is detected by NBI as dark brown. (*C*) Endoscopic ultrasonography findings of this tumor. Scanned mucosal layer appears thickened and mixed hypoechoic, which is representative of the involved area. (*D*) Marking. Circumferential marking around the tumor margin. Marking should be made at 3 to 5 mm outside apart from imaginary border. (*E*) Submucosal injection. During submucosal injection of saline mixed with a small amount of methylene blue, tumor area can be

0.88–1.80; P = .203). The number of clinicians in centers outside of Asia who have expertise and experience in performing ESD have increased, and ESD is the preferred endoscopic treatment for patients with EGC based on certain published guidelines.

Clinical Management After Endoscopic Resection

When a lesion without lymphovascular invasion (LVI) and a negative surgical margin meeting the absolute and expanded indication criteria is resected en bloc, it is considered a curative lesion.[16,30,31] Metachronous gastric cancer may possibly develop following ER, and the cumulative 3-year risk is approximately 5.9%.[32] Regular surveillance endoscopy every 6 to 12 months was recommended for patients who underwent curative ER of EGC based on the absolute or expanded criteria for early detection of metachronous gastric cancer. In addition, regular abdominopelvic computed tomography scans at 6- to 12-month intervals were performed after curative ER of EGC for the detection of extragastric recurrence based on absolute and expanded criteria. The patients were tested for *Helicobacter pylori* infection; if the test yielded a positive result, appropriate treatment was provided to eradicate the infection.[33–35]

Resected tumors that do not fulfill the following criteria were considered for noncurative resection: (1) differentiated (well or moderately differentiated tubular or papillary) intramucosal cancer measuring greater than 2 cm in diameter without ulcers (active or scar), (2) differentiated mucosal cancer measuring less than 3 cm with ulcers (active or scar), (3) undifferentiated (poorly differentiated tubular or poorly cohesive) mucosal cancer measuring less than 2 cm without ulcers (active or scar), and (4) differentiated mucosal cancer measuring less than 3 cm with subtle submucosal invasion (<500 μm).[16] LVI and positive vertical margins, which are confirmed after ER, are also important reasons for the recommendation of an additional gastrectomy.[16,31] Most studies that have investigated the long-term outcomes with or without additional surgery in patients who did not meet the curative criteria for ER of EGC showed a significant survival benefit.[36–38]

clearly seen as brown. This change is originated from the thickness of the tumor. (*F*) Precutting. Circumferential cutting of the mucosa, including the marking spots. As can be appreciated, there is sufficient free margin along the precut. (*G–I*) Submucosal dissection. (*G*) After circumferential precutting, the submucosal layer is dissected from the oral side for the distal location. If the tumor location is the proximal or middle stomach, dissection begins from the anal side. (*H*) The direction of dissection is usually from the posterior wall side to the dependent position. (*I*) It would be more comfortable to dissect the last submucosa located in the dependent position. (*J*) Completion of submucosal dissection. (*K*) Hemostasis. Coagulation of bleeding and nonbleeding exposed vessels to prevent delayed bleeding. (*L*) Pinning of resected specimen. The retrieved specimen should be fixed using pins, and all the marking spots and tissue orientation should be confirmed. The image shows different numbers at the right side to keep proper orientation after resection. The total procedure time for ESD was 37 min. The specimen size was 80 × 55 mm. (*M*) Specimen after fixation in the formalin bag. The tumor margin usually can be seen after formalin fixation. This lesion is a superficially depressed lesion, including several nondepressed foci. (*N*) Mapping of specimen. Resected specimen is sliced at every 2- to 3-mm interval to make a histopathological map. The final diagnosis was a 57 × 32-mm sized EGC, 2c+2b, moderately differentiated adenocarcinoma. The depth of invasion extends to the muscularis mucosae (M3). All lateral and deep margins are free of tumor with no lymphovascular tumor embolism.

Based on the updated 2018 JGCA guidelines, the technical terms related to the curability of ER of EGC were revised: endoscopic curability (eCura) A to C-2. Curative resection and expanded curative resection were changed to eCuraA and B. Noncurative resection was divided into eCuraC-1 and C-2.[11] The resection is classified as endoscopic curability A (eCuraA) when all of the following conditions are fulfilled, provided that the cancer does not have ulcerative findings: en bloc resection, any tumor size, histologically differentiated type-dominant, pT1a, negative horizontal and vertical margins, and absence of LVI. The resection is classified as endoscopic curability B (eCuraB) for histologically undifferentiated dominant type tumors when all of the following conditions are fulfilled: no ulcerative findings, en bloc resection, pT1a, negative horizontal and vertical margins, no LVI, and tumor size $\leq$2 cm. The resection is classified as endoscopic curability C-1 (eCuraC-1) when it is of histologically differentiated type and fulfills the criteria for either eCuraA or eCuraB classification but was not used to resect tumors en bloc or has positive horizontal margins. All other eCuraC resections were subclassified as endoscopic curability C-2 (eCuraC-2). An exception applies if cancer invasion is observed only at the horizontal resection margin (eCuraC-1). Additional endoscopic management rather than SR is applied if histopathological evaluation of endoscopically resected EGC specimen shows positive involvement at the horizontal resection margin without any other findings compatible with noncurative resection. Repeat ESD, close observation expecting a burn effect of the initial ESD, and endoscopic coagulation using a laser or argon-plasma coagulator rather than surgical gastrectomy fall under the category of eCuraC-1. The standard management of eCuraC-2 is additional surgery; however, the clinicians' decision should consider the patient's physical condition.[11]

Long-Term Outcomes

Many studies with long-term follow-up have identified ER as a favorable method for curative resection of EGC with absolute indication.[39] In the case of EGC with absolute indication, the 5-year disease-specific survival rate is almost 100%. Therefore, the data comparing outcomes in patients who underwent ER with those who had a gastrectomy suggest similar clinical outcomes.[5] Several studies investigated the long-term outcomes of ESD in EGC that met the expanded indication criteria, and the results were comparable with those in patients meeting the absolute indication criteria (**Table 1**).

No randomized trials have compared endoscopic and surgical management of EGC. Recently, to validate the expanded indication criteria of ER, several studies

Table 1
Long-term outcomes of endoscopic resection for early gastric cancer

Author, Publication Year	Number of Patients (EMR/ESD)	FU Period (mo)	En Bloc Resection (%)	5-y DFS (%)	5-y OS (%)	5-y DSS (%)
Shichijo et al,[45] 2020	0/214	88.8	99	NA	99.5	93.9
Kim et al,[40] 2018	0/697	59	99.1	87.9	96.6	90.6
Choi et al,[41] 2015	33/928	48.3	88.7	99.1	94.8	NA
Kosaka et al,[42] 2014	0/438	73	97.7	NA	83.1	100
Ahn et al,[43] 2011	534/833	32	86.1	NA	96.8	NA

Abbreviations: DFS, disease-free survival; DSS, disease-specific survival; FU, follow-up; NA, not available.

compared the long-term outcomes of ER and SR, which reported favorable results for ER (**Table 2**). Compared with SR, the benefits of ER included fewer complications and a shorter length of hospital stay. ER preserves the stomach, thereby improving patients' quality of life compared with SR.[47] In a single-center prospective study by Kim and colleagues,[47] ER can provide better health-related quality-of-life benefits for EGC patients than can SR, especially during the early posttreatment period. However, the 5-year cumulative metachronous recurrence rates after ER (5.8%–10.9%) were significantly higher than those after SR (0.9%–1.1%).[5,6] Metachronous gastric cancer or local recurrence could be treated by ER if the lesion is detected early. Therefore, more attention should be paid during surveillance endoscopy after ER.

The indications for ER include undifferentiated-type intramucosal EGC ≤2 cm in diameter without ulceration or LVI.[11,15] Instrumental and technical advancements, such as the development of ESD, have enabled the resection of larger tumors. Consequently, ER for undifferentiated EGC often results in the complete resection of the undifferentiated intramucosal EGC greater than 2 cm in diameter with negative resection margins and the absence of ulceration and LVI. In a recent multicenter study in Korea conducted by Yang and colleagues,[48] the risk of LNM or distant metastasis was 1% for patients undergoing noncurative ER for undifferentiated EGC, with the tumor size of greater than 2 cm as the only noncurative factor. The results of previous studies were obtained by retrospective assessment of the patients' medical records. Thus, a prospective multicenter study with a high follow-up rate is required for a more precise evaluation of the long-term outcomes of gastric ESD.

Treatment Strategy for Noncurative Resection

The indication for endoscopic treatment of EGC is gradually expanding. Various other factors may cause "noncurative resection," unintended by the practitioner. According to various previous studies, the incidence of noncurative resection after ER of EGC was approximately 11.9% to 18.5%.[49] The aim of ER for EGC is curative resection, but unintended noncurative resection may occur because of various factors. Several previous studies have analyzed the risk factors affecting noncurative resection in the ER of EGC, including large tumor size, tumor location, and presence of ulcers and undifferentiated tumors. In the case of noncurative resection, additional treatment is required considering the risk of local recurrence and LNM, and the standard treatment

Table 2
Comparison of long-term outcomes between endoscopic resection and surgical resection for early gastric cancer

Author, Publication Year	No. of Patients ER/SR	FU Period (mo) ER/SR	R0 Resection (%) ER/SR	5-y DFS (%) ER/SR	5-y OS (%) ER/SR	5-y DSS (%) ER/SR
Lee et al,[46] 2018	522/522	52.7/59.2	NA	92.7/96.7	98.1/96.4	99.6/98.9
Quero et al,[9] 2020	64/73	23/21	88.1/100	74.9/72	77.7/71.8	NA
Fukunaga et al,[44] 2017	181/127	42.9/64.2	NA	NA	97.1/85.8	NA
Gong et al,[10] 2017	40/39	60.9	92.5/NA	NA	93.9/97.3	NA
Pyo et al,[8] 2016	1290/1273	46	82.7/96.4	98/96.9	97.1/96.3	99.6/99.4
Choi et al,[6] 2015	261/114	74.9/78.1	85.8/NA	94.8/99.1	95.7/93.6	100/100
Choi et al,[5] 2011	172/379	81	NA	NA	93.6/94.2	98.7/99.7

Abbreviation: No., number.

is gastrectomy with lymphadenectomy. Additional gastrectomy with lymph node dissection is the standard treatment after noncurative ER.[11,15,16,37] The rate of LNM in patients who underwent additional gastrectomy after noncurative resection of ER for EGC is 7.5% to 16.7%.[50–52] Furthermore, if recurrence is observed when no additional treatment was provided after a noncurative ER, most patients do not achieve long-term survival. In a recent study by Kim and colleagues,[53] they developed a nomogram to predict the status of LNM with the aim of avoiding unnecessary surgery. Multivariate analyses revealed that age, tumor size, lymphatic invasion, depth of invasion, and histologic differentiation were all significant prognostic factors for LNM. Patients with LVI or vertical margin positivity showed a survival benefit with additional curative surgery.[36,54] Thus, additional surgery should be selected in healthy, nonelderly patients.

Otherwise, in some elderly patients and/or those with severe underlying diseases, the advantages and disadvantages of additional surgery should be considered when selecting the treatment strategy after noncurative ER.[55] In elderly patients with gastric cancer, it is necessary to evaluate not only the risk for LNM but also the underlying conditions of the patient because heterogeneity in the aging process leads to a diverse range of age-related declines in health and physical status among the elderly.[56,57] For reasons such as an increase in elderly patients because of the increase in average life expectancy, underlying disease, poor general condition, or patient's refusal of a gastrectomy, patients with noncurative resection may be treated with redo ESD, argon plasma coagulation, or careful observation without further treatment.[58,59]

Adverse Event

Bleeding

Post-ESD bleeding is difficult to predict and can be a potentially life-threatening complication. Bleeding is the most common major complication of ER. Bleeding is classified into immediate bleeding during ER and delayed bleeding after ER. Immediate bleeding can be defined as cases requiring blood transfusion, emergency surgery, or vasopressor therapy in which the rate is less than 1%.[60] The major factors affecting intraoperative bleeding were tumor location (more often in the upper and middle thirds than in the lower third) and tumor size (more often >2 cm in size).[61] However, bleeding can be successfully treated in most cases through coagulation of the bleeding vessels, or placement of metallic clips for severe bleeding. In terms of postoperative bleeding, the most acceptable definition is marked bleeding from the ER-related ulcers requiring special measures for hemostasis; it is clinically noticed before endoscopy when the hemoglobin level decreases by 2 g/dL, vital signs change, or either hematochezia or massive melena is seen. It is reported that delayed bleeding occurs in 1.8% to 15.6% of cases.[62–64] Delayed bleeding is associated with tumor location, larger tumors (>40 mm), recurrent lesions, presence of ulcers, old age (≥80 years), longer procedure time, chronic kidney disease, liver cirrhosis, and the use of antithrombotic agents.[65–68] Delayed bleeding was reported to occur more frequently after ESD for lesions in the lower and middle thirds of the stomach compared with the upper third of the stomach.[69,70] Antral active peristalsis, and bile reflux might lead to a high incidence of post-ESD bleeding in the lower stomach. Prophylactic hemostasis of visible vessels on the postresection ulcer caused by ER of EGC may lower the risk of delayed bleeding.[70] In addition, proton pump inhibitors decrease the risk of symptoms and complications associated with iatrogenic ulcers caused by ER of EGC.[71,72] Several randomized trials and a meta-analysis indicated that administering proton pump inhibitors significantly reduced the incidence of delayed bleeding compared with using a histamine-2 receptor antagonist.[71] A second-look endoscopy after ER may contribute little to the prevention of delayed bleeding.[73,74] The preventive coagulation of non-bleeding visible vessels in second-look endoscopy after gastric ESD may contribute little to the prevention of late delayed bleeding.[70]

With the increase in the use of antithrombotic agents, the management of these drugs during the perioperative period remains a great concern. Patients receiving antithrombotic agents have an increased risk of bleeding. However, discontinuing the use of antithrombotic agents may lead to unexpected thrombotic events. In a recent Korean propensity score matching study, So and colleagues[65] reported conflicting results on the risk of bleeding after ESD for gastric neoplasms: delayed bleeding rate in the continued use of antithrombotic agents group was higher than that of the matched control group (15.9% vs 5.1%; OR: 3.55; 95% CI: 1.24–10.14; $P = .018$). No thromboembolic events were observed in patients in the continuation of antithrombotic agents group. In another study in Japan by Koh and colleagues,[75] oral antithrombotic drug treatment was selected as an independent risk factor for delayed but not early bleeding, according to the multivariate analysis (OR: 2.667; 95% CI: 1.231–5.776; $P = .013$). Interruption of antithrombotic drug treatment may be adequate for preventing early post-ER bleeding; however, reinitiating antithrombotic agents is a significant independent risk factor for delayed post-ER bleeding. Therefore, the post-ER bleeding risk for each agent must be analyzed individually.

Perforation

Perforation during ER with rates reportedly ranging from 1.2% to 9.6% can be conservatively treated by complete endoscopic closure with endoclips.[76,77] Delayed perforation because of artificial ulcers following ER is rare, reportedly 0.06% to 0.45% after gastric ER; however, it can lead to serious conditions that often require emergency operations.[78] Perforations that occur in relation to ESD are classified into macroperfusions and microperforations. A perforation is diagnosed when mesenteric fat or intra-abdominal space is directly observed during the procedure (macroperforation) or free air is found on a radiograph after the procedure without a visible stomach wall defect during the procedure (microperforation). Immediate small perforations can be successfully treated without surgery with a combination of endoscopic clipping and broad-spectrum antibiotics.[79] However, large perforations would require immediate surgery. Delayed perforation after ER may occur because of various factors, such as tumor state (tumor depth, invasion status, and upper stomach), lesions in the gastric tube, and the patient's condition. The essential mechanism of delayed perforation after ESD was suggested to be electrical cautery during submucosal dissection or repeated coagulation that caused ischemic change to the gastric wall, resulting in necrosis.[80] Recognizing delayed perforation in the differential diagnosis is important when patients who have previously undergone ER for EGC show signs of peritoneal irritation. Patients with delayed perforation who recovered with conservative management were mostly those who developed adverse events before dietary intake and/or received endoscopic intervention within 24 hours after onset.[81]

Other adverse events

The circumferential extent of the mucosal defect of greater than 75% of the circumference of the lumen and longitudinal extent of greater than 5 cm were related to post-ER stenosis with both cardiac and pyloric resections.[82] Stenosis after gastric ER has been reported to range from 0.7% to 1.9%.[83] Several studies described the use of a steroid (triamcinolone) solution for submucosal injection during ER.[84] Balloon dilation is a recognized standard treatment for benign strictures and is used as the primary treatment for post-ER stenosis.[85]

According to a prospective study in Japan, ER procedures carry a moderate risk for venous thromboembolism.[86] In this study, D-dimer measurements were higher in patients with deep vein thrombosis (DVT) than in patients without DVT. D-dimer levels on the day after ESD, in particular, may be associated with DVT in patients with ESD. According to the receiver operating characteristic curve analysis, the resulting cutoff value of the D-dimer level on the day after ER was 1.9 μg/mL for ESD patients, with superior association to pre-ESD or immediate post-ESD levels (sensitivity 83.3%; specificity 79.6%).

The possibility of sedation-related adverse events, including pulmonary complications, may be increased when performing therapeutic endoscopy. In a single-center retrospective study in Korea conducted by Gong and colleagues,[87] the incidence of aspiration pneumonia after ER for gastric neoplasms was 0.62%. In addition, old age, smoking, and a longer hemostasis time were risk factors for the occurrence of aspiration pneumonia after ER.

SUMMARY

ER is an effective treatment for EGC without metastasis because of the high en bloc and complete resection and low local recurrence rate. With regard to its safety and efficacy, the indications for ER have broadened in the field of therapeutic endoscopy. Long-term outcomes in terms of recurrence and death are excellent using both the absolute and the expanded criteria. ER can preserve organ function with excellent maintenance of the patient's quality of life. Therefore, ER may be positioned as a primary treatment modality, replacing radical gastrectomy. To obtain these results, accurate diagnosis, selection of patients, proper appreciation of technical aspects, and rational strategy for follow-up are necessary. Thus, further technological advances in treatment and outcomes of long-term follow-up under the expanded indications of ER for EGC owing to the risk of LNM are expected in the next decade.

CLINICS CARE POINTS

- Endoscopic resection is recommended an established first-line treatment modality in both absolute and selected expanded indication for early gastric cancer.
- The meticulous pathologic evaluation is needed to confirm the curability and to decide the candidates taking additional gastrectomy with regional lymphadenectomy in the patients with noncurative resection.
- To determine additional treatment strategy for noncurative resection, both aspects of the underlying medical condition of the patient and the risk factors for lymph node metastasis should be considered.

DISCLOSURE

The authors have nothing to disclose.

SUPPLEMENTARY DATA

Supplementary data to this article can be found online at https://doi.org/10.1016/j.giec.2021.03.008.

REFERENCES

1. Draganov PV, Wang AY, Othman MO, et al. AGA Institute Clinical Practice Update: endoscopic submucosal dissection in the United States. Clin Gastroenterol Hepatol 2019;17:16–25.e1.
2. Ribeiro-Mourao F, Pimentel-Nunes P, Dinis-Ribeiro M. Endoscopic submucosal dissection for gastric lesions: results of an European inquiry. Endoscopy 2010; 42:814–9.
3. Ngamruengphong S, Ferri L, Aihara H, et al. Efficacy of endoscopic submucosal dissection for superficial gastric neoplasia in a large cohort in North America [published online ahead of print Jun 18, 2020]. Clin Gastroenterol Hepatol 2020. https://doi.org/10.1016/j.cgh.2020.06.023.
4. Nagahama T, Yao K, Maki S, et al. Usefulness of magnifying endoscopy with narrow-band imaging for determining the horizontal extent of early gastric cancer when there is an unclear margin by chromoendoscopy (with video). Gastrointest Endosc 2011;74:1259–67.
5. Choi KS, Jung HY, Choi KD, et al. EMR versus gastrectomy for intramucosal gastric cancer: comparison of long-term outcomes. Gastrointest Endosc 2011; 73:942–8.
6. Choi IJ, Lee JH, Kim YI, et al. Long-term outcome comparison of endoscopic resection and surgery in early gastric cancer meeting the absolute indication for endoscopic resection. Gastrointest Endosc 2015;81:333–341 e1.
7. Kim YI, Kim YW, Choi IJ, et al. Long-term survival after endoscopic resection versus surgery in early gastric cancers. Endoscopy 2015;47:293–301.
8. Pyo JH, Lee H, Min BH, et al. Long-term outcome of endoscopic resection vs. surgery for early gastric cancer: a non-inferiority-matched cohort study. Am J Gastroenterol 2016;111:240–9.
9. Quero G, Fiorillo C, Longo F, et al. Propensity score-matched comparison of short- and long-term outcomes between surgery and endoscopic submucosal dissection (ESD) for intestinal type early gastric cancer (EGC) of the middle and lower third of the stomach: a European Tertiary Referral Center experience [published online ahead of print Jun 1, 2020]. Surg Endosc 2020. https://doi.org/10.1007/s00464-020-07677-3.
10. Gong EJ, Kim DH, Ahn JY, et al. Comparison of long-term outcomes of endoscopic submucosal dissection and surgery for esophagogastric junction adenocarcinoma. Gastric Cancer 2017;20:84–91.
11. Japanese Gastric Cancer Association. Japanese gastric cancer treatment guidelines 2018 (5th edition) [published online ahead of print Feb 14, 2020]. Gastric Cancer 2020. https://doi.org/10.1007/s10120-020-01042-y.
12. Gotoda T, Yanagisawa A, Sasako M, et al. Incidence of lymph node metastasis from early gastric cancer: estimation with a large number of cases at two large centers. Gastric Cancer 2000;3:219–25.
13. Yamao T, Shirao K, Ono H, et al. Risk factors for lymph node metastasis from intramucosal gastric carcinoma. Cancer 1996;77:602–6.
14. Park CH, Yang DH, Kim JW, et al. Clinical practice guideline for endoscopic resection of early gastrointestinal cancer. Clin Endosc 2020;53:142–66.
15. Japanese Gastric Cancer Association. Japanese Gastric Cancer Treatment guidelines 2014 (ver. 4). Gastric Cancer 2017;20:1–19.
16. Guideline Committee of the Korean Gastric Cancer Association (KGCA), Development Working Group & Review Panel. Korean Practice Guideline for Gastric

Cancer 2018: an evidence-based, multi-disciplinary approach. J Gastric Cancer 2019;19:1–48.
17. Gotoda T. Endoscopic resection of early gastric cancer. Gastric Cancer 2007; 10:1–11.
18. Takeuchi Y, Uedo N, Iishi H, et al. Endoscopic submucosal dissection with insulated-tip knife for large mucosal early gastric cancer: a feasibility study (with videos). Gastrointest Endosc 2007;66:186–93.
19. Oka S, Tanaka S, Kaneko I, et al. Advantage of endoscopic submucosal dissection compared with EMR for early gastric cancer. Gastrointest Endosc 2006;64: 877–83.
20. Hasuike N, Ono H, Boku N, et al. A non-randomized confirmatory trial of an expanded indication for endoscopic submucosal dissection for intestinal-type gastric cancer (cT1a): the Japan Clinical Oncology Group study (JCOG0607). Gastric Cancer 2018;21:114–23.
21. Tada M, Murakami A, Karita M, et al. Endoscopic resection of early gastric cancer. Endoscopy 1993;25:445–50.
22. Inoue H, Takeshita K, Hori H, et al. Endoscopic mucosal resection with a cap-fitted panendoscope for esophagus, stomach, and colon mucosal lesions. Gastrointest Endosc 1993;39:58–62.
23. Soehendra N, Seewald S, Groth S, et al. Use of modified multiband ligator facilitates circumferential EMR in Barrett's esophagus (with video). Gastrointest Endosc 2006;63:847–52.
24. Choi IJ, Kim CG, Chang HJ, et al. The learning curve for EMR with circumferential mucosal incision in treating intramucosal gastric neoplasm. Gastrointest Endosc 2005;62:860–5.
25. Min BH, Lee JH, Kim JJ, et al. Clinical outcomes of endoscopic submucosal dissection (ESD) for treating early gastric cancer: comparison with endoscopic mucosal resection after circumferential precutting (EMR-P). Dig Liver Dis 2009; 41:201–9.
26. Tanabe S, Koizumi W, Mitomi H, et al. Clinical outcome of endoscopic aspiration mucosectomy for early stage gastric cancer. Gastrointest Endosc 2002;56: 708–13.
27. Kim JJ, Lee JH, Jung HY, et al. EMR for early gastric cancer in Korea: a multicenter retrospective study. Gastrointest Endosc 2007;66:693–700.
28. Gotoda T, Kondo H, Ono H, et al. A new endoscopic mucosal resection procedure using an insulation-tipped electrosurgical knife for rectal flat lesions: report of two cases. Gastrointest Endosc 1999;50:560–3.
29. Noda M, Kodama T, Atsumi M, et al. Possibilities and limitations of endoscopic resection for early gastric cancer. Endoscopy 1997;29:361–5.
30. Tao M, Zhou X, Hu M, et al. Endoscopic submucosal dissection versus endoscopic mucosal resection for patients with early gastric cancer: a meta-analysis. BMJ Open 2019;9:e025803.
31. Ono H, Yao K, Fujishiro M, et al. Guidelines for endoscopic submucosal dissection and endoscopic mucosal resection for early gastric cancer. Dig Endosc 2016;28:3–15.
32. Nakajima T, Oda I, Gotoda T, et al. Metachronous gastric cancers after endoscopic resection: how effective is annual endoscopic surveillance? Gastric Cancer 2006;9:93–8.
33. Choi IJ, Kook MC, Kim YI, et al. Helicobacter pylori therapy for the prevention of metachronous gastric cancer. N Engl J Med 2018;378:1085–95.

34. Bae SE, Jung HY, Kang J, et al. Effect of Helicobacter pylori eradication on metachronous recurrence after endoscopic resection of gastric neoplasm. Am J Gastroenterol 2014;109:60–7.
35. Choi JM, Kim SG, Choi J, et al. Effects of Helicobacter pylori eradication for metachronous gastric cancer prevention: a randomized controlled trial. Gastrointest Endosc 2018;88:475–485 e2.
36. Suzuki H, Oda I, Abe S, et al. Clinical outcomes of early gastric cancer patients after noncurative endoscopic submucosal dissection in a large consecutive patient series. Gastric Cancer 2017;20:679–89.
37. Eom BW, Kim YI, Kim KH, et al. Survival benefit of additional surgery after noncurative endoscopic resection in patients with early gastric cancer. Gastrointest Endosc 2017;85:155–163 e3.
38. Kusano C, Iwasaki M, Kaltenbach T, et al. Should elderly patients undergo additional surgery after non-curative endoscopic resection for early gastric cancer? Long-term comparative outcomes. Am J Gastroenterol 2011;106:1064–9.
39. Min BH, Kim ER, Kim KM, et al. Surveillance strategy based on the incidence and patterns of recurrence after curative endoscopic submucosal dissection for early gastric cancer. Endoscopy 2015;47:784–93.
40. Kim SG, Park CM, Lee NR, et al. Long-term clinical outcomes of endoscopic submucosal dissection in patients with early gastric cancer: a prospective multicenter cohort study. Gut Liver 2018;12:402–10.
41. Choi J, Kim SG, Im JP, et al. Long-term clinical outcomes of endoscopic resection for early gastric cancer. Surg Endosc 2015;29:1223–30.
42. Kosaka T, Endo M, Toya Y, et al. Long-term outcomes of endoscopic submucosal dissection for early gastric cancer: a single-center retrospective study. Dig Endosc 2014;26:183–91.
43. Ahn JY, Jung HY, Choi KD, et al. Endoscopic and oncologic outcomes after endoscopic resection for early gastric cancer: 1370 cases of absolute and extended indications. Gastrointest Endosc 2011;74:485–93.
44. Fukunaga S, Nagami Y, Shiba M, et al. Long-term prognosis of expandedindication differentiated-type early gastric cancer treated with endoscopic submucosal dissection or surgery using propensity score analysis. Gastrointest Endosc 2017; 85:143–52.
45. Shichijo S, Uedo N, Kanesaka T, et al. Long-term outcomes after endoscopic submucosal dissection for differentiated-type early gastric cancer that fulfilled expanded indication criteria: a prospective cohort study [published online ahead of print Jul 14, 2020]. J Gastroenterol Hepatol 2020. https://doi.org/10.1111/jgh.15182.
46. Lee S, Choi KD, Han M, et al. Long-term outcomes of endoscopic submucosal dissection versus surgery in early gastric cancer meeting expanded indication including undifferentiated-type tumors: a criteria-based analysis. Gastric Cancer 2018;21:490–9.
47. Kim SG, Ji SM, Lee NR, et al. Quality of life after endoscopic submucosal dissection for early gastric cancer: a prospective multicenter cohort study. Gut Liver 2017;11:87–92.
48. Yang HJ, Nam SY, Min BH, et al. Clinical outcomes of endoscopic resection for undifferentiated intramucosal early gastric cancer larger than 2 cm [published online ahead of print Aug 24, 2020]. Gastric Cancer 2020. https://doi.org/10.1007/s10120-020-01115-y.
49. Oda I, Gotoda T, Sasako M, et al. Treatment strategy after non-curative endoscopic resection of early gastric cancer. Br J Surg 2008;95:1495–500.

50. Kim ER, Lee H, Min BH, et al. Effect of rescue surgery after non-curative endoscopic resection of early gastric cancer. Br J Surg 2015;102:1394–401.
51. Yang HJ, Kim SG, Lim JH, et al. Predictors of lymph node metastasis in patients with non-curative endoscopic resection of early gastric cancer. Surg Endosc 2015;29:1145–55.
52. Toyokawa T, Ohira M, Tanaka H, et al. Optimal management for patients not meeting the inclusion criteria after endoscopic submucosal dissection for gastric cancer. Surg Endosc 2016;30:2404–14.
53. Kim SM, Min BH, Ahn JH, et al. Nomogram to predict lymph node metastasis in patients with early gastric cancer: a useful clinical tool to reduce gastrectomy after endoscopic resection. Endoscopy 2020;52:435–43.
54. Kawata N, Kakushima N, Takizawa K, et al. Risk factors for lymph node metastasis and long-term outcomes of patients with early gastric cancer after non-curative endoscopic submucosal dissection. Surg Endosc 2017;31:1607–16.
55. Toya Y, Endo M, Nakamura S, et al. Long-term outcomes and prognostic factors with non-curative endoscopic submucosal dissection for gastric cancer in elderly patients aged $\geq$ 75 years. Gastric Cancer 2019;22:838–44.
56. Sekiguchi M, Oda I, Suzuki H, et al. Clinical outcomes and prognostic factors in gastric cancer patients aged $\geq$85 years undergoing endoscopic submucosal dissection. Gastrointest Endosc 2017;85:963–72.
57. Abe N, Gotoda T, Hirasawa T, et al. Multicenter study of the long-term outcomes of endoscopic submucosal dissection for early gastric cancer in patients 80 years of age or older. Gastric Cancer 2012;15:70–5.
58. Han JP, Hong SJ, Kim HK, et al. Risk stratification and management of non-curative resection after endoscopic submucosal dissection for early gastric cancer. Surg Endosc 2016;30:184–9.
59. Choi JY, Jeon SW, Cho KB, et al. Non-curative endoscopic resection does not always lead to grave outcomes in submucosal invasive early gastric cancer. Surg Endosc 2015;29:1842–9.
60. Fujishiro M, Chiu PW, Wang HP. Role of antisecretory agents for gastric endoscopic submucosal dissection. Dig Endosc 2013;25(Suppl 1):86–93.
61. Jeon SW, Jung MK, Cho CM, et al. Predictors of immediate bleeding during endoscopic submucosal dissection in gastric lesions. Surg Endosc 2009;23:1974–9.
62. Muraki Y, Enomoto S, Iguchi M, et al. Management of bleeding and artificial gastric ulcers associated with endoscopic submucosal dissection. World J Gastrointest Endosc 2012;4:1–8.
63. Chung IK, Lee JH, Lee SH, et al. Therapeutic outcomes in 1000 cases of endoscopic submucosal dissection for early gastric neoplasms: Korean ESD Study Group multicenter study. Gastrointest Endosc 2009;69:1228–35.
64. Park YM, Cho E, Kang HY, et al. The effectiveness and safety of endoscopic submucosal dissection compared with endoscopic mucosal resection for early gastric cancer: a systematic review and metaanalysis. Surg Endosc 2011;25:2666–77.
65. So S, Ahn JY, Kim N, et al. Comparison of the effects of antithrombotic therapy on delayed bleeding after gastric endoscopic resection: a propensity score-matched case-control study. Gastrointest Endosc 2019;89:277–285 e2.
66. Choi YK, Ahn JY, Na HK, et al. Outcomes of endoscopic submucosal dissection for gastric epithelial neoplasm in chronic kidney disease patients: propensity score-matched case-control analysis. Gastric Cancer 2019;22:164–71.

67. Mukai S, Cho S, Kotachi T, et al. Analysis of delayed bleeding after endoscopic submucosal dissection for gastric epithelial neoplasms. Gastroenterol Res Pract 2012;2012:875323.
68. Choi YK, Ahn JY, Kim DH, et al. Efficacy and safety of endoscopic submucosal dissection for gastric neoplasms in patients with compensated liver cirrhosis: a propensity score-matched case-control study. Gastrointest Endosc 2018;87: 1423–14231 e3.
69. Tsuji Y, Ohata K, Ito T, et al. Risk factors for bleeding after endoscopic submucosal dissection for gastric lesions. World J Gastroenterol 2010;16:2913–7.
70. Takizawa K, Oda I, Gotoda T, et al. Routine coagulation of visible vessels may prevent delayed bleeding after endoscopic submucosal dissection–an analysis of risk factors. Endoscopy 2008;40:179–83.
71. Uedo N, Takeuchi Y, Yamada T, et al. Effect of a proton pump inhibitor or an H2-receptor antagonist on prevention of bleeding from ulcer after endoscopic submucosal dissection of early gastric cancer: a prospective randomized controlled trial. Am J Gastroenterol 2007;102:1610–6.
72. Ye BD, Cheon JH, Choi KD, et al. Omeprazole may be superior to famotidine in the management of iatrogenic ulcer after endoscopic mucosal resection: a prospective randomized controlled trial. Aliment Pharmacol Ther 2006;24:837–43.
73. Park CH, Park JC, Lee H, et al. Second-look endoscopy after gastric endoscopic submucosal dissection for reducing delayed postoperative bleeding. Gut Liver 2015;9:43–51.
74. Na S, Ahn JY, Choi KD, et al. Delayed bleeding rate according to the Forrest classification in second-look endoscopy after endoscopic submucosal dissection. Dig Dis Sci 2015;60:3108–17.
75. Koh R, Hirasawa K, Yahara S, et al. Antithrombotic drugs are risk factors for delayed postoperative bleeding after endoscopic submucosal dissection for gastric neoplasms. Gastrointest Endosc 2013;78:476–83.
76. Ohta T, Ishihara R, Uedo N, et al. Factors predicting perforation during endoscopic submucosal dissection for gastric cancer. Gastrointest Endosc 2012;75: 1159–65.
77. Yoo JH, Shin SJ, Lee KM, et al. Risk factors for perforations associated with endoscopic submucosal dissection in gastric lesions: emphasis on perforation type. Surg Endosc 2012;26:2456–64.
78. Yano T, Tanabe S, Ishido K, et al. Delayed perforation after endoscopic submucosal dissection for early gastric cancer: clinical features and treatment. World J Gastrointest Endosc 2016;8:368–73.
79. Jeon SW, Jung MK, Kim SK, et al. Clinical outcomes for perforations during endoscopic submucosal dissection in patients with gastric lesions. Surg Endosc 2010; 24:911–6.
80. Kang SH, Lee K, Lee HW, et al. Delayed perforation occurring after endoscopic submucosal dissection for early gastric cancer. Clin Endosc 2015;48:251–5.
81. Suzuki H, Oda I, Sekiguchi M, et al. Management and associated factors of delayed perforation after gastric endoscopic submucosal dissection. World J Gastroenterol 2015;21:12635–43.
82. Coda S, Oda I, Gotoda T, et al. Risk factors for cardiac and pyloric stenosis after endoscopic submucosal dissection, and efficacy of endoscopic balloon dilation treatment. Endoscopy 2009;41:421–6.
83. Oda I, Suzuki H, Nonaka S, et al. Complications of gastric endoscopic submucosal dissection. Dig Endosc 2013;25(Suppl 1):71–8.

84. Nishiyama N, Mori H, Kobara H, et al. Novel method to prevent gastric antral strictures after endoscopic submucosal dissection: using triamcinolone. World J Gastroenterol 2014;20:11910–5.
85. Na HK, Choi KD, Ahn JY, et al. Outcomes of balloon dilation for the treatment of strictures after endoscopic submucosal dissection compared with peptic strictures. Surg Endosc 2013;27:3237–46.
86. Kusunoki M, Miyake K, Shindo T, et al. The incidence of deep vein thrombosis in Japanese patients undergoing endoscopic submucosal dissection. Gastrointest Endosc 2011;74:798–804.
87. Gong EJ, Kim DH, Jung HY, et al. Pneumonia after endoscopic resection for gastric neoplasm. Dig Dis Sci 2014;59:2742–8.

Surgical Treatment for Gastric Cancer

Ian Solsky[a], Haejin In, MD, MPH, MBA[a,b,c,*]

KEYWORDS

• Gastric cancer • Gastrectomy • Lymphadenectomy • Staging laparoscopy

KEY POINTS

- Staging laparoscopy is an important modality for patients with gastric cancer with stages T1b or greater to evaluate for peritoneal spread when chemoradiation or surgery is considered.
- The appropriate surgical procedure for gastric cancer is based on the lesion's location: subtotal gastrectomy is generally the procedure of choice for distal tumors, whereas total gastrectomy is generally performed for proximal lesions in the upper third of the stomach.
- D2 lymphadenectomy is now supported as a critical part of a curative intent resection given that gastric cancer spreads through lymphatics to regional lymph nodes.

Video content accompanies this article at http://www.giendo.theclinics.com.

INTRODUCTION

Regionality is an important theme when it comes to the surgical management of gastric cancer. Not only does the location of gastric cancer and its extent of spread dictate the operative plan but also, historically, the management of gastric cancer is often thought of in terms of "Eastern versus Western" approaches. Incidence rates in Eastern Asia are significantly higher than they are in North America.[1] The greater experience in treating gastric cancer in Asian institutions has led to differing management practices in terms of screening and prevention as well as in treatment.[2] In terms of surgical management, Eastern surgeons have been pioneers and proponents of minimally invasive techniques and more extensive lymph node dissections, which have been controversial in Western institutions but are now being performed with greater frequency. Despite some ongoing debate about the details of gastric cancer management, what is agreed on is that surgery is an essential component of

[a] Department of Surgery, Montefiore Medical Center, Albert Einstein College of Medicine, 1300 Morris Park Avenue Block Building #112, New York, NY 10461, USA; [b] Department of Surgery, Albert Einstein College of Medicine, New York, NY, USA; [c] Department of Epidemiology and Population Health, Albert Einstein College of Medicine, New York, NY, USA
* Corresponding author. Department of Surgery, Montefiore Medical Center, Albert Einstein College of Medicine, 1300 Morris Park Avenue #112, New York, NY 10461.
E-mail address: hin@montefiore.org

Gastrointest Endoscopy Clin N Am 31 (2021) 581–605
https://doi.org/10.1016/j.giec.2021.04.001
giendo.theclinics.com

curative-intent treatment strategies. However, the care of each patient with gastric cancer must be individualized and may require additional neoadjuvant or adjuvant therapies, such as chemotherapy or radiation therapy. With the ongoing development of new therapeutics, such as immunotherapy, and technologies, such as robotic surgery, the future of gastric cancer care will continue to evolve and require the coordinated teamwork of physicians with different medical and surgical expertise to optimize patient outcomes. It is important that all physicians who will be caring for patients with gastric cancer understand the current best practices of surgical management to provide patients with the highest quality of care. This article aims to provide this information while acknowledging areas of surgical management that are still controversial.

STAGING LAPAROSCOPY AS PART OF THE STAGING EVALUATION

Conventional staging for gastric cancer usually includes a physical examination, a computed tomographic (CT) scan of the chest/abdomen/pelvis, and an endoscopic ultrasound, which is performed in accordance with the TNM staging system of the combined American Joint Committee on Cancer/Union for International Cancer Control (**Table 1**).[3] Per National Comprehensive Cancer Network (NCCN) guidelines, the performance of a staging laparoscopy with peritoneal washings is also indicated for clinical stages ≥T1b to evaluate for peritoneal spread when chemoradiation or surgery is considered.[4] Many experts follow these guidelines and support its use for locally advanced disease and for patients being considered for neoadjuvant therapy but not for those with early-stage disease.[5] A staging laparoscopy is performed to directly visualize the liver surface, peritoneum, and lymph nodes while allowing for the biopsy of any worrisome lesions and the collection of peritoneal fluid for cytologic analysis. Staging laparoscopy, with reported sensitivity of 86% and specificity of 100%, is superior to radiographic studies for detecting metastatic disease and may detect radiographically occult disease that can alter management in approximately 9% to greater than 50% of patients with only localized disease on imaging.[6–9] If metastatic disease is identified, a patient may be spared from the performance of an unnecessary laparotomy, which has a morbidity of 13% to 23% and a mortality of 10% to 21%, whereas staging laparoscopy has a morbidity of 0% to 2.5% and no reported mortality.[7,10–13] During laparoscopy, peritoneal fluid can be collected and sent for cytology, which if positive, upstages a patient to stage IV disease and is a poor prognostic sign predictive of disease recurrence.[9,14] Studies are ongoing to further delineate the role of surgery and neoadjuvant strategies for individuals with positive cytology.[15,16]

When a patient is selected to undergo staging laparoscopy, it can be performed as a one- or a 2-stage approach. In a one-stage approach, the staging laparoscopy is performed concurrently at the same time as the planned surgical resection. In a 2-stage approach, the staging laparoscopy is the only procedure performed to be followed at a later date by a separate surgical resection if no metastatic disease is identified during the staging laparoscopy. The advantage of the one-stage approach is that it involves only 1 procedure and 1 anesthetic exposure. However, the disadvantage is that it can add additional time and complexity to the case if there is uncertainty with a frozen section biopsy or if there is a need for final pathology to confirm a worrisome finding. It is also not possible to have cytology examined during a one-stage procedure. The advantage of performing the staging laparoscopy separately in a 2-stage approach is that it may identify patients who are more suited for a neoadjuvant approach. Although a 2-stage approach requires the patient to be exposed a second time to anesthesia for a definitive cancer operation, it is a more robust approach for ensuring

Table 1
Eighth American Joint Committee on Cancer staging system for gastric adenocarcinoma

Primary tumor	TX	Primary tumor cannot be assessed		
	T0	No evidence of primary tumor		
	Tis	Carcinoma in situ: intraepithelial tumor without invasion of the lamina propria, high-grade dysplasia		
	T1	Tumor invades the lamina propria, muscularis mucosae, or submucosa		
	T1a	Tumor invades the lamina propria or muscularis mucosae		
	T1b	Tumor invades the submucosa		
	T2	Tumor invades the muscularis propria		
	T3	Tumor penetrates the subserosal connective tissue without invasion of the visceral peritoneum or adjacent structures		
	T4	Tumor invades the serosa (visceral peritoneum) or adjacent structures		
	T4a	Tumor invades the serosa (visceral peritoneum)		
	T4b	Tumor invades adjacent structures/organs		
Regional nodes	NX	Regional lymph nodes cannot be assessed		
	N0	No regional lymph node metastasis		
	N1	Metastasis in 1 or 2 regional lymph nodes		
	N2	Metastasis in 3 to 6 regional lymph nodes		
	N3	Metastasis in 7 or more regional lymph nodes		
	N3a	Metastasis in 7 to 15 regional lymph nodes		
	N3b	Metastasis in 16 or more regional lymph nodes		
Metastases	M0	No distant metastasis		
	M1	Distant metastasis		
Stage groupings (pathologic)	0	TisN0M0	IIIB	T1N3bM0
	IA	T1N0M0		T2N3bM0
	IB	T1N1M0		T3N3aM0
		T2N0M0		T4aN3aM0
	IIA	T1N2M0		T4bN1M0
		T2N1M0		T4bN2M0
		T3N0M0	IIIC	T3N3bM0
	IIB	T1N3aM0		T4aN3bM0
		T2N2M0		T4bN3aM0
		T3N1M0		T4bN3bM0
		T4aN0M0	IV	Any T, any N, M1
	IIIA	T2N3aM0		
		T3N2M0		
		T4aN1M0		
		T4aN2M0		
		T4bN0M0		

From Cameron J and Cameron A 2019. Current surgical therapy. 13th edition. p.102.

accurate staging. As the role of staging laparoscopy continues to be defined, it remains underused in the United States: 1 study suggested that it was only performed in 8% of older patients with gastric cancer.[17]

The uptake is likely higher at major cancer centers, where staging laparoscopy is acknowledged as an important aspect of accurate staging.[18] As further research elucidates the value of neoadjuvant approaches and as more surgeons learn of its utility, there may be a greater uptake of staging laparoscopy to rule out metastatic disease and to obtain cytology to guide specific therapy (Video 1).

SURGICAL APPROACH

Anatomy

Knowledge of the surgical anatomy of the stomach is important not only for the technical performance of gastric cancer surgery but also to help all providers understand the physiologic changes that may be seen in patients after gastrectomy. **Fig. 1** shows the important anatomic structures and the relevant blood supply. Located in the left upper quadrant of the abdomen, the stomach is adjacent to many important structures, including the left lateral lobe of the liver, the transverse colon, omentum, pancreas, spleen, left kidney, left adrenal gland, and the diaphragm. The stomach can be divided into 5 anatomic sections based on histology and function: (1) cardia and gastroesophageal junction, (2) fundus, (3) body, (4) antrum, and (5) pylorus. The cardia, the proximal stomach next to the lower esophageal sphincter, contains mucus and endocrine cells. The fundus, adjacent to and rising above the cardiac opening, contains parietal cells, chief cells, endocrine cells, and mucus cells. The body, between the fundus and antrum, contains cells similar to the fundus. The antrum, the distal stomach separated from the body by the angular incisura, contains pyloric glands, endocrine cells, mucus cells, and G cells. The pyloric sphincter, a muscular valve separating the antrum from the duodenum, contains mucus cells and endocrine cells. The lesser curve of the stomach is supplied by the left and right gastric arteries, which branch off the celiac and common hepatic arteries, respectively. The greater curvature is supplied by the right and left gastroepiploic arteries, which arise from the gastroduodenal and splenic arteries, respectively. The fundus of the stomach is supplied by the short gastric arteries, which also come off the splenic artery. Veins parallel the arterial supply.[19,20] The lymph node stations of the stomach have been defined by the Japanese Research Society for the Study of Gastric Cancer and are grouped into 16 stations according to location: 1 to 6 are perigastric and the others are adjacent to major blood vessels, along the aorta, or behind the pancreas.[21] **Table 2** contains description of the lymph node stations.

Indicators of Resectability

Resection offers patients with gastric cancer the best chance for cure, but patients must be appropriately referred for what can be a major procedure. Patients being considered for resection must not have severe comorbidities that would prevent the safe receipt of anesthesia. A gastric cancer is generally considered unresectable if there are distant metastases, invasion of major vasculature such as the aorta, or encasement of the hepatic artery or celiac axis. Involvement of the distal splenic artery

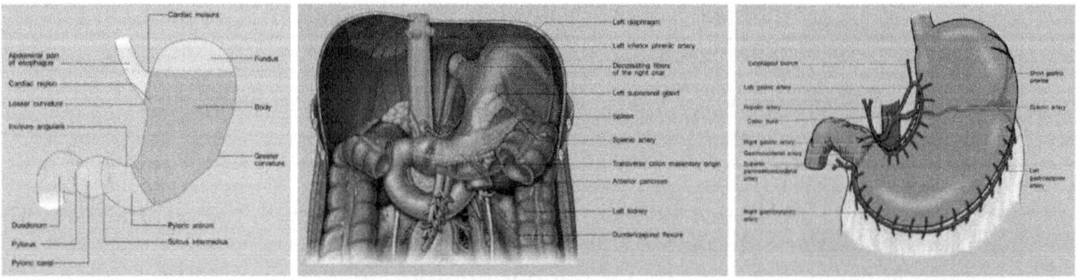

The borders and regions of the stomach — Posterior topographical relations of the stomach — Arterial supply of the stomach

Fig. 1. Stomach anatomy and vasculature. (*From* Vishy Mahadevan, Anatomy of the stomach, Surgery (Oxford), Volume 35, Issue 11, 2017, Pages 608-611, ISSN 0263-9319, https://doi.org/10.1016/j.mpsur.2017.08.004. Accessed via https://www.sciencedirect.com/science/article/pii/S0263931917301850.)

Table 2
Anatomic definitions of lymph node stations

No.	Definition
1	Right paracardial lymph nodes (LNs), including those along the first branch of the ascending limb of the left gastric artery
2	Left paracardial LNs, including those along the esophagocardiac branch of the left subphrenic artery
3a	Lesser curvature LNs along the branches of the left gastric artery
3b	Lesser curvature LNs along the 2nd branch and distal part of the right gastric artery
4sa	Left greater curvature LNs along the short gastric arteries (perigastric area)
4sb	Left greater curvature LNs along the left gastroepiploic artery (perigastric area)
4d	Right greater curvature LNs along the 2nd branch and distal part of the right gastroepiploic artery
5	Suprapyloric LNs along the 1st branch and proximal part of the right gastric artery
6	Infrapyloric LNs along the first branch and proximal part of the right gastroepiploic artery down to the confluence of the right gastroepiploic vein and the anterior superior pancreatoduodenal vein
7	LNs along the trunk of left gastric artery between its root and the origin of its ascending branch
8a	Anterosuperior LNs along the common hepatic artery
8p	Posterior LNs along the common hepatic artery
9	Celiac artery LNs
10	Splenic hilar LNs, including those adjacent to the splenic artery distal to the pancreatic tail, and those on the roots of the short gastric arteries and those along the left gastroepiploic artery proximal to its 1st gastric branch
11p	Proximal splenic artery LNs from its origin to halfway between its origin and the pancreatic tail end
11d	Distal splenic artery LNs from halfway between its origin and the pancreatic tail end to the end of the pancreatic tail
12a	Hepatoduodenal ligament LNs along the proper hepatic artery, in the caudal half between the confluence of the right and left hepatic ducts and the upper border of the pancreas
12b	Hepatoduodenal ligament LNs along the bile duct, in the caudal half between the confluence of the right and left hepatic ducts and the upper border of the pancreas
12p	Hepatoduodenal ligament LNs along the portal vein in the caudal half between the confluence of the right and left hepatic ducts and the upper border of the pancreas
13	LNs on the posterior surface of the pancreatic head cranial to the duodenal papilla
14v	LNs along the superior mesenteric vein
15	LNs along the middle colic vessels
16a1	Paraaortic LNs in the diaphragmatic aortic hiatus
16a2	Paraaortic LNs between the upper margin of the origin of the celiac artery and the lower border of the left renal vein

(*continued on next page*)

Table 2
(*continued*)

No.	Definition
16b1	Paraaortic LNs between the lower border of the left renal vein and the upper border of the origin of the inferior mesenteric artery
16b2	Paraaortic LNs between the upper border of the origin of the inferior mesenteric artery and the aortic bifurcation
17	LNs on the anterior surface of the pancreatic head beneath the pancreatic sheath
18	LNs along the inferior border of the pancreatic body
19	Infradiaphragmatic LNs predominantly along the subphrenic artery
20	Paraesophageal LNs in the diaphragmatic esophageal hiatus
110	Paraesophageal LNs in the lower thorax
111	Supradiaphragmatic LNs separate from the esophagus
112	Posterior mediastinal LNs separate fro

Adapted from Japanese Gastric Cancer Association. Japanese classification of gastric carcinoma: 3rd English edition. Gastric Cancer 14, 101–112 (2011). https://doi.org/10.1007/s10120-011-0041-5.

is not a contraindication to resection, as the vessel can be taken en bloc along with the stomach, spleen, and distal pancreas. The presence of bulky lymph nodes in the aortocaval region, mediastinum, or the porta hepatis is considered distant disease and is classified as stage IV.[6] Concerning linitis plastica, extensive tumor infiltration of the stomach resulting in a rigid thickened stomach, which is associated with poor prognosis, there is some controversy as to whether this should be considered resectable or not; however, in the era of neoadjuvant therapy, many surgeons would elect to proceed with resection if negative margins can be obtained.[22–24] Of note, although patients with metastatic gastric cancer generally are not eligible for curative surgery, this does not mean that these patients are excluded from surgical treatments, which may be of benefit to some patients with complications, such as obstruction, bleeding, or perforation (see later section on Palliative Interventions).

Preoperative Planning

The decision to pursue gastric cancer resection should occur with consultation of a multidisciplinary tumor board to ensure that an appropriate multimodality treatment strategy is planned. In the United States, neoadjuvant therapy is advocated by NCCN guidelines and is increasingly pursued before surgical resection.[4] Furthermore, given that most resections will be performed under elective situations, it is critical for patients to undergo preoperative medical assessments, as most of these patients are older and present with comorbidities.[25] As part of the workup, genetic counseling may be indicated in cases whereby any genetic syndrome, such as hereditary diffuse gastric cancer, familial adenomatous polyposis, or Peutz-Jeghers, is suspected.[26] During the consent process for surgery, patients should be made aware not only of the risks of surgery and its complications but also of complications related to anesthesia, the possibility of a prolonged intensive care unit course, and the potential need for additional therapies, such as chemotherapy or radiation depending on the surgical pathology.[27] Before surgery, some surgeons will give patients a mechanical bowel preparation or antibiotics for oral enteral decontamination, but there currently are not enough data to support these practices as routine.[28,29] At the time of surgery, patients will receive antibiotic and venous thromboembolism prophylaxis.

Total versus Partial Gastrectomy

Although endoscopic resection is proving to be a promising technique for early cancers, surgical gastrectomy remains the most frequently performed procedure for the treatment of invasive gastric cancer. Currently, there are 2 main approaches that can be used based on the gastric cancer's location and characteristics: total gastrectomy and partial gastrectomy, which is a broad term referring to any procedure not removing the entire stomach (**Fig. 2**). It is important to note that these procedures are sometimes performed for reasons outside of gastric cancer. However, in the setting of gastric cancer, they must be performed adhering to oncologic principles, including attention to surgical margins and appropriate lymph node dissection. As such, for gastric adenocarcinoma in the distal stomach, smaller resections, such as wedge resections or distal gastrectomy, generally are not appropriate, as they do not allow for adequate lymphadenectomy.[6] Subtotal gastrectomy, in which only the fundus of the stomach is retained, is required to ensure the lymph nodes of the lesser curvature are fully removed, and only well-vascularized viable stomach is remaining because the ligation of the left gastric artery is required for a proper lymph node dissection. Total gastrectomy, the removal of the entire stomach, is generally performed for proximal lesions in the upper third of the stomach. Although proximal gastric cancers can technically be approached with either a total gastrectomy or a proximal partial gastrectomy, total gastrectomy is currently preferred because it is associated with a much lower rate of reflux esophagitis when performed with a Roux-en-Y reconstruction (2% vs >30%), a more complete lymph node dissection, and fewer complications.[30,31] However, the preference for total over proximal partial gastrectomy is based on older data, and there are ongoing studies to further evaluate these approaches (randomized clinical trial ongoing, KLASS 05 trial).[32] Regarding distal tumors, the literature has shown that there is no added survival benefit for total gastrectomy compared with subtotal gastrectomy, which is why the latter less aggressive approach is preferred.[33,34] In some cases of local invasion, the removal of adjacent organs may also be needed in order to perform a curative intent procedure.

The general surgical steps involved in partial or total gastrectomy include the following (Video 2):

1. Mobilization of the greater curvature with division of the left gastroepiploic. The short gastric vessels are also divided for total gastrectomy, and omentectomy is considered for advanced cancers.[35]
2. Infrapyloric mobilization with ligation of the right gastroepiploic vessels

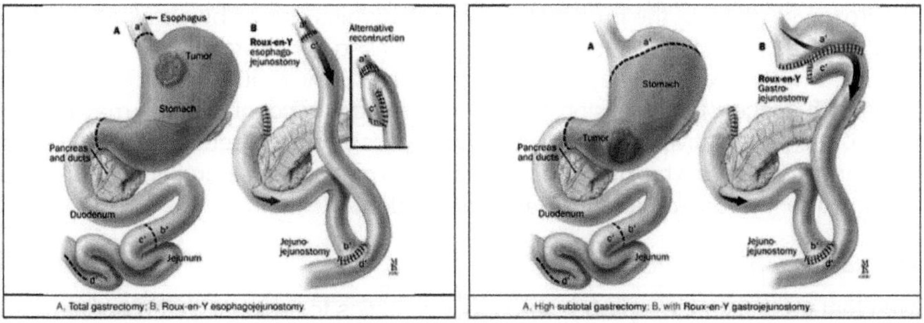

Fig. 2. Total versus subtotal gastrectomy. (Illustrations by Michael Linkinhoker © 2013 Johns Hopkins University. All rights reserved)

3. Suprapyloric mobilization with ligation of the right gastric vessels
4. Duodenal transection
5. D2 or D1+ lymphadenectomy, with dissection of the porta hepatis, common hepatic artery, left gastric artery, celiac axis, and splenic artery, and ligation of left gastric vessels (based on location)
6. Gastric (or esophageal) transection
7. Reconstruction by loop or Roux-en-Y gastrojejunostomy (or Roux-en-Y esophagojejunostomy)[36]

When preparing patients for total gastrectomy, it is important to prepare and drape the chest in addition to the abdomen because of the possibility of needing to perform a thoracotomy to obtain a clear proximal margin. For both procedures, intraoperative frozen sections are generally performed to ensure that the cancer is fully removed. Regarding partial gastrectomy, there are some variations developed by the Japanese that are sometimes performed to limit postoperative syndromes that result from altered gastric anatomy and physiology (see later discussion under Complications).[37–40] Function-preserving techniques include those that preserve the pylorus (pylorus-preserving segmental gastrectomy) and those that preserve the distal named branches of the vagus nerves.[37–40] These techniques are not widely described in North American literature.

Optimal Surgical Margin

The goal of gastric resection for adenocarcinoma is to obtain a tumor-free resection margin (R0) on pathologic examination because positive margins have been associated with worse outcomes.[41] Another consideration is that gastric cancer has a tendency for intramural spread.[42] Although it was previously thought that a gross margin of at least 5 cm was needed to obtain an R0 resection, this was based on older data, and thus, there is ongoing debate as to the optimal margin, particularly in light of increased use of neoadjuvant chemotherapy before resection.[6] NCCN guidelines previously endorsed obtaining a margin ≥4 cm from the gross tumor, but now they simply recommend "adequate gastric resection to achieve negative microscopic margins."[4] Although there are no randomized data to guide margin management, retrospective studies have been performed and have suggested obtaining margins ranging from 2 to 6 cm.[43,44] The 2018 Japanese Gastric Cancer Treatment Guidelines recommend a gross resection margin of 2 cm for T1 tumors, 3 cm margin for T2 or deeper tumors with an expansive growth pattern, and 5 cm for T2 or deeper tumors with an infiltrative growth pattern.[45] Ultimately, the operating surgeon must determine the appropriate margin considering whether the risk of morbidity from further resection outweighs the potential oncologic benefit. To identify whether the margin is adequate, intraoperative frozen sections of the proximal and distal margins should be obtained in all patients undergoing potentially curative surgery. Based on the results of these frozen sections, a wider excision may be necessary, as improved outcomes have been reported with successful reexcision.[46] However, experts recognize that it may be difficult to obtain a negative margin even with successive frozen sections.[47] There is no gold standard of care when it comes to positive frozen section margins, and management is currently surgeon and institution dependent.

Extent of Lymph Node Dissection

Given that gastric cancer spreads through lymphatics to regional lymph nodes, curative intent resections must focus on adequate control of the lymph nodes for staging, minimizing recurrence, and improving overall survival. The 16 lymph node stations defined by the Japanese Research Society for the Study of Gastric Cancer have been grouped into a broader classification scheme that is used to describe the extent of lymph node dissection based on the nodal stations to be removed. The extent of lymphadenectomy is categorized into D1, D1+, D2, or D3, ranging from the minimal required lymph nodes to a more extensive lymph node dissection. A D3 lymphadenectomy is referred to as a superextended lymphadenectomy and includes a D2 lymphadenectomy plus the removal of nodes within the root of mesentery and periaortic regions (stations 1–16). The nodal stations that make up each lymph node removal degree are defined by the type of gastrectomy conducted, which is in turn driven by the location of the tumor (**Fig. 3**).[6,45]

The extent of lymph node dissection (D1 vs D2 vs D3) needed during a gastric cancer resection has been a topic of controversy. In Eastern countries, D2 lymphadenectomy is considered standard of care. Western institutions have also started to adopt

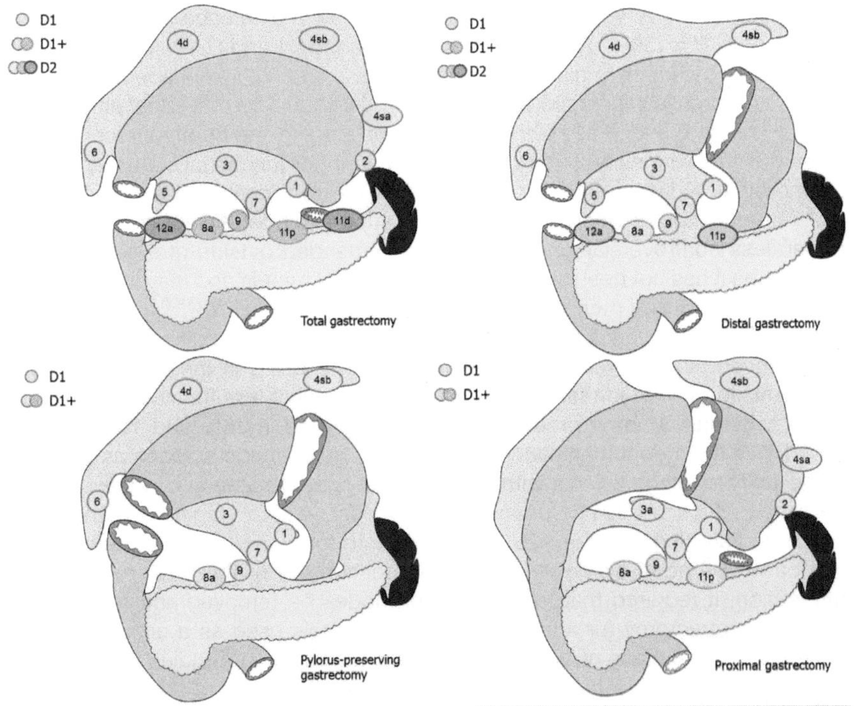

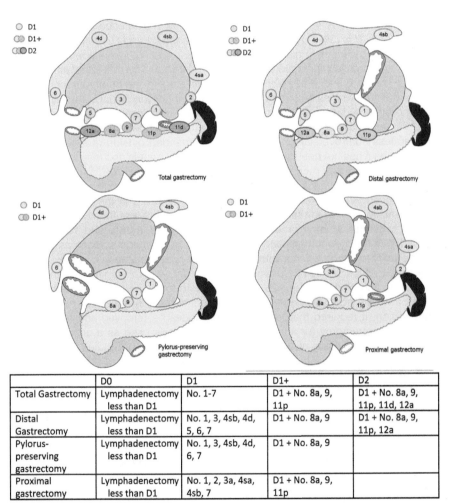

	D0	D1	D1+	D2
Total Gastrectomy	Lymphadenectomy less than D1	No. 1-7	D1 + No. 8a, 9, 11p	D1 + No. 8a, 9, 11p, 11d, 12a
Distal Gastrectomy	Lymphadenectomy less than D1	No. 1, 3, 4sb, 4d, 5, 6, 7	D1 + No. 8a, 9	D1 + No. 8a, 9, 11p, 12a
Pylorus-preserving gastrectomy	Lymphadenectomy less than D1	No. 1, 3, 4sb, 4d, 6, 7	D1 + No. 8a, 9	
Proximal gastrectomy	Lymphadenectomy less than D1	No. 1, 2, 3a, 4sa, 4sb, 7	D1 + No. 8a, 9, 11p	

Fig. 3. Lymph node stations. (*From* Japanese Gastric Cancer Association. Japanese gastric cancer treatment guidelines 2018, 5th edition. Gastric Cancer 24, 1–21 (2021). https://doi.org/10.1007/s10120-020-01042-y.)

the recommendation that a D2 lymphadenectomy be performed. Current treatment guidelines published by the NCCN, Cancer Care Ontario, and the European Society of Surgical Oncology support the performance of a D2 lymph node dissection and acknowledge that it is preferred over a D1 dissection when it can be safely performed.[4,48,49] Western institutions were slow adopters of the D2 dissection largely because of the initial outcomes of 2 Western trials—the Dutch Gastric Cancer Group Trial and the British Cooperative trial conducted by the Medical Research Council trial—which showed that there was no improvement in overall survival with D2 as compared with D1 lymph node dissection, but there was increased morbidity.[50,51] However, these trials were criticized for including institutions lacking expertise in performing D2 dissection as well as for incorporating routine splenectomy and distal pancreatectomy as part of their procedures, which were thought to have impacted the outcomes. Furthermore, 15-year data from the Dutch trial showed that a D2 lymph node dissection as compared with a D1 dissection was associated with lower local recurrence (12% vs 22%), regional recurrence (13 vs 19%), and gastric cancer–related deaths (37% vs 48%) while still failing to show a difference in overall survival (21% and 29%, $P = .34$).[52] A meta-analysis comparing D1 and D2 lymphadenectomy showed an improvement in disease-specific survival after D2 lymphadenectomy, but there was an increase in postoperative mortality.[53] It should be noted that although D2 is generally recommended as standard for optimal staging and treatment for most patients, in patients with early tumors, advanced age, poor functional status, and multiple comorbidities, D1 or D1+ dissections can be considered on a case-by-case basis.[6] The question of whether to perform a superextended D3 lymphadenectomy has been less controversial, and it is not recommended outside of a select subset of patients, as it has not been shown to have a survival benefit and may increase perioperative morbidity and mortality given its aggressive approach.[53–55]

Although D2 dissection is now supported by major institutions like the NCCN, this does not mean that this recommendation is being followed in the United States. A US randomized trial noted that 54% of patients underwent less than a D1 lymphadenectomy, whereas D1 or ≥ procedures were performed in 36% and 10%, respectively.[56] Difficulty in documentation of removal by lymph node stations as well as a desire to unify staging systems with other cancer sites resulted in changes to the N stage of the American Joint Committee on Cancer (AJCC) staging system, which was changed starting with the AJCC fifth edition to follow a numeric system instead of one based on node distance from tumor location. As of the most recent AJCC eighth edition, it required that least 16 lymph nodes be removed and examined at the time of gastrectomy for adequate staging, which is used as a quality metric in the United States in place of documentation of D2 dissection. Studies using number of lymph nodes examined have similarly shown the inadequacy of US lymphadenectomies reporting that less than one-third of US patients had 15 or more lymph nodes removed during their procedures as was the recommendation in the AJCC fifth through seventh editions.[57,58]

Failure to perform an adequate lymphadenectomy may not simply be due to a difference in philosophy, but it may also be that Western surgeons have not been adequately trained how to do this complex procedure and may not be comfortable performing it. The technical demands of performing a D2 lymphadenectomy are well documented, and the literature points to a steep learning curve. Although Western surgeons have reported the feasibility of performing this technique with good outcomes, they have also acknowledged the importance of having these procedures performed in specialized centers by individuals who have been adequately supervised during the steep learning curve.[59,60] In 1 study from Korea, it was reported that the learning curve for gastric cancer survival did not plateau until after a surgeon had performed 100 operations.[61]

Thus, even though D2 dissection is now supported by Western institutions, training will be required for surgeons to be proficient at this technique. Until that time, these procedures should be performed at selected centers with surgeons with expertise in performing this procedure, which is supported by a meta-analysis that shows the relationship of outcomes after gastric cancer surgery with hospital and surgeon factors.[62] Although there is still significant work that needs to be done in the West to improve rates of D2 dissections, in the future, there may be other advancements in the management of regional lymph nodes that will also have to be adopted. There is growing interest in the use of sentinel lymph node biopsies for patients with early gastric cancer as has been done for other types of cancer; however, this technique has not been refined enough yet, and the data cannot yet support its use.[63–67]

Reconstructive Options

After a partial or total gastrectomy, it is necessary to reconstruct the gastrointestinal (GI) tract. Different procedures have been devised to preserve duodenal continuity, important for preventing loss of fat-soluble vitamins, and jejunal continuity, important for preventing retrograde flow of jejunal contents that can occur when there is disruption in electrical activity initiated by the duodenal pacemaker.[68] Some procedures also include the construction of a gastric pouch to serve as a functional reservoir after gastrectomy. These different reconstructions have been devised to try to limit the effects of postgastrectomy syndromes, but each generally has some degree of early or late dumping because the pylorus is typically removed (see Complications in later discussion).

After a partial gastrectomy, the most common reconstructive procedures are the Billroth and Roux-en-Y reconstructions (**Fig. 4**). The Billroth I reconstruction anastomoses the remnant stomach to the duodenal stump in a primary end-to-end fashion, which in turn preserves duodenal and jejunal continuity. This procedure, which requires a tension-free anastomosis, is not feasible after subtotal gastrectomy or total gastrectomy, which is commonly required for adequate tumor resection. The Billroth II reconstruction anastomoses the remnant stomach to the proximal jejunum in an end-to-side fashion, which preserves jejunal but not duodenal continuity. Gastritis and dumping can be seen after this reconstruction, and it also tends to have some degree of malabsorption of fat-soluble vitamins because of the loss of duodenal continuity. The Roux-en-Y reconstruction anastomoses the remnant stomach to an

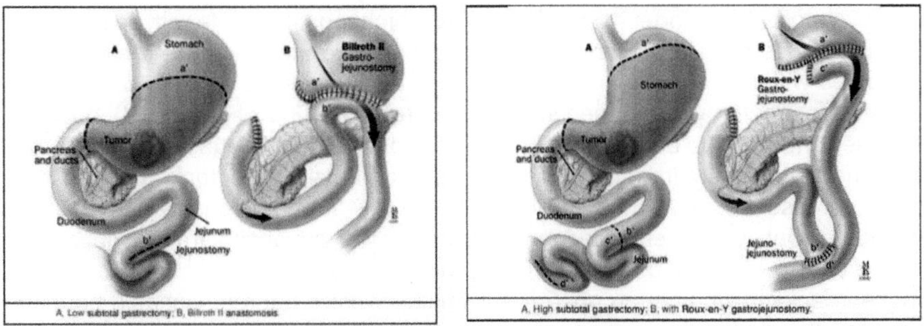

Fig. 4. Reconstruction options. (Illustrations by Michael Linkinhoker © 2013 Johns Hopkins University. All rights reserved.)

isoperistaltic roux limb of jejunum, whereas the proximal jejunum is anastomosed to the distal roux limb in an end-to-side fashion; it is performed to divert the bilious drainage away from the gastric remnant. The Roux-en-Y reconstruction results in less reflux than in the Billroth reconstructions, but it can lead to gastric atony along with the adverse effects of jejunal transection, which contributes to the "Roux syndrome" in which patients develop abdominal pain and vomiting.[6,36] Although the patient's anatomy and surgeon preference often dictate the type of reconstruction that is performed, randomized trials seem to suggest that the Roux-en-Y reconstruction is better tolerated overall and is associated with an improved quality of life compared with the Billroth reconstructions.[69–71]

After a total gastrectomy, GI continuity can be restored with either a Roux-en-Y reconstruction or a bowel interposition technique (jejunal or colon interposition). For a Roux-en-Y approach, a surgeon may elect to perform a straight esophagojejunal anastomosis, a looped esophagojejunal anastomosis, or a jejunal pouch construction, which can be brought behind the colon (Hunt) or in front of the colon (Rodino).[72] The most prevalent reconstruction strategy and the one that is generally recommended is the Roux-en-Y reconstruction.[73,74] Despite some limited data, the literature also seems to favor a jejunal pouch reconstruction, especially in patients who are anticipated to have a longer survival, as it has been associated with better functional outcomes and improved quality of life.[6,75–80]

ADDITIONAL TECHNICAL CONSIDERATIONS

Minimally Invasive Techniques

Like all of surgery, gastric cancer surgery is trending toward the development of more minimally invasive approaches. In addition to endoscopic techniques as described previously, there are also laparoscopic and robotic approaches to gastrectomy, which are gaining in popularity. Like most of gastric surgery, advances are primarily reported in literature from Eastern institutions, but the benefits of these approaches are starting to find their way into the practices and literature of Western institutions. Although an open approach is still widely performed around the world, laparoscopic gastric resection when performed in experienced centers has been associated with a faster recovery with less pain and fewer complications while allowing for comparable lymph node retrieval.[81–84] Laparoscopic gastrectomy is a well-established technique for treating gastric cancer in Eastern countries and, in 2009, accounted for approximately one-quarter of all gastric surgeries performed for cancer in Japan and South Korea.[85] Many Eastern studies have been performed that show the benefit of a laparoscopic technique to early gastric cancer[81,83,86–89] and locally advanced gastric cancer.[82,90–94] A 2016 meta-analysis concluded that laparoscopic gastrectomy resulted in less postoperative morbidity, shorter hospitalization, and higher quality of life with no difference in lymph nodes retrieved, mortality, cancer recurrence, and disease-free survival.[95] Compared with Eastern countries, Western countries have less experience with laparoscopic gastrectomy (performed in approximately 8%–23% of cases[96,97]), but it has also been shown to be beneficial in Western cohorts.[97–99] Although most of the aforementioned studies are in regards to laparoscopic partial gastrectomy, total gastrectomy can also be performed minimally invasively. It is a technically demanding procedure, but when performed by a surgeon with advanced training in a high-volume center, short- and longer-term outcomes are satisfactory.[100–102]

When deciding whether an open or minimally invasive approach should be taken, ultimately the choice depends on several provider and patient factors. Laparoscopic gastrectomy is a technically demanding procedure, especially when a D2 lymphadenectomy and GI reconstruction are also performed, which requires an experienced surgeon who can be supported by staff and hospital resources to assist not only intraoperatively but also in postoperative management. Studies suggest that 40 to 100 cases must be performed for a surgeon to be proficient in this technique.[103–106] Regarding patient factors, the ideal patient is one with early gastric cancer who does not have significant cardiopulmonary comorbidities, obesity, or previous upper abdominal surgery, which may complicate a patient's ability to receive pneumoperitoneum and to have a safe dissection without encountering extensive intra-abdominal adhesions. In addition, many bulky gastric cancers with local invasion into other organs may not be best suited for a laparoscopic procedure. All these factors have to be taken into consideration when deciding what type of surgery should be performed, but the presence of these factors do not necessarily exclude a patient from a minimally invasive approach.

Although Western countries are still catching up to their Eastern colleagues in terms of laparoscopic gastric cancer management, the future of gastric cancer surgery may trend toward robotic surgery, which has been an alternative minimally invasive technique since the early 2000s, yet still remains an emerging technology. In a meta-analysis, robotic surgery was associated with less blood loss, less time to first flatus, and greater lymph node yield than conventional laparoscopic gastrectomy, although this study included no randomized trials.[107] It also found that both approaches had similar postoperative morbidity and mortality. As robotic technology becomes cheaper and more prevalent, it is anticipated that it will take up a larger percentage of the procedures performed for gastric cancer.

Drains and Feeding Tubes

Intraoperatively, some surgeons may elect to place drains and feeding tubes in gastrectomy patients, but in general, the literature does not support this practice, having found no improvement in outcomes and a possible increase in complications with their placement. However, there are some select patients in whom the placement of a small bowel feeding tube can be justified: patients at the highest risk of anastomotic leak and/or malnutrition, such as those undergoing total gastrectomy, and in those patients in whom additional enteral feeding may decrease the time to adjuvant therapy.[6] Although there are no strong recommendations regarding these feeding tubes (the NCCN guidelines only recommend that they may be considered in select patients), their placement still occurs in 24% to 32% of patients.[4,108,109]

Surgical Approach to Metastatic Disease

As new treatments emerge, providers are starting to question the oncologic dogma that metastatic disease should only be treated with systemic therapy. There is some evidence emerging to suggest that in some select patients a more aggressive surgical approach may have some value. In recent years, literature has started to show that a select group of patients with metastatic gastric cancer limited only to the peritoneum without solid organ metastases may achieve a survival benefit by undergoing aggressive cytoreductive surgery and heated intraperitoneal chemotherapy, but further research is needed.[110–113] Furthermore, when it comes to isolated solid organ metastases, such as hepatic and pulmonary, there is some evidence to support the practice of metastasectomy. Hepatic metastasectomy has been reported, but the occurrence of isolated liver metastases is a rare event (only 0.5% in Asian populations). There is currently a lack of consensus as to the appropriate patient selection for this procedure and to whether it should be performed at all given the poor prognosis.[114–116] Similarly, there are little data to guide the performance of pulmonary metastasectomy, which can potentially result in a benefit for patients, but it is a rare event.

Palliative Interventions

When decision between provider and patient is no longer to pursue cure or life-prolonging treatments, surgery still may have a role in a palliative sense and can include options, such as stenting, palliative gastrectomy, and gastrojejunostomy. Although chemotherapy is the cornerstone of effective treatment for metastatic disease, it often is insufficient to address local symptoms secondary to obstruction, perforation, or bleeding. Patients who present with bleeding may require endoscopy, angiography, or radiotherapy.[117] Patients who present with an obstruction may be managed with endoscopic stent placement, a venting gastrostomy, and in some select patients, a gastrojejunostomy or palliative gastrectomy can be considered.[118] Studies have compared endoscopic stenting with palliative gastrojejunostomy and have found that although there was no difference in efficacy or complications, stenting was associated with shorter hospital stays and faster relief of symptoms, which could be of critical importance to patients with limited remaining time; however, there was a need for more frequent reintervention in those who received stents.[119] Therefore, palliative gastrojejunostomy is generally used in cases where stenting is not deemed to be feasible. It is also considered when longer survival is anticipated. An even more aggressive procedure, a palliative gastrectomy, in general cannot be recommended given its high morbidity, and it is reserved for extremely symptomatic cases where there are no other options. The REGATTA randomized controlled trial examined whether the addition of gastrectomy to chemotherapy improved survival for patients with advanced gastric cancer with a single noncurable factor; however, the study was closed on the basis of futility and found that gastrectomy followed by chemotherapy did not show any survival benefit compared with chemotherapy alone (overall survival at 2 years was 25.1% vs 31.7%, respectively).[120] The decision to pursue any of these interventions must take into account the patient's prognosis and goals in order to limit aggressive therapy at the end of life that is not aligned with the patient's wishes.

POSTOPERATIVE MANAGEMENT, SURVEILLANCE, AND RECURRENT DISEASE

Postoperatively, patients with gastric cancer will be admitted to the surgical floor or a monitored setting based on what is necessary. When possible, enhanced recovery after surgery, and fast-track protocols may be able to be followed,[121,122] particularly for minimally invasive procedures, which emphasize early mobilization and nonnarcotic analgesia. These protocols may improve time to ambulation and oral intake while decreasing length of hospital stay.[123] Although there are no true gold-standard guidelines for postoperative care, patients are started on enteral nutrition as soon as possible, and the involvement of a dietician can be helpful to assist patients in adjusting to their new dietary regimen. Patients are advised to eat small frequent meals high in protein, inclusive of fat, and supplemented by vitamins while avoiding carbohydrates to try to avoid weight loss and nutritional deficiencies.[124] There is some controversy in the literature as to whether routine nasogastric decompression should be performed postoperatively[122,125] and as to whether patients need a postoperative upper GI swallow study.[36]

After patients make it out of the acute postoperative period, they will need to continue to be followed to monitor for recurrent disease. Although NCCN guidelines acknowledge that there are sparse data to guide surveillance strategies, they in general recommend the following: (1) a complete history and physical examination every 3 to 6 months for the first 2 years, every 6 to 12 months for years 3 to 5, and annually thereafter; (2)

complete blood count and chemistry laboratory tests when clinically indicated; (3) Esophagogastroduodenoscopy (EGD) for patients with early-stage disease (TiS or T1a) who underwent endoscopic resection every 6 months for the first year and then annually for either 3 years (Tis) or 5 years (T1a); (4) EGD for patients who underwent surgery as clinically indicated; (5) CT scan with oral and intravenous (IV) contrast based on stage of disease (stage I: as clinically indicated; stage II–III: every 6–12 months for the first 2 years, then annually for up to 5 years).[4] Guidelines from the European Society for Medical Oncology are also somewhat limited in their guidance, suggesting regular posttreatment follow-up with dietary support without providing specifics as to other testing or the frequency of follow-up.[126] When gastric cancer does recur, it can be classified as local or distant recurrence. In general, curative resection is not attempted in patients with locally recurrent disease, although it has been described.[127] Instead, most patients with recurrent disease are offered systemic chemotherapy.

COMPLICATIONS

Despite surgery offering the best chance of cure for patients with gastric cancer, it is not without its risks, and several patients will have complications. Complications can include surgical site infections, intra-abdominal bleeding, anastomotic complications, duodenal/pancreatic/lymphatic fistulas, cardiopulmonary complications, delayed gastric emptying, and postgastrectomy syndromes.[21] The perioperative surgical complications after total gastrectomy are primarily due to anastomotic leak, and long-term complications can include esophageal stricture and the postgastrectomy syndromes. The most worrisome complication in the early postoperative period after total gastrectomy is a breakdown of the esophagojejunal anastomosis, which has been reported to occur in 5% to 7% of patients.[128,129] Although minor leaks without sepsis can be controlled nonoperatively with antibiotics, intestinal decompression, and percutaneous drainage, interventions may be needed for more significant disruptions. Covered stents have been reported to have some success, but major disruptions will need reoperation, and this is associated with increased mortality, which has been reported to be about 30%.[129,130] Anastomotic leak can also result in esophageal stricture, reported in approximately 4% of patients, which usually can be managed with serial endoscopic dilations.[131] The jejunojejunal anastomosis rarely leaks.

Less worrisome but still problematic are the postgastrectomy syndromes.[132,133] Following gastric resection, the motility of the stomach can be affected, resulting in rapid or delayed transit. Rapid transit can be seen with dumping syndrome, which is a phenomenon caused by destruction or bypass of the pyloric sphincter. It can present with symptoms of diarrhea, nausea, vomiting, diaphoresis, sweating, and palpitations. When these symptoms develop early after a meal, it is attributed to the rapid emptying of hyperosmolar chyme into the small bowel; when it occurs late, it is thought to be owing to hypoglycemia that occurs following an insulin peak after eating. Most patients' symptoms will improve with dietary changes.[134] After gastrectomy, some patients may also have delayed gastric emptying, which can be associated with epigastric fullness and emesis. The degree of postsurgical gastroparesis depends on several factors, including whether vagotomy was performed, the extent of stomach and intestinal resection, the extent of lymphatic dissection, and the type of reconstruction performed.[135] Longstanding untreated gastroparesis has significant nutritional and metabolic consequences, which can generally be managed with dietary and behavioral modification in addition to the use of oral prokinetic and antiemetic medications but could potentially require hospitalization in the setting of severe fluid and electrolyte imbalances.[136]

PERIOPERATIVE OUTCOMES

Over the past 2 decades, prognosis for gastric cancer has only improved modestly in the United States, which is indicative of the fact that US gastric cancers are diagnosed at later stages.[137] Regarding perioperative mortality following partial gastric resection, it is low and ranges from 1% to greater than 10% depending on patient age and medical comorbidities.[138–140] For total gastrectomy, perioperative death is reported in trials as ranging from 2% to 13%.[50,141] Regarding longer-term prognosis, it is dependent on patient, tumor, and treatment factors, including histologic type, status of resection margins, age and sex, the stage of disease, its location, the treatment received, and the population studied. In general, Asian populations have been found to have better outcomes than Western populations even when stratified by stage.[142–146] Hypotheses to explain these differences have included differences in treatment (particularly surgical techniques), patient characteristics and behavior, and race-related differences in tumor biology. Although long-term data on quality of life after gastrectomy are limited, studies suggest that these procedures can be performed while maintaining a satisfactory quality of life, which generally improves after the short-term perioperative period.[147–152]

SUMMARY

The management of gastric cancer has evolved over the last several decades and will continue to do so as new therapeutics are developed. At the heart of all gastric cancer treatment has been surgery, and it is likely to stay this way for the time-being. All providers must continue to work together clinically and in research to continue to determine the best types of treatment, their sequence, and timing to achieve the best outcomes for our patients.

CLINICS CARE POINTS

- Staging laparoscopy with peritoneal washings should be performed for gastric cancer clinical stages ≥T1b to evaluate for peritoneal spread when chemoradiation or surgery is considered.
- The decision to pursue gastric cancer resection should occur with consultation of a multidisciplinary tumor board to ensure that an appropriate multimodality treatment strategy is planned.
- The goal of gastric resection for adenocarcinoma is to obtain a tumor-free resection margin (R0) on pathologic examination.
- A D2 lymphadenectomy is recognized as the optimal approach to lymph node dissection and should accompany gastric resection when it can be safely performed.
- After gastric resection, Roux-en-Y reconstruction is better tolerated overall and associated with an improved quality of life compared with the Billroth reconstructions.

DISCLOSURE

The authors have no disclosures.

SUPPLEMENTARY DATA

Supplementary data related to this article can be found online at https://doi.org/10.1016/j.giec.2021.04.001.

REFERENCES

1. Jemal A, Bray F, Center MM, et al. Global cancer statistics. CA Cancer J Clin 2011;61(2):69–90.
2. Kim GH, Liang PS, Bang SJ, et al. Screening and surveillance for gastric cancer in the United States: is it needed? Gastrointest Endosc 2016;84(1):18–28.
3. Amin MB, Edge S, Greene F, et al, editors. AJCC cancer staging manual. 8th edition. Chicago: Springer; 2017.
4. National Comprehensive Cancer Network. NCCN clinical practice guidelines in oncology. Gastric cancer. Version 3.2020. Available at: https://www.nccn.org/professionals/physician_gls/pdf/gastric.pdf. Accessed August 22, 2020.
5. Power DG, Schattner MA, Gerdes H, et al. Endoscopic ultrasound can improve the selection for laparoscopy in patients with localized gastric cancer. J Am Coll Surg 2009;208(2):173–8.
6. The American College of Surgeons and the Alliance for Clinical Trials in Oncology. Gastrectomy. In: Katz, Matthew HG, editors. Operative standards for cancer care. Volume 2: thyroid, gastric, rectum, esophagus, melanoma. Philadelphia: LWW; 2019. p. 77–178.
7. Muntean V, Mihailov A, Iancu C, et al. Staging laparoscopy in gastric cancer. Accuracy and impact on therapy. J Gastrointest Liver Dis 2009;18(2):189–95.
8. Yano M, Tsujinaka T, Shiozaki H, et al. Appraisal of treatment strategy by staging laparoscopy for locally advanced gastric cancer. World J Surg 2000;24(9):1130–5, discussion 1135-1136.
9. Leake PA, Cardoso R, Seevaratnam R, et al. A systematic review of the accuracy and indications for diagnostic laparoscopy prior to curative-intent resection of gastric cancer. Gastric Cancer 2012;15(Suppl 1):S38–47.
10. Muntean V, Oniu T, Lungoci C, et al. Staging laparoscopy in digestive cancers. J Gastrointest Liver Dis 2009;18(4):461–7.
11. Irvin TT, Bridger JE. Gastric cancer: an audit of 122 consecutive cases and the results of R1 gastrectomy. Br J Surg 1988;75(2):106–9.
12. Viste A, Haùgstvedt T, Eide GE, et al. Postoperative complications and mortality after surgery for gastric cancer. Ann Surg 1988;207(1):7–13.
13. Valen B, Viste A, Haugstvedt T, et al. Treatment of stomach cancer, a national experience. Br J Surg 1988;75(7):708–12.
14. Burke EC, Karpeh MS Jr, Conlon KC, et al. Peritoneal lavage cytology in gastric cancer: an independent predictor of outcome. Ann Surg Oncol 1998;5(5):411–5.
15. Leake PA, Cardoso R, Seevaratnam R, et al. A systematic review of the accuracy and utility of peritoneal cytology in patients with gastric cancer. Gastric Cancer 2012;15(Suppl 1):S27–37.
16. Badgwell B, Cormier JN, Krishnan S, et al. Does neoadjuvant treatment for gastric cancer patients with positive peritoneal cytology at staging laparoscopy improve survival? Ann Surg Oncol 2008;15(10):2684–91.
17. Karanicolas PJ, Elkin EB, Jacks LM, et al. Staging laparoscopy in the management of gastric cancer: a population-based analysis. J Am Coll Surg 2011;213(5):644–51, 651.e641.
18. Badgwell B, Das P, Ajani J. Treatment of localized gastric and gastroesophageal adenocarcinoma: the role of accurate staging and preoperative therapy. J Hematol Oncol 2017;10(1):149.
19. Soybel DI. Anatomy and physiology of the stomach. Surg Clin North Am 2005;85(5):875–94, v.

20. Daniels IR, Allum WH. The anatomy and physiology of the stomach. In: Lumley J, editor. Upper gastrointestinal surgery. Springer specialist surgery series. London: Springer; 2005. p. 17–37.
21. Chang-Ming H, Chao-Hui Z. Laparoscopic gastrectomy for gastric cancer. New York: Springer; 2015.
22. Henning GT, Schild SE, Stafford SL, et al. Results of irradiation or chemoirradiation following resection of gastric adenocarcinoma. Int J Radiat Oncol Biol Phys 2000;46(3):589–98.
23. Liang C, Chen G, Zhao B, et al. Borrmann type IV gastric cancer: focus on the role of gastrectomy. J Gastrointest Surg 2020;24(5):1026–32.
24. Blackham AU, Swords DS, Levine EA, et al. Is linitis plastica a contraindication for surgical resection: a multi-institution study of the U.S. gastric cancer collaborative. Ann Surg Oncol 2016;23(4):1203–11.
25. Birkmeyer JD, Sun Y, Wong SL, et al. Hospital volume and late survival after cancer surgery. Ann Surg 2007;245(5):777–83.
26. van der Post RS, Vogelaar IP, Carneiro F, et al. Hereditary diffuse gastric cancer: updated clinical guidelines with an emphasis on germline CDH1 mutation carriers. J Med Gent 2015;52(6):361–74.
27. Woodfield CA, Levine MS. The postoperative stomach. Eur J Radiol 2005;53(3): 341–52.
28. Schardey HM, Joosten U, Finke U, et al. The prevention of anastomotic leakage after total gastrectomy with local decontamination. A prospective, randomized, double-blind, placebo-controlled multicenter trial. Ann Surg 1997;225(2): 172–80.
29. Farran L, Llop J, Sans M, et al. Efficacy of enteral decontamination in the prevention of anastomotic dehiscence and pulmonary infection in esophagogastric surgery. Dis Esophagus 2008;21(2):159–64.
30. Buhl K, Schlag P, Herfarth C. Quality of life and functional results following different types of resection for gastric carcinoma. Eur J Surg Oncol 1990; 16(4):404–9.
31. Pu YW, Gong W, Wu YY, et al. Proximal gastrectomy versus total gastrectomy for proximal gastric carcinoma. A meta-analysis on postoperative complications, 5-year survival, and recurrence rate. Saudi Med J 2013;34(12):1223–8.
32. Lee JH. Ongoing surgical clinical trials on minimally invasive surgery for gastric cancer: Korea. Transl Gastroenterol Hepatol 2016;1:40.
33. Bozzetti F, Marubini E, Bonfanti G, et al. Subtotal versus total gastrectomy for gastric cancer: five-year survival rates in a multicenter randomized Italian trial. Italian Gastrointestinal Tumor Study Group. Ann Surg 1999;230(2):170–8.
34. Gouzi JL, Huguier M, Fagniez PL, et al. Total versus subtotal gastrectomy for adenocarcinoma of the gastric antrum. A French prospective controlled study. Ann Surg 1989;209(2):162–6.
35. Sato Y, Yamada T, Yoshikawa T, et al. Randomized controlled phase III trial to evaluate omentum preserving gastrectomy for patients with advanced gastric cancer (JCOG1711, ROAD-GC). Jpn J Clin Oncol 2020;50(11):1321–4.
36. Mullen JT. Gastric cancer. In: Fischer J, editor. Fischer's mastery of surgery. 7th edition. Philadelphia: Wolters Kluwer; 2019. p. 1127–40.
37. Katai H. Function-preserving surgery for gastric cancer. Int J Clin Oncol 2006; 11(5):357–66.
38. Park DJ, Lee HJ, Jung HC, et al. Clinical outcome of pylorus-preserving gastrectomy in gastric cancer in comparison with conventional distal gastrectomy with Billroth I anastomosis. World J Surg 2008;32(6):1029–36.

39. Ishikawa K, Arita T, Ninomiya S, et al. Outcome of segmental gastrectomy versus distal gastrectomy for early gastric cancer. World J Surg 2007;31(11): 2204–7.
40. Ando S, Tsuji H. Surgical technique of vagus nerve-preserving gastrectomy with D2 lymphadenectomy for gastric cancer. ANZ J Surg 2008;78(3):172–6.
41. Bria E, De Manzoni G, Beghelli S, et al. A clinical-biological risk stratification model for resected gastric cancer: prognostic impact of Her2, Fhit, and APC expression status. Ann Oncol 2013;24(3):693–701.
42. Hashimoto T, Arai K, Yamashita Y, et al. Characteristics of intramural metastasis in gastric cancer. Gastric Cancer 2013;16(4):537–42.
43. Dikken JL, Baser RE, Gonen M, et al. Conditional probability of survival nomogram for 1-, 2-, and 3-year survivors after an R0 resection for gastric cancer. Ann Surg Oncol 2013;20(5):1623–30.
44. Shin D, Park SS. Clinical importance and surgical decision-making regarding proximal resection margin for gastric cancer. World J Gastrointest Oncol 2013;5(1):4–11.
45. Japanese Gastric Cancer Association. Japanese gastric cancer treatment guidelines 2018 (5th edition). Gastric Cancer 2021;24(1):1–21.
46. Chen JD, Yang XP, Shen JG, et al. Prognostic improvement of reexcision for positive resection margins in patients with advanced gastric cancer. Eur J Surg Oncol 2013;39(3):229–34.
47. Brar S, Law C, McLeod R, et al. Defining surgical quality in gastric cancer: a RAND/UCLA appropriateness study. J Am Coll Surg 2013;217(2):347–57.e341.
48. Coburn N, Cosby R, Klein L, et al. Staging and surgical approaches in gastric cancer: a clinical practice guideline. Curr Oncol 2017;24(5):324–31.
49. Waddell T, Verheij M, Allum W, et al. Gastric cancer: ESMO-ESSO-ESTRO clinical practice guidelines for diagnosis, treatment and follow-up. Eur J Surg Oncol 2014;40(5):584–91.
50. Hartgrink HH, van de Velde CJ, Putter H, et al. Extended lymph node dissection for gastric cancer: who may benefit? Final results of the randomized Dutch gastric cancer group trial. J Clin Oncol 2004;22(11):2069–77.
51. Cuschieri A, Weeden S, Fielding J, et al. Patient survival after D1 and D2 resections for gastric cancer: long-term results of the MRC randomized surgical trial. Surgical Co-operative Group. Br J Cancer 1999;79(9–10):1522–30.
52. Songun I, Putter H, Kranenbarg EM, et al. Surgical treatment of gastric cancer: 15-year follow-up results of the randomised nationwide Dutch D1D2 trial. Lancet Oncol 2010;11(5):439–49.
53. Mocellin S, McCulloch P, Kazi H, et al. Extent of lymph node dissection for adenocarcinoma of the stomach. Cochrane Database Syst Rev 2015;2015(8): Cd001964.
54. Yonemura Y, Wu CC, Fukushima N, et al. Randomized clinical trial of D2 and extended paraaortic lymphadenectomy in patients with gastric cancer. Int J Clin Oncol 2008;13(2):132–7.
55. Maeta M, Yamashiro H, Saito H, et al. A prospective pilot study of extended (D3) and superextended para-aortic lymphadenectomy (D4) in patients with T3 or T4 gastric cancer managed by total gastrectomy. Surgery 1999;125(3):325–31.
56. Hundahl SA, Macdonald JS, Benedetti J, et al. Surgical treatment variation in a prospective, randomized trial of chemoradiotherapy in gastric cancer: the effect of undertreatment. Ann Surg Oncol 2002;9(3):278–86.
57. Baxter NN, Tuttle TM. Inadequacy of lymph node staging in gastric cancer patients: a population-based study. Ann Surg Oncol 2005;12(12):981–7.

58. Bilimoria KY, Talamonti MS, Wayne JD, et al. Effect of hospital type and volume on lymph node evaluation for gastric and pancreatic cancer. Arch Surg 2008; 143(7):671–8, discussion 678.
59. Luna A, Rebasa P, Montmany S, et al. Learning curve for D2 lymphadenectomy in gastric cancer. ISRN Surg 2013;2013:508719.
60. Parikh D, Johnson M, Chagla L, et al. D2 gastrectomy: lessons from a prospective audit of the learning curve. Br J Surg 1996;83(11):1595–9.
61. Kim CY, Nam BH, Cho GS, et al. Learning curve for gastric cancer surgery based on actual survival. Gastric Cancer 2016;19(2):631–8.
62. Mahar AL, McLeod RS, Kiss A, et al. A systematic review of the effect of institution and surgeon factors on surgical outcomes for gastric cancer. J Am Coll Surg 2012;214(5):860–8.e812.
63. Kitagawa Y, Fujii H, Mukai M, et al. Intraoperative lymphatic mapping and sentinel lymph node sampling in esophageal and gastric cancer. Surg Oncol Clin N Am 2002;11(2):293–304.
64. Ohdaira H, Nimura H, Mitsumori N, et al. Validity of modified gastrectomy combined with sentinel node navigation surgery for early gastric cancer. Gastric Cancer 2007;10(2):117–22.
65. Takeuchi H, Kitagawa Y. Sentinel lymph node biopsy in gastric cancer. Cancer J 2015;21(1):21–4.
66. Wang Z, Dong ZY, Chen JQ, et al. Diagnostic value of sentinel lymph node biopsy in gastric cancer: a meta-analysis. Ann Surg Oncol 2012;19(5):1541–50.
67. Ryu KW, Eom BW, Nam BH, et al. Is the sentinel node biopsy clinically applicable for limited lymphadenectomy and modified gastric resection in gastric cancer? A meta-analysis of feasibility studies. J Surg Oncol 2011;104(6): 578–84.
68. Sharma D. Choice of digestive tract reconstructive procedure following total gastrectomy: a critical reappraisal. Indian J Surg 2004;66:270–6.
69. Zong L, Chen P. Billroth I vs. Billroth II vs. Roux-en-Y following distal gastrectomy: a meta-analysis based on 15 studies. Hepatogastroenterology 2011; 58(109):1413–24.
70. Hirao M, Takiguchi S, Imamura H, et al. Comparison of Billroth I and Roux-en-Y reconstruction after distal gastrectomy for gastric cancer: one-year postoperative effects assessed by a multi-institutional RCT. Ann Surg Oncol 2013;20(5): 1591–7.
71. Csendes A, Burgos AM, Smok G, et al. Latest results (12-21 years) of a prospective randomized study comparing Billroth II and Roux-en-Y anastomosis after a partial gastrectomy plus vagotomy in patients with duodenal ulcers. Ann Surg 2009;249(2):189–94.
72. Lehnert T, Buhl K. Techniques of reconstruction after total gastrectomy for cancer. Br J Surg 2004;91(5):528–39.
73. Wang G, Ceng G, Zhou B, et al. Meta-analysis of two types of digestive tract reconstruction modes after total gastrectomy. Hepatogastroenterology 2013; 60(127):1817–21.
74. Naum C, Bîrlă R, Marica DC, et al. In search of the optimal reconstruction method after total gastrectomy. Is Roux-en-Y the Best? A review of the randomized clinical trials. Chirurgia (Bucur) 2020;115(1):12–22.
75. El Halabi HM, Lawrence W Jr. Clinical results of various reconstructions employed after total gastrectomy. J Surg Oncol 2008;97(2):186–92.

76. Syn NL, Wee I, Shabbir A, et al. Pouch versus no pouch following total gastrectomy: meta-analysis of randomized and non-randomized studies. Ann Surg 2019;269(6):1041–53.
77. Menon P, Sunil I, Chowdhury SK, et al. Hunt-Lawrence pouch after total gastrectomy: 4 years follow up. Indian Pediatr 2003;40(3):249–51.
78. Hunt CJ. Construction of food pouch from segment of jejunum as substitute for stomach in total gastrectomy. AMA Arch Surg 1952;64(5):601–8.
79. Lawrence W Jr. Reservoir construction after total gastrectomy: an instructive case. Ann Surg 1962;155(2):191–8.
80. Lawrence W Jr. Reconstruction after total gastrectomy: what is preferred technique? J Surg Oncol 1996;63(4):215–20.
81. Kim W, Kim HH, Han SU, et al. Decreased morbidity of laparoscopic distal gastrectomy compared with open distal gastrectomy for stage i gastric cancer: short-term outcomes from a multicenter randomized controlled trial (KLASS-01). Ann Surg 2016;263(1):28–35.
82. Hu Y, Huang C, Sun Y, et al. Morbidity and mortality of laparoscopic versus open D2 distal gastrectomy for advanced gastric cancer: a randomized controlled trial. J Clin Oncol 2016;34(12):1350–7.
83. Honda M, Hiki N, Kinoshita T, et al. Long-term outcomes of laparoscopic versus open surgery for clinical stage I gastric cancer: the LOC-1 study. Ann Surg 2016;264(2):214–22.
84. Best LM, Mughal M, Gurusamy KS. Laparoscopic versus open gastrectomy for gastric cancer. Cochrane Database Syst Rev 2016;3(3):Cd011389.
85. Son SY, Kim HH. Minimally invasive surgery in gastric cancer. World J Gastroenterol 2014;20(39):14132–41.
86. Kitano S, Shiraishi N, Uyama I, et al. A multicenter study on oncologic outcome of laparoscopic gastrectomy for early cancer in Japan. Ann Surg 2007;245(1):68–72.
87. Kim HH, Han SU, Kim MC, et al. Effect of laparoscopic distal gastrectomy vs open distal gastrectomy on long-term survival among patients with stage I gastric cancer: the KLASS-01 randomized clinical trial. JAMA Oncol 2019;5(4):506–13.
88. Katai H, Mizusawa J, Katayama H, et al. Short-term surgical outcomes from a phase III study of laparoscopy-assisted versus open distal gastrectomy with nodal dissection for clinical stage IA/IB gastric cancer: Japan Clinical Oncology Group Study JCOG0912. Gastric Cancer 2017;20(4):699–708.
89. Hyung WJ, Yang HK, Han SU, et al. A feasibility study of laparoscopic total gastrectomy for clinical stage I gastric cancer: a prospective multi-center phase II clinical trial, KLASS 03. Gastric Cancer 2019;22(1):214–22.
90. Li Z, Shan F, Wang Y, et al. Laparoscopic versus open distal gastrectomy for locally advanced gastric cancer after neoadjuvant chemotherapy: safety and short-term oncologic results. Surg Endosc 2016;30(10):4265–71.
91. Hu Y, Ying M, Huang C, et al. Oncologic outcomes of laparoscopy-assisted gastrectomy for advanced gastric cancer: a large-scale multicenter retrospective cohort study from China. Surg Endosc 2014;28(7):2048–56.
92. Yu J, Huang C, Sun Y, et al. Effect of laparoscopic vs open distal gastrectomy on 3-year disease-free survival in patients with locally advanced gastric cancer: the CLASS-01 randomized clinical trial. JAMA 2019;321(20):1983–92.
93. Hur H, Lee HY, Lee HJ, et al. Efficacy of laparoscopic subtotal gastrectomy with D2 lymphadenectomy for locally advanced gastric cancer: the protocol of the

KLASS-02 multicenter randomized controlled clinical trial. BMC Cancer 2015; 15:355.
94. Inaki N, Etoh T, Ohyama T, et al. A multi-institutional, prospective, phase II feasibility study of laparoscopy-assisted distal gastrectomy with D2 lymph node dissection for locally advanced gastric cancer (JLSSG0901). World J Surg 2015;39(11):2734–41.
95. Li HZ, Chen JX, Zheng Y, et al. Laparoscopic-assisted versus open radical gastrectomy for resectable gastric cancer: systematic review, meta-analysis, and trial sequential analysis of randomized controlled trials. J Surg Oncol 2016; 113(7):756–67.
96. Glenn JA, Turaga KK, Gamblin TC, et al. Minimally invasive gastrectomy for cancer: current utilization in US academic medical centers. Surg Endosc 2015; 29(12):3768–75.
97. Greenleaf EK, Sun SX, Hollenbeak CS, et al. Minimally invasive surgery for gastric cancer: the American experience. Gastric Cancer 2017;20(2):368–78.
98. Kelly KJ, Selby L, Chou JF, et al. Laparoscopic versus open gastrectomy for gastric adenocarcinoma in the west: a case-control study. Ann Surg Oncol 2015;22(11):3590–6.
99. Hendriksen BS, Brooks AJ, Hollenbeak CS, et al. The impact of minimally invasive gastrectomy on survival in the USA. J Gastrointest Surg 2020;24(5):1000–9.
100. Lee MS, Lee JH, Park DJ, et al. Comparison of short- and long-term outcomes of laparoscopic-assisted total gastrectomy and open total gastrectomy in gastric cancer patients. Surg Endosc 2013;27(7):2598–605.
101. Kim HS, Kim BS, Lee IS, et al. Comparison of totally laparoscopic total gastrectomy and open total gastrectomy for gastric cancer. J Laparoendosc Adv Surg Tech A 2013;23(4):323–31.
102. Shinohara T, Satoh S, Kanaya S, et al. Laparoscopic versus open D2 gastrectomy for advanced gastric cancer: a retrospective cohort study. Surg Endosc 2013;27(1):286–94.
103. Kim HG, Park JH, Jeong SH, et al. Totally laparoscopic distal gastrectomy after learning curve completion: comparison with laparoscopy-assisted distal gastrectomy. J Gastric Cancer 2013;13(1):26–33.
104. Moon JS, Park MS, Kim JH, et al. Lessons learned from a comparative analysis of surgical outcomes of and learning curves for laparoscopy-assisted distal gastrectomy. J Gastric Cancer 2015;15(1):29–38.
105. Kim HH, Han SU, Kim MC, et al. Long-term results of laparoscopic gastrectomy for gastric cancer: a large-scale case-control and case-matched Korean multicenter study. J Clin Oncol 2014;32(7):627–33.
106. Jung DH, Son SY, Park YS, et al. The learning curve associated with laparoscopic total gastrectomy. Gastric Cancer 2016;19(1):264–72.
107. Hu LD, Li XF, Wang XY, et al. Robotic versus laparoscopic gastrectomy for gastric carcinoma: a meta-analysis of efficacy and safety. Asian Pac J Cancer Prev 2016;17(9):4327–33.
108. Patel SH, Kooby DA, Staley CA 3rd, et al. An assessment of feeding jejunostomy tube placement at the time of resection for gastric adenocarcinoma. J Surg Oncol 2013;107(7):728–34.
109. Dann GC, Squires MH 3rd, Postlewait LM, et al. An assessment of feeding jejunostomy tube placement at the time of resection for gastric adenocarcinoma: a seven-institution analysis of 837 patients from the U.S. gastric cancer collaborative. J Surg Oncol 2015;112(2):195–202.

110. Yang XJ, Huang CQ, Suo T, et al. Cytoreductive surgery and hyperthermic intraperitoneal chemotherapy improves survival of patients with peritoneal carcinomatosis from gastric cancer: final results of a phase III randomized clinical trial. Ann Surg Oncol 2011;18(6):1575–81.
111. Bonnot PE, Piessen G, Kepenekian V, et al. Cytoreductive surgery with or without hyperthermic intraperitoneal chemotherapy for gastric cancer with peritoneal metastases (CYTO-CHIP study): a propensity score analysis. J Clin Oncol 2019;37(23):2028–40.
112. The Chicago consensus on peritoneal surface malignancies: management of gastric metastases. Ann Surg Oncol 2020;27(6):1768–73.
113. Gill RS, Al-Adra DP, Nagendran J, et al. Treatment of gastric cancer with peritoneal carcinomatosis by cytoreductive surgery and HIPEC: a systematic review of survival, mortality, and morbidity. J Surg Oncol 2011;104(6):692–8.
114. Shirabe K, Wakiyama S, Gion T, et al. Hepatic resection for the treatment of liver metastases in gastric carcinoma: review of the literature. HPB (Oxford) 2006; 8(2):89–92.
115. Cheon SH, Rha SY, Jeung HC, et al. Survival benefit of combined curative resection of the stomach (D2 resection) and liver in gastric cancer patients with liver metastases. Ann Oncol 2008;19(6):1146–53.
116. Linhares E, Monteiro M, Kesley R, et al. Major hepatectomy for isolated metastases from gastric adenocarcinoma. HPB (Oxford) 2003;5(4):235–7.
117. Hashimoto K, Mayahara H, Takashima A, et al. Palliative radiation therapy for hemorrhage of unresectable gastric cancer: a single institute experience. J Cancer Res Clin Oncol 2009;135(8):1117–23.
118. Ejaz ARB, Johnston F. Management of gastric adenocarcinoma. In: Cameron JCA, editor. Current surgical therapy. 13th Edition. Elsevier; 2020.
119. Jeurnink SM, van Eijck CH, Steyerberg EW, et al. Stent versus gastrojejunostomy for the palliation of gastric outlet obstruction: a systematic review. BMC Gastroenterol 2007;7:18.
120. Fujitani K, Yang HK, Mizusawa J, et al. Gastrectomy plus chemotherapy versus chemotherapy alone for advanced gastric cancer with a single non-curable factor (REGATTA): a phase 3, randomised controlled trial. Lancet Oncol 2016; 17(3):309–18.
121. Chen S, Zou Z, Chen F, et al. A meta-analysis of fast track surgery for patients with gastric cancer undergoing gastrectomy. Ann R Coll Surg Engl 2015; 97(1):3–10.
122. Li YJ, Huo TT, Xing J, et al. Meta-analysis of efficacy and safety of fast-track surgery in gastrectomy for gastric cancer. World J Surg 2014;38(12):3142–51.
123. Abdikarim I, Cao XY, Li SZ, et al. Enhanced recovery after surgery with laparoscopic radical gastrectomy for stomach carcinomas. World J Gastroenterol 2015;21(47):13339–44.
124. Dorcaratto D, Grande L, Pera M. Enhanced recovery in gastrointestinal surgery: upper gastrointestinal surgery. Dig Surg 2013;30(1):70–8.
125. Yang Z, Zheng Q, Wang Z. Meta-analysis of the need for nasogastric or nasojejunal decompression after gastrectomy for gastric cancer. Br J Surg 2008; 95(7):809–16.
126. Smyth EC, Verheij M, Allum W, et al. Gastric cancer: ESMO clinical practice guidelines for diagnosis, treatment and follow-up. Ann Oncol 2016;27(suppl 5):v38–49.
127. Badgwell B, Cormier JN, Xing Y, et al. Attempted salvage resection for recurrent gastric or gastroesophageal cancer. Ann Surg Oncol 2009;16(1):42–50.

128. Sierzega M, Kolodziejczyk P, Kulig J. Impact of anastomotic leakage on long-term survival after total gastrectomy for carcinoma of the stomach. Br J Surg 2010;97(7):1035–42.
129. Lang H, Piso P, Stukenborg C, et al. Management and results of proximal anastomotic leaks in a series of 1114 total gastrectomies for gastric carcinoma. Eur J Surg Oncol 2000;26(2):168–71.
130. Lee SR, Kim HO, Park JH, et al. Clinical outcomes of endoscopic metal stent placement for esophagojejunostomy leakage after total gastrectomy for gastric adenocarcinoma. Surg Laparosc Endosc Percutan Tech 2018;28(2):113–7.
131. Fukagawa T, Gotoda T, Oda I, et al. Stenosis of esophago-jejuno anastomosis after gastric surgery. World J Surg 2010;34(8):1859–63.
132. Svedlund J, Sullivan M, Liedman B, et al. Quality of life after gastrectomy for gastric carcinoma: controlled study of reconstructive procedures. World J Surg 1997;21(4):422–33.
133. Liedman B, Andersson H, Bosaeus I, et al. Changes in body composition after gastrectomy: results of a controlled, prospective clinical trial. World J Surg 1997; 21(4):416–20, discussion 420-411.
134. Berg P, McCallum R. Dumping syndrome: a review of the current concepts of pathophysiology, diagnosis, and treatment. Dig Dis Sci 2016;61(1):11–8.
135. Shafi MA, Pasricha PJ. Post-surgical and obstructive gastroparesis. Curr Gastroenterol Rep 2007;9(4):280–5.
136. Parkman HP, Hasler WL, Fisher RS. American Gastroenterological Association technical review on the diagnosis and treatment of gastroparesis. Gastroenterology 2004;127(5):1592–622.
137. Siegel RL, Miller KD, Jemal A. Cancer statistics, 2020. CA Cancer J Clin 2020; 70(1):7–30.
138. Kurita N, Miyata H, Gotoh M, et al. Risk model for distal gastrectomy when treating gastric cancer on the basis of data from 33,917 Japanese patients collected using a nationwide web-based data entry system. Ann Surg 2015;262(2): 295–303.
139. Damhuis RA, Tilanus HW. The influence of age on resection rates and postoperative mortality in 2773 patients with gastric cancer. Eur J Cancer 1995; 31a(6):928–31.
140. Bo T, Peiwu Y, Feng Q, et al. Laparoscopy-assisted vs. open total gastrectomy for advanced gastric cancer: long-term outcomes and technical aspects of a case-control study. J Gastrointest Surg 2013;17(7):1202–8.
141. Cuschieri A, Fayers P, Fielding J, et al. Postoperative morbidity and mortality after D1 and D2 resections for gastric cancer: preliminary results of the MRC randomised controlled surgical trial. The Surgical Cooperative Group. Lancet 1996; 347(9007):995–9.
142. Verdecchia A, Mariotto A, Gatta G, et al. Comparison of stomach cancer incidence and survival in four continents. Eur J Cancer 2003;39(11):1603–9.
143. Markar SR, Karthikesalingam A, Jackson D, et al. Long-term survival after gastrectomy for cancer in randomized, controlled oncological trials: comparison between West and East. Ann Surg Oncol 2013;20(7):2328–38.
144. Wanebo HJ, Kennedy BJ, Chmiel J, et al. Cancer of the stomach. A patient care study by the American College of Surgeons. Ann Surg 1993;218(5):583–92.
145. Gill S, Shah A, Le N, et al. Asian ethnicity-related differences in gastric cancer presentation and outcome among patients treated at a Canadian cancer center. J Clin Oncol 2003;21(11):2070–6.

146. Davis PA, Sano T. The difference in gastric cancer between Japan, USA and Europe: what are the facts? What are the suggestions? Crit Rev Oncol Hematol 2001;40(1):77–94.
147. Anderson ID, MacIntyre IM. Symptomatic outcome following resection of gastric cancer. Surg Oncol 1995;4(1):35–40.
148. Wu CW, Chiou JM, Ko FS, et al. Quality of life after curative gastrectomy for gastric cancer in a randomised controlled trial. Br J Cancer 2008;98(1):54–9.
149. Shan B, Shan L, Morris D, et al. Systematic review on quality of life outcomes after gastrectomy for gastric carcinoma. J Gastrointest Oncol 2015;6(5):544–60.
150. Karanicolas PJ, Graham D, Gönen M, et al. Quality of life after gastrectomy for adenocarcinoma: a prospective cohort study. Ann Surg 2013;257(6):1039–46.
151. Iivonen MK, Mattila JJ, Nordback IH, et al. Long-term follow-up of patients with jejunal pouch reconstruction after total gastrectomy. A randomized prospective study. Scand J Gastroenterol 2000;35(7):679–85.
152. Tyrväinen T, Sand J, Sintonen H, et al. Quality of life in the long-term survivors after total gastrectomy for gastric carcinoma. J Surg Oncol 2008;97(2):121–4.

Advances in Systemic Therapy for Gastric Cancer

Andrew Hsu, MD, Alexander G. Raufi, MD*

KEYWORDS

• Gastric cancer • Targeted therapy • Immunotherapy • Cytotoxic chemotherapy

KEY POINTS

- Multiple randomized controlled trials have shown benefit with adjuvant and perioperative chemotherapy with or without radiation therapy in resected stage I to III gastric adenocarcinoma.
- Several standard-of-care options exist for resectable disease, and practices vary depending on region.
- Standard-of-care treatment options for metastatic gastric cancer is guided by performance status, and multiple 2- and 3-drug regimens, with or without immunotherapy, have shown efficacy.
- In human epidermal growth factor 2–overexpressing metastatic gastric cancer, trastuzumab combined with chemotherapy is considered the standard of care.
- Several second- and third-line treatment options have recently been approved, including the vascular endothelial growth factor antibody, ramucirumab, with or without paclitaxel, as well TAS-102.
- Immunotherapy has been approved in the second- and third-line settings for select patients.

INTRODUCTION

Although the global incidence of gastric cancer is declining, it continues to represent a major health problem and leading cause of cancer-related mortality. Many cases are diagnosed late, with unresectable or metastatic disease. For the approximately 50% of patients diagnosed with early stage disease, characterized by disease localized to the stomach or surrounding lymph nodes, systemic chemotherapy, with or without radiotherapy, has proved to improve outcomes in select patients undergoing surgery.[1]

The prognosis remains poor for those patients diagnosed with metastatic or unresectable gastric cancer, with standard-of-care therapies having a modest impact on

The Warren Alpert Medical School of Brown University, Lifespan Cancer Institute, Rhode Island Hospital/The Miriam Hospital, 164 Summit Avenue, Fain Building, Third Floor, Providence, RI 02906, USA
* Corresponding author.
E-mail address: alex.raufi@gmail.com

Gastrointest Endoscopy Clin N Am 31 (2021) 607–623
https://doi.org/10.1016/j.giec.2021.03.009
giendo.theclinics.com

patient survival and quality of life. Currently, the median survival ranges from 4 months with best supportive care (BSC), to 12 months with traditional cytotoxic chemotherapy.[2,3] Over the past few decades, improved understanding of the molecular pathogenesis and biology of cancer has led to the development of novel targeted therapeutic strategies that have led to improvements in survival in select settings. These targeted therapies are currently available as monoclonal antibodies (mAbs) and small molecule inhibitors, most of which are tyrosine kinase inhibitors (TKIs). As a result, current systemic treatments for metastatic gastric cancer consists of combination cytotoxic chemotherapy, with targeted therapies such as trastuzumab and ramucirumab being incorporated in combination with cytotoxic chemotherapy in first- and second-line treatment, respectively, in select settings.[4,5] Furthermore, the discovery of immune checkpoint inhibition in the past decade has been considered a major medical and scientific breakthrough in the treatment of cancer; however, trials examining the use of immunotherapy either as a monotherapy or in combination with cytotoxic chemotherapy in gastric cancers have only led to limited approval in the second-line setting, after failure of initial therapy, with relatively low response rates ranging between 5% and 30%.[6,7] The aim of this chapter is to summarize the currently studied and approved treatments for gastric cancer and to briefly highlight some of the most promising future treatments currently under investigation.

RESECTABLE DISEASE

Patients with early disease (ie, those with in situ or T1a tumors) can often be cured with either endoscopic or surgical resection alone. However, in patients with more advanced disease, those with invasion into or beyond the muscularis propria (≥T2 lesions) or those with regional lymph node involvement, recurrence rates are significantly higher. For these patients, chemotherapy with or without radiotherapy plays an important role in reducing recurrence and has been integrated into standard of care treatment approaches. **Table 1** summarizes several landmark trials that investigated systemic and radiotherapies for the treatment of resectable gastric cancer.

The first study to demonstrate benefit with adjuvant therapy was the US Southwest Oncology Group/Intergroup study (SWOG 9008/INT-0116) reported in 2001. This phase III trial randomized 556 patients with adenocarcinoma of the stomach or gastroesophageal junction (GEJ) to receive surgery followed by adjuvant chemoradiotherapy or surgery alone. Patients who received chemoradiotherapy were administered adjuvant fluorouracil with leucovorin, followed by chemoradiotherapy with 45 Gy of radiation with fluorouracil with leucovorin as a radiosensitizer, and radiation, followed by fluorouracil with leucovorin. The addition of adjuvant chemoradiotherapy led to an improvement in median overall survival (mOS) (36 vs 27 months; hazard ratio [HR] 1.35; CI 95% 1.09 to 1.66; P = .005).[1] Although this was a practice changing trial, a major criticism of this study was the low rate of D2 lymph node dissections performed during surgery. Approximately 90% of patients underwent either a D0 or D1 lymph node dissection, suggesting that adjuvant treatment primarily benefits those patients receiving a less extensive lymph node dissection.[16] A retrospective analysis of the Dutch Gastric Cancer Group Trial (DGCT) in which patients were randomly assigned to undergo either a D1 or D2 dissection followed by chemoradiotherapy have led further support to this notion. The investigators found that adjuvant chemoradiotherapy significantly benefited those patients who received a D1 dissection but had a more limited impact on those who received a D2 dissection.[17]

The phase III CLASSIC trial sought to investigate the potential role for postoperative chemotherapy in patients who underwent a curative D2 gastrectomy. In this study,

Table 1
Landmark trials in the treatment of resectable gastric cancer

Author (Date), Study Name	Treatment Regimen	Total Patients	DFS, HR, *P*-value	mOS, HR, *P*-value
MacDonald et al,[1] 2001, SWOG 9008/INT-0116	Adjuvant chemoradiotherapy (fluorouracil) vs surgery alone	556	48% vs 31%, HR 1.52, $P < .001$	36 vs 27 mo, HR 1.35, $P = .005$
Noh et al,[8] 2014, CLASSIC	Adjuvant chemotherapy (capecitabine + oxaliplatin) vs surgery alone	1035	74% vs 59%, HR 0.58, $P < .0001$	78% vs 69%, HR 0.66
Lee et al,[9] 2012, ARTIST	Adjuvant chemotherapy (XP) vs chemoradiotherapy	458	78.2% vs 74.2%, $P = .862$	NR
Park et al,[10] 2019, ARTIST II	Adjuvant chemotherapy vs chemoradiotherapy in D2 node positive disease	538	78% vs 73%, $P = .667$	NR
Cunningham et al, [11] 2006, MAGIC	Perioperative chemotherapy (ECF) vs surgery alone	506	NR HR 0.66, $P < .001$	36% vs 23%, HR 0.75, $P = .009$
Ychou et al,[12] 2011, FNCLCC/FFCD	Perioperative chemotherapy (CF) vs surgery alone	224	34% vs 19%, HR 0.65, 0 = 0.003	38% vs 24%, HR 0.69, $P = .02$
Alderson et al,[13] 2017, UK MRCOE05	Neoadjuvant chemotherapy ECX vs CF	897	14.4 vs 11.6, HR 0.86, $P = .051$	26.1 vs 23.4, $P = .19$
Cats et al,[14] 2018, CRITICS	Perioperative chemotherapy (ECX) vs neoadjuvant chemotherapy + adjuvant chemoradiotherapy	788	NR	43 vs 37 mo, HR 1.01, $P = .90$
Al-Batran et al,[15] 2019, FLOT4-AIO	Perioperative ECX/ECF vs FLOT	716	30 vs 18 mo, HR 0.75, $P < .001$	50 vs 35 mo, HR 0.77, $P = .012$

Abbreviation: NR, not reported.

1035 patients were randomized to receive adjuvant capecitabine and oxaliplatin for 6 months versus observation following surgery. The addition of adjuvant chemotherapy led to a significant improvement in 3-year disease-free survival (DFS; 74% vs 59%; HR 0.58; 95% CI 0.47–0.72; $P < .0001$) and 5-year overall survival (OS; 78% vs 69%; HR 0.66; 95% CI 0.51–0.85). Notably, 56% of patients in the adjuvant chemotherapy arm experienced grade 3 or 4 toxicities primarily in the form of nausea, neutropenia, and decreased appetite.[8]

Multiple studies have also attempted to determine the benefits of radiation therapy when added to adjuvant chemotherapy in patients who achieve a D2 resection. The ARTIST trial randomized 458 patients who had undergone a curative D2 gastrectomy to receive either adjuvant chemotherapy or adjuvant chemoradiotherapy. Patients received 6 cycles of adjuvant capecitabine and cisplatin (XP) versus 2 cycles of XP followed by radiation therapy, then an additional 2 cycles of XP. Interestingly, the addition of radiation therapy did not lead to improvement in 3-year DFS (78.2% vs 74.2%; $P = .862$) or OS. However, a subgroup analysis revealed that in those patients with lymph node positive who received adjuvant chemoradiotherapy there was a 3-year DFS benefit (77.5% vs 72.3%; $P = .0365$).[9] This prompted the subsequent ARTIST II trial, which further examined the role of adjuvant chemoradiotherapy in 538 patients who had undergone curative D2 gastrectomy and were found to have lymph node positive disease. Ultimately, there was no difference in 3-year DFS between adjuvant chemotherapy versus adjuvant chemoradiotherapy (78% vs 73%, respectively; $P = .667$) in this population.[10]

The MAGIC trial investigated the role of perioperative chemotherapy versus surgery alone in 503 patients with potentially resectable gastric adenocarcinoma. Perioperative chemotherapy consisted of 3 cycles of epirubicin, cisplatin, and fluorouracil (ECF) given both before and after resection. The addition of perioperative ECF led to an improvement in 5-year mOS (36% vs 23%; HR 0.75; CI 95% 0.60–0.93; $P = .009$) but was associated with significant toxicities, with 58% of patients being unable to complete all 6 treatments. Of the patients who completed preoperative treatments, 34% were unable to complete postoperative treatments due to disease progression, patient choice, toxicity, or operative complications.[11] In light of these findings, much of the benefit observed on this trial has been attributed to the neoadjuvant treatment received. Given the high rate of toxicity with perioperative chemotherapy in the MAGIC trial, the French FNCLCC/FFCD trial examined the use of perioperative chemotherapy with cisplatin and fluorouracil (CF) versus surgery alone. This study also demonstrated a statistically significant improvement in 5-year mOS (38% vs 24%; HR 0.69; CI 95% 0.50–0.95; $P = .02$), similar to that noted in the MAGIC trial with ECF. Furthermore, the incidence of grade 3 and 4 toxicity was lower, occurring in 38% of patients.[12] Given the improved toxicity profile with a similar survival benefit, the UK Medical Research Council OE05 trial compared the neoadjuvant use of epirubicin, cisplatin, and capecitabine (ECX) with CF. This phase III trial demonstrated a similar mOS (26.1 vs 23.4 months, respectively; $P = .19$) with a lower rate of treatment completion in the ECX arm (81% vs 96%).[13] The CRITICS trial sought to investigate the addition of radiotherapy to perioperative epirubicin, capecitabine, and cisplatin or oxaliplatin (ECX or EOX) in patients with resectable gastric or GEJ adenocarcinoma. In this phase III trial, 788 patients received 3 cycles of preoperative and postoperative ECX/EOX. In the chemoradiotherapy arm, patients also received 3 cycles of preoperative and postoperative ECX/EOX with the addition of postoperative radiotherapy. Ultimately, there was no difference in mOS with perioperative chemoradiotherapy compared with chemotherapy alone (37 vs 43 months, respectively; HR 1.01; 95% CI 0.84–1.22; $P = .90$).[14] This has become widely adopted as the perioperative treatment regimen of choice and has been adopted into major guidelines throughout the United States.

Recently, the phase II/III FLOT4-AIO trial examined an alternative regimen, a combination of fluorouracil with leucovorin plus oxaliplatin and docetaxel (FLOT), as perioperative therapy. In this trial, 716 patients with locally advanced, resectable gastric or GEJ adenocarcinoma were randomized to receive 3 cycles of preoperative and postoperative ECF/ECX or 4 cycles of preoperative and postoperative FLOT. This regimen demonstrated an improved mOS (50 vs 35 months; HR 0.77; 95% CI 0.63–0.94; $P = .012$) and progression-free survival (PFS) (30 vs 18 months; HR 0.75; 95% CI 0.62–0.91; $P < .001$) with a 27% toxicity rate in both arms.[15]

The role of chemotherapy with or without radiation in patients with resectable disease continues to evolve, and this is reflected in differing global treatment practices. Perioperative chemotherapy is becoming widely adopted in the United States and Europe, adjuvant chemoradiotherapy is still used in much of the United states, and adjuvant chemotherapy alone is often favored in Asia.

ADVANCED DISEASE

First-Line Treatment

Cytotoxic chemotherapy has demonstrated modest activity against gastric cancer: anthracyclines (eg, doxorubicin, epirubicin), fluoropyrimidines (eg, fluorouracil, capecitabine, S-1), platinums (eg, cisplatin, oxaliplatin), taxanes (eg, paclitaxel, docetaxel), and topoisomerase inhibitors (eg, irinotecan). These agents have all shown activity when used as a monotherapy. For example, the objective response rates (ORR) with fluoropyrimidines lies between 20% and 40%,[3,18] compared with an ORR of approximately 20% with either taxanes ORR 20% or irinotecan use.[19,20] Furthermore, a Cochrane review showed an improved mOS with combination chemotherapy when compared with single-agent fluorouracil (8.3 vs 6.7 months).[3]

In patients with human epidermal growth factor 2 (HER2)-negative, metastatic gastric adenocarcinoma, deemed fit for multiagent chemotherapy, the current standard of care consists of either 2- or 3-drug regimens. **Table 2** summarizes the landmark trials for first-line treatment of metastatic gastric cancer. The first multiagent chemotherapy was established in 1980, based on the findings of a randomized trial in which 62 patients with advanced gastric cancer were treated with fluorouracil, doxorubicin, and mitomycin (FAM) and resulted in a partial response rate of 42% and an mOS of 5.5 months.[26] In 1991, a randomized phase III trial compared FAM with fluorouracil, doxorubicin, and methotrexate (FAMTX) and demonstrated an improvement in both mOS (9.7 vs 6.7 months; $P < .004$) and an ORR of (41% versus 9%; $P < .001$). Impressively, 6% of patients in the FAMTX arm demonstrated a complete response (CR) compared with 0% in the FAM arm.[21] FAMTX remained the standard front-line regimen until the late 1990s when the ECF demonstrated superiority in the phase III randomized controlled trial. In this trial 274 patients with advanced gastroesophageal cancer were randomized to ECF or FAMTX. ECF demonstrated both an improved ORR (45% vs 21%; $P = .0002$) and mOS (8.9 vs 5.7 months; $P = .0009$).[22] Surprisingly, mOS of FAMTX in this trial was substantially lower as compared with prior studies, and these results remain controversial to this day. Furthermore, the added benefit of epirubicin, which adds substantial toxicity, has been questions, similar to its use in resectable disease.

In 2006, the V325 study group compared the efficacy of a 2- versus 3-drug combination in a multinational phase II/III trial. In total, 445 patients with metastatic or locally recurrent gastric or GEJ adenocarcinoma were randomized to receive either

Table 2
Landmark trials in first-line treatment of metastatic gastric cancer

Author (Date), Study Name	Treatment Regimen	Total Patients	ORR/CR	mPFS (mo) HR, *P*-value	mOS (mo), HR, *P*-value
MacDonald, et al,[26] 1980	Fluorouracil, doxorubicin, & mitomycin (FAM)	62	42%/NR	NR	5.5
Wils, et al,[21] 1991	Fluorouracil, doxorubicin, & methotrexate (FAMTX) vs FAM	160	41%/6% 9%/0%	NR	9.7 vs 6.7
Webb, et al,[22] 1997	Epirubicin, cisplatin, & fluorouracil (ECF) vs FAMTX	219	45%/6% 21%/2%	FFS: 7.4 vs 3.4 $P = .00006$	8.9 vs 5.7, $P = .0009$
Van Cutsem, et al,[23] 2006, V325	Cisplatin & fluorouracil (CF) vs docetaxel, cisplatin, & fluorouracil (DCF)	270	37%/2% 25%/1%	TTP: 5.6 vs 3.7 HR 1.47, $P < .001$	8.2 vs 9.6, HR 1.29, $P = .02$
Shah et al,[24] 2015	DCF + granulocyte stimulating factor (G-CSF) vs modified DCF (mDCF)	85	33%/NR 49%/NR	6.5 vs 9.7 $P = .2$	12.6 vs 18.8, $P = .007$
Cunningham, et al,[25] 2008, REAL2	Epirubicin, cisplatin, & fluorouracil (ECF) vs Epirubicin, cisplatin, & capecitabine (ECX) Epirubicin, oxaliplatin, & fluorouracil (EOF) Epirubicin, oxaliplatin, & capecitabine (EOX)	1002	41%/4% 46%/4% 42%/3% 48%/4%	6.2 vs 6.7 vs 6.5 vs 7.0[a]	9.9 vs 9.9 vs 9.3 vs 11.2[a]
Bang, et al,[5] 2010, ToGA[b]	Fluoropyrimidine, cisplatin, & trastuzumab vs fluoropyrimidine, cisplatin, & placebo	594	47%/5% 35%/2%	6.7 vs 5.5 HR 0.71, $P = .0002$	13.8 vs 11.1 HR 0.74, $P = .0046$

Abbreviation: NR, not reported.
[a] Noninferior
[b] HER2-positive only.

docetaxel, cisplatin, and fluorouracil (DCF) or CF. In this trial, DCF demonstrated an improved mOS (9.2 vs 8.6 months; $P = .02$), ORR (37% vs 25%; $P = .01$), and time to progression (TTP) (5.6 vs 3.7 months; $P < .001$). Furthermore, the addition of docetaxel led to an increased rate of grade 3 and 4 toxicities, particularly neutropenia (29% vs 12%) when compared with CF.[23] Given the increased rate of neutropenia, a subsequent phase III study examined the use of granulocyte colony-stimulating factor (G-CSF) with DCF support versus modified DCF (mDCF), which consisted of a shorter continuous infusion of fluorouracil along with dose-reduced docetaxel and cisplatin. Modified DCF demonstrated an improved toxicity profile when compared with DCF plus G-CSF (22% vs 52% hospitalized) and a markedly improved mOS (18.8 vs 12.6 months; $P = .007$).[24]

In 2008, the results of the randomized phase III REAL2 trial was published. This study evaluated the interchangeability of 2 fluoropyrimidines, fluorouracil and capecitabine, and 2 platinums, cisplatin and oxaliplatin, in the treatment of advanced gastroesophageal cancer. Using a two-by-two design, the investigators evaluated 4 regimens: ECF; ECX; epirubicin, oxaliplatin, fluorouracil; and EOX. The 4 regimens were ultimately found to have noninferior ORR (41% vs 47% vs 42% vs 48%, respectively), PFS (6.2 vs 6.7 vs 6.5 vs 7.0 months, respectively), and mOS (9.9 vs 9.9 vs 9.3 vs 11.2 months, respectively).[25] The investigators concluded that capecitabine and oxaliplatin was as effective as fluorouracil and cisplatin. Notably, in current clinical practice the toxicity profile of epirubicin has limited its use to younger patients with excellent performance status.

S-1 is an oral fluoropyrimidine composed of tegafur (a prodrug of fluorouracil), gimercil (a dihydropyrimidine dehydrogenase inhibitor, which prolongs the half-life of fluorouracil), and oteracil potassium (an inhibitor of phosphorylation of intestinal fluorouracil, which increases gastrointestinal tolerability). It is approved for use in several Asian counties but has yet to be granted approval in the United States. This approval was based on the SPIRITS trial in which cisplatin plus S-1 (CS) was compared with S-1 monotherapy. CS demonstrated an improved mOS (13.0 vs 11 months; $P = .04$) and median PFS (mPFS) (6.0 vs 4.0 months; $P < .0001$).[27]

HER2 is a transmembrane protein of the ErbB family. Dimerization leads to the activation of downstream signaling pathways that ultimately drives cell-cycle progression, cell proliferation, and resistance to apoptosis.[28] As in breast cancer, *HER2* gene amplification is common and estimated to be present in up to 30% of gastric cancer cases.[29] Trastuzumab is an anti-HER2 mAb that represents one of the few successful targeted therapies for metastatic gastric cancer. The ToGA trial was the first randomized controlled trial to show benefit of trastuzumab and led to its approval in combination with chemotherapy for front-line use in the HER2-positive, metastatic gastric and GEJ adenocarcinoma.[5] HER2-positive disease in this trial was defined as 3+ positivity on immunohistochemistry or a HER2:CEP17 ratio of 2 or greater by fluorescence in situ hybridization. This landmark study randomized 584 patients to receive trastuzumab with a fluoropyrimidine and cisplatin versus placebo plus fluoropyrimidine with cisplatin and demonstrated an improved mPFS (6.7 vs 5.5 months; HR 0.71; 95% CI 0.59–0.85; $P = .0002$) and mOS (13.8 vs 11.1 months; HR 0.74; 95% CI 0.60–0.91; $P = .0046$). The addition of trastuzumab also demonstrated an improved duration of response (6.9 vs 4.8 months; HR 0.53; 95% CI 0.40–0.73; $P < .0001$), ORR (47% vs 35%; $P = .0017$), and TTP (7.1 vs 5.6 months; HR 0.70; 95% CI 0.58–0.85; $P = .0003$). The overall rates of all grades or only grade 3 to 4 toxicities were not significantly different between the 2 arms.[5]

In April 2021, nivolumab was approved for use in combination with chemotherapy for metastatic gastric cancer and esophageal adenocarcinoma. As is described later in this chapter, the CHECKMATE-649 trial demonstrated a statistically significant improvement in PFS and OS with the combination of chemotherapy and immunotherapy over chemotherapy alone and is now redefining the standard of care.

Subsequent Lines of Treatment

In the second-line setting and beyond, cytotoxic chemotherapy has had a modest impact on mOS. Ramucirumab, an mAb targeting vascular endothelial growth factors (VEGF), has been examined in the front- and second-line setting. In the phase III RAINFALL trial, 645 patients with HER2-negative, metastatic gastric or GEJ adenocarcinoma were randomized to receive ramucirumab plus a fluoropyrimidine and cisplatin or placebo plus a fluoropyrimidine and cisplatin. When added to chemotherapy in the front-line setting, ramucirumab did not significantly improve mOS (11.7 vs 10.7 months, respectively; P = .6757), and only marginally improved mPFS (5.7 vs 5.4 months; P = .0106).[30] However, in the second-line setting, ramucirumab has demonstrated benefit both as a single agent and in combination with chemotherapy. The phase III REGARD trial compared the use of ramucirumab monotherapy versus BSC in the second-line setting for patients with metastatic gastric or GEJ adenocarcinoma. Ramucirumab monotherapy led to an improvement in mOS (5.2 vs 3.8 months; HR 0.78; 95% CI 0.60–0.99; P = .047) and mPFS (6.7 vs 5.3 months; HR 0.80; 95% CI 0.68–0.93; P = .037).[31] More recently, the landmark RAINBOW trial randomized patients who had progressed on or within 4 months of first-line chemotherapy (fluoropyrimidine-platinum with or without an anthracycline) to receive either ramucirumab plus paclitaxel or placebo plus paclitaxel. Ramucirumab plus paclitaxel demonstrated an improvement in mOS (9.6 vs 7.4 months; HR 0.81, 95% CI 0.68–0.96; P = .0169), leading to the approval of ramucirumab plus paclitaxel in the second-line setting, and this is currently a preferred second-line regimen for patients with metastatic gastric cancer.[4]

Multiple trials have also investigated single-agent chemotherapy in the second-line setting, demonstrating improvements in both quality of life and survival. In 2011, a randomized study compared irinotecan with BSC in the second-line setting and demonstrated a modest improvement in mOS (4.0 vs 2.4 months; HR 0.48, 95% CI 0.25–0.92; P = .012).[32] Another phase III study comparing salvage chemotherapy with either docetaxel or irinotecan with BSC in the second-line setting also demonstrated a modest improvement in mOS (5.3 vs 3.8 months, respectively; HR 0.657, 95% CI 0.485–0.891; P = .007) with salvage chemotherapy.[33] COUGAR-02, an open-labeled phase III study, compared docetaxel with BSC in the second-line setting in patients with esophageal, gastric, or GEJ adenocarcinoma that had progressed on or within 6 months of treatment with a fluoropyrimidine-platinum regimen. This open-labeled phase III study demonstrated that docetaxel led to an improved mOS (5.2 vs 3.6 months; HR 0.67, 95% CI 0.49–0.92; P = .01).[34] Nanoparticle albumin-bound paclitaxel (nab-paclitaxel) was compared with solvent-bound paclitaxel in the phase III ABSOLUTE trial. In this study, nab-paclitaxel was administered either weekly or every 3 weeks compared with solvent-bound paclitaxel, which was administered weekly. This trial demonstrated noninferiority between the weekly nab-paclitaxel and solvent-bound paclitaxel in terms of mOS (11.1 vs 10.9 months; HR 0.97, 97.5% CI 0.76–1.23; noninferiority margin 1.25; one-sided P = .0085). However, when nab-paclitaxel was administered every 3 weeks and compared with the weekly solvent-bound paclitaxel, nab-paclitaxel failed to meet the noninferiority threshold (10.3 vs 10.9 months; HR 1.06, 97.5% CI 0.87–1.31; one-sided P = .062).[35] Together, these trials demonstrate benefit with single-agent chemotherapy in the second-line setting providing clinicians with several options.

Recently, TAS-102, a combination of trifluridine (FTD), a thymidine analogue, and tipiracil (TPI), thymidine phosphorylase inhibitor, has been examined in patients with metastatic gastric and GEJ cancer. The TAGS trial evaluated this agent in patients with or without prior gastrectomy, who had progressed on at least 2 previous lines of chemotherapy. A total of 507 patients were randomized 2:1 to receive TAS-102 or BSC. FTD/TPI demonstrated an improved mOS (6.0 vs 3.4 months; HR 0.57, CI 95% 0.41–0.79) and mPFS (2.2 vs 1.8 months; HR 0.48, 95% CI 0.35–0.65) in the population who had undergone prior gastrectomy and an improved mOS (5.6 vs 3.8 months; HR 0.80, CI 95% 0.60–1.06) and mPFS (1.9 vs 1.8 months; HR 0.65, 95% CI 0.49–0.85) in patients without a prior gastrectomy.[36] These data led to the approval of TAS-102 as a third-line therapy for patients with metastatic gastroesophageal cancer.

Immunotherapy for Gastric Cancer

Several novel classes of agents have also shown promise in advanced gastric cancer. Immune checkpoint inhibitors (ICIs) are among those that have been most developed and have recently been approved in the second- and third-line settings. Response rates are variable and select patient populations derive more benefit, for example, those with microsatellite instability (MSI-H) or deficient mismatch repair (dMMR), and therefore careful selection is necessary.[37]

Pembrolizumab is the most extensively studied ICI in gastric cancer and is the only agent approved for use in the second-line setting, in MSI-H or dMMR disease, and in the third-line setting, for programmed death ligand 1 (PD-L1)-positive disease. In 2017, pembrolizumab gained approval for use in the third-line setting based on the findings of KEYNOTE-059. This phase II trial enrolled 259 patients and administered pembrolizumab every 3 weeks until disease progression and demonstrated an ORR of 11.6% with 2.3% achieving a CR. Furthermore, inpatients whose tumors that were PD-L1 positive had an ORR of 15.5% compared with 6.4% in those with PD-L1–negative tumors. In tumors that were MSI, the ORR was 57% compared with 9% in MSS tumors.[6]

Subsequently, KEYNOTE-062 sought to examine the use of pembrolizumab monotherapy versus cisplatin plus a fluoropyrimidine with or without pembrolizumab in 763 patients with HER-2–negative, advanced or metastatic gastric or GEJ cancer whose tumors expressed PD-L1 (defined as Combined Positive Score [CPS] $\geq$ 1). When chemotherapy alone was compared with pembrolizumab monotherapy, there was noninferior mOS (10.6 vs 11.1 months; HR 0.91, 95% CI 0.69–1.18; noninferiority margin 1.2) although there was a lower ORR (14.5% vs 36.8%). When examining the use of pembrolizumab monotherapy in patients whose tumors strongly expressed PD-L1 (CPS $\geq$ 10), there was significant improvement in mOS (17.4 vs 10.8 months; HR 0.69, 95% CI 0.49–0.97). Unfortunately, the addition of pembrolizumab to chemotherapy did not lead to an improved mOS (12.5 vs 11.1 months; HR 0.85, 95% CI 0.70–1.03) or mPFS (6.9 vs 6.4 months; HR 0.84, 95% CI 0.70–1.02).[38]

Additional cohorts from KEYNOTE-059 have examined the use of pembrolizumab monotherapy or in combination with chemotherapy (fluoropyrimidine and cisplatin) in the front-line setting for advanced gastric and GEJ cancers. Patients who received pembrolizumab monotherapy were required to have PD-L1–positive disease (CPS $\geq$ 1) and demonstrated an ORR of 25.8% with 6.5% achieving a CR and mPFS of 3.3 month. In the patients who received pembrolizumab in combination with chemotherapy, PD-L1 expression was not a requirement, although 64% of patients had PD-L1 expression. In this arm, ORR was 60%, with 4% demonstrating a CR and mPFS of 6.6 months.[39–41]

More recently, based on the results of the CHECKMATE-649 trial, the combination of nivolumab and chemotherapy has been approved for use in patients with unresectable advanced metastatic gastric or gastroesophageal cancer. In this global phase III study, a total of 1,581 patients with untreated, unresectable advanced or metastatic gastric, GEJ or esophageal cancer were randomized to receive nivolumab with chemotherapy versus nivolumab plus ipilimumab versus chemotherapy alone. In patients with a CPS > 5, the addition of nivolumab to chemotherapy led to improvement in mOS (14.4 vs 11.1 months; HR 0.71; 98.4% CI 0.59-0.86; p<0.0001) and mPFS (7.7 vs 6.0 months; HR 0.68; 98% CI 0.56-0.81; p<0.0001). Notably, benefits with combination therapy were also statistically significant for the PD-L1 CPS ≥ 1 population (HR = 0.77; P = .0001) and for all randomly assigned patients (HR = 0.80; P = .0002). Fewer than 5% of patients experienced grade 3 or 4 toxicities, and there were no grade 5 events.[42]

In Asia, nivolumab is approved for monotherapy use based on the results of ATTRACTION-2, which examined 493 patients with unresectable advanced or recurrent gastric or GEJ cancer who progressed after 2 or more previous chemotherapy regimens. Patients from Japan, South Korea, and Taiwan were randomized to nivolumab monotherapy or BSC and demonstrated an improved mOS (5.26 vs 4.14 months; HR 0.63, 95% CI 0.51–0.78; *P* < .0001) and mPFS (1.61 vs 1.45 months; HR 0.60, *P* < .0001).[7] CheckMate-032 examined the use of nivolumab combined with ipilimumab, an anticytotoxic T-lymphocyte–associated protein 4 antibody, in the second-line setting any beyond in patients with locally advanced or metastatic esophageal, gastric, or GEJ cancers regardless of PD-L1 or MSI status. In this phase I/II study, 160 patients were randomized to nivolumab, 3 mg/kg, monotherapy (NIVO3); nivolumab, 1 mg/kg, plus ipilimumab, 3 mg/kg, (NIVO1 + IPI3); and nivolumab, 3 mg/kg, plus ipilimumab, 1 mg/kg, (NIVO3 + IPI1). This trial demonstrated an ORR of 12% versus 24% versus 8%, respectively; mPFS of 1.4 versus 1.4 versus 1.6 months, respectively; and mOS of 6.2 versus 6.9 versus 4.8 months, respectively. Treatment-related grade 3 and 4 toxicities were 17% versus 47% versus 27%, respectively. As would be expected, there were higher rates of toxicity in the arms with combination immunotherapy and particularly higher in the NIVO1 + IPI3 arm.[43] The results of this phase I/II study has led to subsequent larger phase II and III studies investigating nivolumab's role in front-line use either as a monotherapy or in combination with cytotoxic chemotherapy, other immunotherapies, or targeted therapies.

In Europe, avelumab, an mAb targeting PD-L1, is approved as a monotherapy for unresectable or metastatic gastric cancer based on the phase Ib JAVELIN study, which examined its use in patients who had progressed after one or more lines of fluoropyrimidine-platinum chemotherapy. Overall, avelumab demonstrated an ORR of 10%; however, in patient tumors with PD-L1 expression (defined as CPS ≥ 1), ORR was improved to 27.3% with an mOS of 9.1 months and 7.5% grade 3 or 4 toxicities.[44] JAVELIN Gastric 100 evaluated avelumab's role in maintenance therapy after first-line chemotherapy versus continued first-line chemotherapy. This phase III trial failed to demonstrate any improvement of mOS (10.4 vs 10.9 months; HR 0.91, 95% CI 0.74–1.11; *P* = .1779).[45] JAVELIN Gastric 300 is currently evaluating avelumab's role in the third-line setting, comparing it with either paclitaxel or irinotecan monotherapy. Preliminary results suggest no improvement in mOS (4.6 vs 5.0 months; HR 1.1, 95% CI 0.9–1.4; *P* = .81) or mPFS (1.4 vs 2.7 months; HR 1.73, 95% CI 1.4–2.2; *P* > .99) with avelumab.[46]

Response rates to immunotherapy in the treatment of gastric cancer have been modest; however, higher responses are observed in patients whose tumors express PD-L1, are MSI-H, or dMMR. As a result, there has been limited approval of ICIs in the

Table 3
Landmark trials in subsequent lines of treatment for metastatic gastric cancer

Author (Date), Study Name	Treatment Regimen	Total Patients	ORR/CR	mPFS (mo) HR, *P*-value	mOS (mo) HR, *P*-value
Fuchs, et al,[31] 2014, REGARD	Ramucirumab & best supportive care vs placebo & best supportive care	355	3%/<1% 3%/0%	2.1 vs 1.3 HR 0.483, $P < .0001$	5.2 vs 3.8 HR 0.776, $P = .47$
Wilke, et al,[4] 2019, RAINBOW	Ramucirumab & paclitaxel vs placebo & paclitaxel	665	28%/<1% 16%/<1%	4.4 vs 2.9 HR 0.635, $P < .0001$	9.6 vs 7.4 HR 0.807, $P = .017$
Fuchs et al,[6] 2018, KEYNOTE-059	Pembrolizumab	259	11.6%/2.3%	2.0	5.6
Kang et al,[7] 2017, ATTRACTION-2	Nivolumab vs placebo	493	11.2%/0% 0%/0%	1.61 v 1.45 HR 0.60, $P < .0001$	5.26 vs 4.14 HR 0.63, $P < .0001$
Doi et al,[44] 2019, JAVELIN	Avelumab	40	10%/2.5%	2.4	9.1

Abbreviation: NR, not reported.

second-line setting or beyond: pembrolizumab (United States),[6] nivolumab (Asia),[7] and avelumab (Europe).[44] Furthermore, these modest results have resulted in studies combining immunotherapy with other modalities to improve outcomes. **Table 3** summarizes the landmark trials for subsequent lines of treatment of metastatic gastric cancer.

Ongoing Studies for Advanced Gastric Cancer

Currently, there are multiple ongoing trials testing novel agents as well as various combination therapies. Success with trastuzumab in HER2-positive disease has prompted further study with trastuzumab deruxtecan, an antibody-drug conjugate combining trastuzumab with deruxtecan, a topoisomerase I inhibitor. The phase II DESTINY-Gastric01 trial randomized patients with previously treated, advanced gastric cancer to trastuzumab deruxtecan or the physician's choice of cytotoxic chemotherapy and demonstrated an improved ORR (51% vs 14%, $P < .001$) and mOS (12.5 vs 8.4 months; HR 0.59; 95% CI 0.39–0.88; $P = .01$).[47] Given these promising results, DESTINY-Gastric02 is evaluating its use in the second-line setting in patients who have received front-line trastuzumab.[48]

With the introduction of immunotherapy onto the treatment landscape, there has been interest in combining immunotherapy with a trastuzumab-chemotherapy backbone. A recent phase II trial examined the addition of pembrolizumab to trastuzumab and fluoropyrimidine/platinum-based chemotherapy in 37 patients with metastatic esophageal, gastric, or GEJ cancer regardless of PD-L1 expression. Notably, 26 of 37 patients (70%) were progression free at 6 months.[49] These promising data have prompted the ongoing, phase III trial, KEYNOTE-811.[50]

Regorafenib is a small molecular TKI with several targets including VEGF. It has been evaluated in the INTEGRATE trial for use in patients with metastatic gastric or GEJ adenocarcinoma who progressed on one or more lines of chemotherapy. In this phase II trial, regorafenib led to an improvement in mPFS (2.6 vs 0.9 months; HR 0.40; 95% CI 0.28–0.59; $P < .001$) with a trend toward improved mOS (5.8 vs 4.5 months; HR 0.74; $P = .147$).[51] INTEGRATE II is the follow-up phase III trial that is currently examining regorafenib in the refractory setting.[52] Regorafenib has been examined in combination with immunotherapy. The phase Ib REGONIVO trial combined regorafenib with nivolumab in 50 patients with metastatic gastric or colorectal cancer who had received at least 2 lines of prior therapy. In the gastric cancer cohort, the mPFS was 5.6 months (95% CI 2.7–10.4 months) and mOS was 12.3 months (95% CI 5.3-not reached) with few treatment-related adverse effects such as rash (12%), proteinuria, (12%) and palmar-plantar erythrodysesthesia (10%).[53] Similar to the RAINBOW trial, regorafenib is currently being examined in the second-line setting in combination with paclitaxel in the phase Ib REPEAT trial.[54]

Claudins are a family of proteins found in gastric mucosa that are involved with tight cell junctions, controlling the movement of molecules between cells. Isoform 2 of claudin-18 (CLDN18.2) is expressed in 50% to 70% of gastric tumors and is thought to be critical for tumor growth and development.[55] Zolbetuximab is a promising anti-CLDN18.2 mAb that is currently being evaluated for use in metastatic gastric cancer. In the phase II FAST trial, patients with advanced or recurrent, HER2-negative CLDN18.2 expressing tumors (defined as >2+ staining with anti-CLDN18 antibodies) were randomized to receive EOX with or without zolbetuximab. The addition of the anti-CLDN18.2 mAb led to an improved mOS (13.0 vs 8.4 months; HR 0.56, 95% CI 0.40–0.67; $P = .0008$) and mPFS (7.5 vs 5.3 months; HR 0.44, 95% CI 0.29–0.67; $P < .0005$).[56] These results prompted the ongoing phase III SPOTLIGHT trial, which randomizes patients with HER2-negative, advanced or metastatic, CLDN18.2-expressing gastroesophageal cancer to FOLFOX with or without zolbetuximab.[57]

SUMMARY

In resectable, localized gastric cancer, randomized trials have demonstrated that adjuvant and perioperative systemic chemotherapy, with or without radiotherapy, improves patient outcomes. Although controversies regarding choice of regimen, timing of therapy, perioperatively versus adjuvant, and whether or not to incorporate radiotherapy remain, there is strong evidence that surgery alone is insufficient, especially in those cases of locally advanced disease. Currently, there are multiple standard-of-care treatment options including fluoropyrimidine/platinum doublet therapies and, for those with strong performance status, a triplicate therapy with FLOT should be considered.[15]

In metastatic disease, traditional cytotoxic chemotherapy has led to modest improvements in patient outcomes. In the front-line setting for HER2-negative, metastatic gastric cancer, standard chemotherapy regimens consist of a combination of a fluoropyrimidine/platinum doublet with the addition of a third chemotherapeutic agent for patients who are medically eligible with good performance status. In HER2-positive disease, trastuzumab is added to a fluoropyrimidine-platinum doublet, which is the standard first-line treatment.[5] In PD-L1 positive disease, nivolumab is added to a fluoropyrimidine-platinum doublet. In the second-line setting, ramucirumab with paclitaxel is a recommended regimen; however, in patients with PD-L1 expressing tumors, pembrolizumab is a reasonable alternative for select patients.[4,6] Currently, several promising targeted therapies and immunotherapies are being investigated and will likely further improve outcomes for patients in the near future.

DISCLOSURE

The authors have nothing to disclose.

REFERENCES

1. Macdonald JS, Smalley SR, Benedetti J, et al. Chemoradiotherapy after surgery compared with surgery alone for adenocarcinoma of the stomach or gastroesophageal junction. N Engl J Med 2001;345:725–30.
2. Glimelius B, Ekström K, Hoff man K, et al. Randomized comparison between chemotherapy plus best supportive care with best supportive care in advanced gastric cancer. Ann Oncol 1997;8:163–8.
3. Wagner A, Unverzagt S, Grothe W, et al. Chemotherapy for advanced gastric cancer. Cochrane Database Syst Rev 2010;3:CD004064.
4. Wilke H, Muro K, Van Cutsem E, et al. Ramucirumab plus paclitaxel versus placebo plus paclitaxel in patients with previously treated advanced gastric or gastro-oesophageal junction adenocarcinoma (RAINBOW): a double-blind, randomised phase 3 trial. Lancet Oncol 2014;15(11):1224–35.
5. Bang YJ, Van Cutsem E, Feyereislova A, et al. Trastuzumab in combination with chemotherapy versus chemotherapy alone for treatment of HER2-positive advanced gastric or gastro-oesophageal junction cancer (ToGA): a phase 3, open-label, randomised controlled trial. Lancet 2010;376:687–97.
6. Fuchs CS, Doi T, Jang RW, et al. Safety and efficacy of pembrolizumab monotherapy in patients with previously treated advanced gastric and gastroesophageal junction cancer: Phase 2 Clinical KEYNOTE-059 Trial. JAMA Oncol 2018;4(5): e180013.
7. Kang YK, Boku N, Satoh T, et al. Nivolumab in patients with advanced gastric or gastro-oesophageal junction cancer refractory to, or intolerant of, at least two

previous chemotherapy regimens (ONO-4538–12, ATTRACTION-2): a randomised, double-blind, placebo-controlled, phase 3 trial. Lancet 2017; 390(10111):2461–71.
8. Dikken JL, Jansen EP, Cats A, et al. Impact of the extent of surgery and postoperative chemoradiotherapy on recurrence patterns in gastric cancer. J Clin Oncol 2010;28:2430–6.
9. Songun I, Putter H, Kranenbarg EM, et al. Surgical treatment of gastric cancer: 15-year follow-up results of the randomised nationwide Dutch D1D2 trial. Lancet Oncol 2010;11(5):439.
10. Noh SH, Park SR, Yang HK, et al. Adjuvant capecitabine plus oxaliplatin for gastric cancer after D2 gastrectomy (CLASSIC): 5-year follow-up of an open-label, randomised phase 3 trial. Lancet Oncol 2014;15:1389–96.
11. Lee J, Lim DH, Kim S, et al. Phase III trial comparing capecitabine plus cisplatin versus capecitabine plus cisplatin with concurrent capecitabine radiotherapy in completely resected gastric cancer with D2 lymph node dissection: the ARTIST trial. J Clin Oncol 2012;30:268–73.
12. Park SH, Zang DY, Han B, et al. *ARTIST 2: Interim results of a phase III trial involving adjuvant chemotherapy and/or chemoradiotherapy after D2-gastrectomy in stage II/III gastric cancer (GC)*. J Clin Oncol 2019;37:4001.
13. Cunningham D, Allum WH, Stenning SP, et al. Perioperative chemotherapy versus surgery alone for resectable gastroesophageal cancer. N Engl J Med 2006;355: 11–20.
14. Ychou M, Boige V, Pignon JP, et al. Perioperative chemotherapy compared with surgery alone for resectable gastroesophageal adenocarcinoma: an FNCLCC and FFCD Multicenter Phase III Trial. J Clin Oncol 2011;29:1715–21.
15. Alderson D, Cunningham D, Nankivell M, et al. Neoadjuvant cisplatin and fluorouracil versus epirubicin, cisplatin, and capecitabine followed by resection in patients with oesophageal adenocarcinoma (UK MRC OE05): an open-label, randomised phase 3 trial. Lancet Oncol 2017;18:1249–60.
16. Cats A, Jansen EPM, van Grieken NCT, et al. Chemotherapy versus chemoradiotherapy after surgery and preoperative chemotherapy for resectable gastric cancer (CRITICS): an international, open-label, randomised phase 3 trial. Lancet Oncol 2018;19:616–28.
17. Al-Batran SE, Homann N, Pauligk C, et al. Perioperative chemotherapy with fluorouracil plus leucovorin, oxaliplatin, and docetaxel versus fluorouracil or capecitabine plus cisplatin and epirubicin for locally advanced, resectable gastric or gastro-oesophageal junction adenocarcinoma (FLOT4): a randomised, phase 2/3 trial. Lancet 2019;393:1948–57.
18. Hong Y, Song S, Lee S, et al. A phase II trial of capecitabine in previously untreated patients with advanced and/or metastatic gastric cancer. Ann Oncol 2004;15:1344–7.
19. Sulkes A, Smyth J, Sessa C, et al. Docetaxel (Taxotere) in advanced gastric cancer: results of a phase II clinical trial. Br J Cancer 1994;70:380–3.
20. Köhne C, Catane R, Klein B, et al. Irinotecan is active in chemonaive patients with metastatic gastric cancer: a phase II multicentric trial. Br J Cancer 2003;89: 997–1001.
21. MacDonald JS, Schein PS, Woolley PV, et al. 5-fluorouracil, doxorubicin, and mitomycin (FAM) combination chemotherapy for advanced gastric cancer. Ann Intern Med 1980;93:533–6.
22. Wils J, Klein H, Wagener D, et al. Sequential high-dose methotrexate and fluorouracil combined with doxorubicin—a step ahead in the treatment of advanced

gastric cancer: a trial of the European Organization for Research and Treatment of Cancer Gastrointestinal Tract Cooperative Group. J Clin Oncol 1991;9:827–31.
23. Webb A, Cunningham D, Scarffe JH, et al. Randomized trial comparing epirubicin, cisplatin, and fluorouracil versus fluorouracil, doxorubicin, and methotrexate in advanced esophagogastric cancer. J Clin Oncol 1997;15:261–7.
24. Van Cutsem E, Moiseyenko V, Tjulandin S, et al. Phase III study of docetaxel and cisplatin plus fluorouracil compared with cisplatin and fluorouracil as first-line therapy for advanced gastric cancer: a report of the V325 Study Group. J Clin Oncol 2006;24:4991–7.
25. Shah MA, Janjigian YY, Stoller R, et al. Randomized multicenter phase II study of modified Docetaxel, Cisplatin, and Fluorouracil (DCF) versus DCF plus growth factor support in patients with metastatic gastric adenocarcinoma: a study of the us gastric cancer consortium. J Clin Oncol 2010;33:3874–9.
26. Cunningham D, Starling N, Rao S, et al. Capecitabine and oxaliplatin for advanced esophagogastric cancer. N Engl J Med 2008;358:36–46.
27. Koizumi W, Narahara H, Hara T, et al. S-1 plus cisplatin versus S-1 alone for first-line treatment of advanced gastric cancer (SPIRITS trial): a phase III trial. Lancet Oncol 2008;9:215–21.
28. Baselga J, Swain SM. Novel anticancer targets: revisiting ERBB2 and discovering ERBB3. Nat Rev Cancer 2009;9:463–75.
29. Kim KC, Koh YW, Chang HM, et al. Evaluation of HER2 protein expression in gastric carcinomas: comparative analysis of 1,414 cases of whole-tissue sections and 595 cases of tissue microarrays. Ann Surg Oncol 2011;18:2833–40.
30. Fuchs CS, Shitara K, Di Bartolomeo M, et al. Ramucirumab with cisplatin and fluoropyrimidine as first-line therapy in patients with metastatic gastric or junctional adenocarcinoma (RAINFALL): a double-blind, randomised, placebo-controlled, phase 3 trial. Lancet Oncol 2019;20(3):420–35.
31. Fuchs CS, Tomasek J, Yong CJ, et al. Ramucirumab monotherapy for previously treated advanced gastric or gastrooesophageal junction adenocarcinoma (REGARD): an international, randomised, multicentre, placebo-controlled, phase 3 trial. Lancet 2014;383(9911):31–9.
32. Thuss-Patience P, Kretzschmar A, Bichev D, et al. *Survival advantage for irinotecan versus best supportive care as second-line chemotherapy in gastric cancer—a randomised phase III study of the Arbeitsgemeinschaft Internistische Onkologie (AIO)*. Eur J Cancer 2011;47:2306–14.
33. Kang J, Lee SI, Lim Do H, et al. Salvage chemotherapy for pretreated gastric cancer: a randomized phase III trial comparing chemotherapy plus best supportive care with best supportive care alone. J Clin Oncol 2012;30:1513–8.
34. Ford H, Marshall A, Bridgewater J, et al. Docetaxel versus active symptom control for refractory oesophagogastric adenocarcinoma (COUGAR-02): an open-label, phase 3 randomised controlled trial. Lancet Oncol 2014;15:78–86.
35. Shitara K, Takashima A, Fujitani K. *Nab-paclitaxel versus solvent-based paclitaxel in patients with previously treated advanced gastric cancer (ABSOLUTE): an open-label, randomised, non-inferiority, phase 3 tria*l. Lancet Gastroenterol Hepatol 2017;2(4):277–87.
36. Ilson DH, Tabernero J, Prokharau A, et al. Efficacy and safety of trifluridine/tipiracil treatment in patients with metastatic gastric cancer who had undergone gastrectomy: subgroup analyses of a randomized clinical trial. JAMA Oncol 2019. https://doi.org/10.1001/jamaoncol.2019.3531.
37. Le DT, Durham JN, Smith KN, et al. Mismatch repair deficiency predicts response of solid tumors to PD-1 blockade. Science 2017;357(6349):409–13.

38. Tabernero J, Cutsem EV, Bang YJ, et al. Pembrolizumab with or without chemotherapy versus chemotherapy for advanced gastric or gastroesophageal junction (G/GEJ) adenocarcinoma: The phase III KEYNOTE-062 study. J Clin Oncol 2019; 37:LBA4007.
39. A Study of Pembrolizumab (MK-3475) in participants with recurrent or metastatic gastric or gastroesophageal junction adenocarcinoma (MK-3475-059/KEYNOTE-059). Available at: https://ClinicalTrials.gov/show/NCT02335411. Accessed November 15, 2020.
40. Bang YJ, Kang YK, Catenacci DV, et al. Pembrolizumab alone or in combination with chemotherapy as firstline therapy for patients with advanced gastric or gastroesophageal junction adenocarcinoma: results from the phase II non-randomized KEYNOTE-059 study. Gastric Cancer 2019;22:828–37.
41. Wainberg ZA, Yoon HH, Catenacci DVT, et al. Efficacy and safety of pembrolizumab (pembro) alone or in combination with chemotherapy (chemo) in patients (pts) with advanced gastric or gastroesophageal (G/GEJ) cancer: long-term follow up from KEYNOTE-059. J Clin Oncol 2019;37:4009.
42. Moehler M, Shitara K, Garrido M, et al. LBA6_PR Nivolumab (nivo) plus chemotherapy (chemo) versus chemo as first-line (1L) treatment for advanced gastric cancer/gastroesophageal junction cancer (GC/GEJC)/esophageal adenocarcinoma (EAC): First results of the CheckMate 649 study. Ann Oncol. 2020;31S:ESMO #S1142.
43. Janjigian YY, Ott PA, Calvo E, et al. Nivolumab $\pm$ ipilimumab in pts with advanced (adv)/metastatic chemotherapy-refractory (CTx-R) gastric (G), esophageal (E), or gastroesophageal junction (GEJ) cancer: CheckMate 032 study. J Clin Oncol 2017;35(15_suppl):4014.
44. Doi T, Iwasa S, Muro K, et al. Phase 1 trial of avelumab (anti-PD-L1) in Japanese patients with advanced solid tumors, including dose expansion in patients with gastric or gastroesophageal junction cancer: the JAVELIN Solid Tumor JPN trial. Gastric Cancer 2019;22(4):817–27.
45. Moehler MH, Dvorkin M, Ozguroglu M, et al. *Results of the JAVELIN Gastric 100 phase 3 trial: avelumab maintenance following first-line (1L) chemotherapy (CTx) vs continuation of CTx for HER2– advanced gastric or gastroesophageal junction cancer (GC/GEJC*). J Clin Oncol 2020;38(4_suppl):278.
46. Bang YJ, Ruiz EY, Van Cutsem E, et al. Phase III, randomised trial of avelumab versus physician's choice of chemotherapy as third-line treatment of patients with advanced gastric or gastro-oesophageal junction cancer: primary analysis of JAVELIN Gastric 300. Ann Oncol 2018;29(10):2052–60.
47. Shitara K, Bang YJ, Iwasa S, et al. *Trastuzumab deruxtecan in previously treated HER2-positive gastric cance*r. N Engl J Med 2020;382:2419–30.
48. DS-8201a in HER2-positive gastric cancer that cannot be surgically removed or has spread (DESTINY-Gastric02). Available at: https://clinicaltrials.gov/ct2/show/NCT04014075. Accessed November 15, 2020.
49. Janjigian YY, Maron SB, Chatila WK, et al. First-line pembrolizumab and trastuzumab in HER2-positive oesophageal, gastric, or gastro-oesophageal junction cancer: an open-label, single-arm, phase 2 trial. Lancet Oncol 2020;21(6):821–31.
50. Pembrolizumab/Placebo Plus Trastuzumab Plus Chemotherapy in Human Epidermal Growth Factor Receptor 2 Positive (HER2+) Advanced Gastric or Gastroesophageal Junction (GEJ) Adenocarcinoma (MK-3475-811/KEYNOTE-811). Available at: https://www.clinicaltrials.gov/ct2/show/NCT03615326. Accessed November 15, 2020.

51. Pavlakis N, Sjoquist KM, Martin AJ, et al. Regorafenib for the treatment of advanced gastric cancer (INTEGRATE): a multinational placebo-controlled phase II Trial. J Clin Oncol 2016;34(23):2728–35.
52. A Study of Regorafenib in Refractory Advanced Gastro-Oesophageal Cancer (INTEGRATEII). Available at: https://clinicaltrials.gov/ct2/show/NCT02773524. Accessed November 15, 2020.
53. Fukuoka S, Hara H, Takahashi N, et al. *Regorafenib Plus nivolumab in patients with advanced gastric or colorectal cancer: an open-label, dose-escalation, and dose-expansion phase Ib Trial (REGONIVO, EPOC1603)*. J Clin Oncol 2020;38(18):2053–61.
54. Regorafenib in combination with paclitaxel in advanced oesophagogastric carcinoma (REPEAT). Available at: https://clinicaltrials.gov/ct2/show/NCT02406170. Accessed November 15, 2020.
55. Sahin U, Koslowski M, Dhaene K, et al. Claudin-18 splice variant 2 is a pan-cancer target suitable for therapeutic antibody development. Clin Cancer Res 2008;14(23):7624–34.
56. Sahin U, Tureci Ö, Manikhas GM, et al. Zolbetuximab combined with EOX as first-line therapy in advanced CLDN18.2+ gastric (G) and gastroesophageal junction (GEJ) adenocarcinoma: updated results from the FAST trial. J Clin Oncol 2019; 37(4_suppl):16.
57. A Phase 3 efficacy, safety, and tolerability study of Zolbetuximab (Experimental Drug) Plus mFOLFOX6 Chemotherapy Compared to Placebo Plus mFOLFOX6 as Treatment for Gastric and Gastroesophageal Junction (GEJ) Cancer (SPOTLIGHT). Available at: https://ClinicalTrials.gov/show/NCT03504397. Accessed November 15, 2020.

Printed and bound by CPI Group (UK) Ltd, Croydon, CR0 4YY
08/05/2025
01864694-0001